For my Nonno Angelo,
who first saw the writer
in the lonely and frightened little girl he loved,
and for Bob, Kristen Angela, and Tommy,
who keep the faith.

Contents

Foreword

SARAH WAS BARREN. She had no child." These terse, stark sentences appear in the eleventh chapter of Genesis, yet it was the imagination-inspiring technical wizardry of a "test-tube" baby, reflected in millions of television and magazine-cover images, that brought infertility out of the shadows of shame and into the aseptic glare of the operating room.

I am a reproductive endocrinologist, trained in both clinical skills and research, certified in two medical specialties. I have access to most of the medical knowledge and tools available for the understanding of human reproduction as we know it today. Yet I cannot help but feel that technical validation alone is neither adequate nor sufficient to the task of treating infertility. The "disease" of infertility is not experienced as an infirmity of the body, but as an unrequited longing of the human heart.

I met Carla Harkness ten years ago at an infertility symposium presented by RESOLVE of Northern California. During our conversation we were struck that of the conditions for which people seek medical consultation, infertility is unique in that the "patient" is a man and a woman. We agreed that only from a shared medical and emotional perspective could two people fully sustain themselves and each other through what is viewed by most as a life crisis. This book is an effort to provide that perspective.

Infertility has no symptoms, causes no disability, and is invisible to the naked eye. It is defined in textbooks as the failure to conceive after one year of unprotected intercourse, yet in reality, infertility starts when a couple begins to fear that something may be wrong. It is the effect of this deepening apprehension that is the "disease" of infertility. Whether expressed as a melancholic wistfulness or as a life-consuming rage is individual, but feelings of anger, guilt, sadness, isolation, loneliness, frustration, and remorse are universal. It is critical to understand that infertility causes stress, *not* the other way around. Even well-meaning friends and family may infuriate with suggestions to "relax," implying that your feelings are the cause of your problem, not the result. Past life decisions based upon educational, career, or personal opportunities may be rehashed or ignored in the vain search for a "reason" for a dilemma which is intrinsically, inherently, and blamelessly unfair.

Time becomes the enemy. Whether it is the incessant ticking of the biologic clock, or the endlessness of waiting for the next menstrual period in a life whose pace is marked by daily temperature dots, no infertile couple accepts the passage of time with equanimity. There are unavoidable medical realities here—

diagnosis is still as much art as science, and treatments often require months of evaluation before they are altered or abandoned. There is no way to measure progress—you are either pregnant or not. There is no "partial credit," no "getting warmer." It is important to recognize that you will feel that things are not going well right up to the moment that you conceive.

My advice is brief. Take control of what you can. Educate yourself about what is known and what is not. Find a physician who is sufficiently experienced and interested in the treatment of infertility and establish a rational plan with defined time intervals for each step. Support your partner with as much openness as possible and seek out others who can be relied on for sympathetic and non-judgmental understanding. Recognize that the outcome is not under your control but your choices and actions are.

Finally, take hope in the fact that the majority of you reading this book will become pregnant, and that all of you can be successful in establishing a family that satisfies the longings in your heart.

Robert D. Nachtigall, M.D.
San Francisco, California
September, 1992

Acknowledgments

REALIZING THE DREAMS of birthing my children and creating both editions of this book was a ten-year effort, accomplished with the support and assistance of many people.

I would like to give special thanks and recognition to:

Robert D. Nachtigall, M.D., for devoting countless hours to reviewing the medical chapters and discussing the psychological and emotional issues of infertility, for sharing his own writings, and for encouraging and taking a chance on a fledgling author;

Robert P. Neff, M.D., for bringing his knowledge, steady hands, and dedicated soul to a dozen hours of meticulous surgery, and for more than a decade of friendship, insights, and compassion that helped me find my babies and heal my body and heart;

Cindy Renshaw, for her role in the creation of this book and her living example of determination and extraordinary courage;

Nancy Whitney, a most special, wise, and loving friend for her perspective on loss and healing;

Linda Palmer, for her unfailing good humor and friendship, practical suggestions, and many hours of careful editing;

Sheri Glucoft Wong, for her wisdom, compassion, and healing insights and friendship;

Joan Hangarter for helping to bring balance to my body and sharing the dream of motherhood;

David Pettee and Mindy Scharlin and Lisa and Roger Howland for generously sharing their perspectives and exhaustive medical and legal research, and to Carol and Mark Simons, Catherine and Tom Knipper, Jed Somit and Toni Maines, Anne Marie Whisman, Lynne Klein, Glenna Seeley, Toni and Richard Corelli, Liz Goodrich, Diane Roddy, and Maris Myerson for graciously lending their insights and experiences to this edition;

Alida Allison and Roberta Rosenbaum for believing in both the subject matter and the author, and for finding the right home for the first edition;

Ruth Gottstein, publisher and friend, for her commitment to creating the best book possible, for her gentle instruction in quality writing and editing, and for her belief in miracles, and to David Hinds and Sal Glynn of Celestial Arts for honoring and continuing the commitment;

Leigh Dickerson Davidson and Colleen Paretty for their diligence, objective perspectives, and editing skills in both editions;

The Board of Directors and members of RESOLVE of Northern California and to RESOLVE's National Office for their support, assistance, and written contributions to both editions;

And most important, to my family — Bob, Kristen, and Tommy — for their unwavering confidence, love, and patience with an often overbusy wife and mommy.

I also wish to thank the following contributors and friends, and those who wish to remain anonymous, for sharing their professional expertise and personal experiences, reviewing numerous chapter drafts, lending their voices to this text, and in many cases, for encouraging and helping me through my own infertility and two editions of this book.

Advisory Panel of Medical Specialists

G. David Adamson, M.D.
Assistant Clinical Professor of Obstetrics and Gynecology
Stanford University School of Medicine and
Director, Fertility and Reproductive Health Institute
Palo Alto, California

Donald Galen, M.D.
Director, The Center for Reproductive Medicine and
In Vitro Fertilization
San Ramon Regional Medical Center
San Ramon, California

Robert Glass, M.D.
Professor of Obstetrics and Gynecology
University of California, San Francisco

Ira Golditch, M.D.
Chief of Obstetrics and Gynecology
Kaiser Permanente Medical Center
San Francisco, California

Simon Henderson, M.D.
Assistant Clinical Professor of Obstetrics and Gynecology
University of California, San Francisco

Kristen A. Ivani, Ph.D.
Laboratory Director,
The Center for Reproductive Medicine and In Vitro Fertilization
San Ramon Regional Medical Center
San Ramon, California

Arnold Jacobson, M.D.
Director, The Center for Reproductive Medicine and In Vitro Fertilization
San Ramon Regional Medical Center
San Ramon, California

Howard W. Jones, Jr., M.D.
Professor of Obstetrics and Gynecology
Eastern Virginia Medical School
and Chairman, Jones Institute for Reproductive Medicine
Norfolk, Virginia

Andrew A. Knight, M.D.
Chief of Anesthesiology
San Ramon Regional Medical Center
San Ramon, California

Emmett Lamb, M.D.
Professor of Obstetrics and Gynecology
University of California, San Francisco

Hovey Lambert, Ph.D.
San Francisco Center for Reproductive Medicine
San Francisco, California

Carl Levinson, M.D.
Professor of Obstetrics and Gynecology
University of California, San Francisco

Larry Lipschultz, M.D.
Professor of Urology
Baylor College of Medicine
Houston, Texas

Mary Martin, M.D.
Associate Professor of Obstetrics and Gynecology
and Director, In Vitro Fertilization Program
University of California, San Francisco

R. Dale McClure, M.D.
Director, Male Infertility and Microsurgical Unit
Virginia Mason Medical Center
Seattle, Washington

Robert D. Nachtigall, M.D.
Associate Clinical Professor of Obstetrics and Gynecology
University of California, San Francisco
and San Francisco Center for Reproductive Medicine
San Francisco, California

Robert P. Neff, M.D.
Assistant Professor of Obstetrics and Gynecology
University of California
San Francisco, California

Camran Nezhat, M.D.
Professor of Clinical Obstetrics and Gynecology
Mercer University School of Medicine
and Director, Center for Special Pelvic Surgery, Fertility
and Endoscopy Center, and Endometriosis Clinic
Atlanta, Georgia

Ira Sharlip, M.D.
Assistant Professor of Urology
University of California, San Francisco

Alex Steinleitner, M.D.
San Francisco Center for Reproductive Medicine
San Francisco, California

Louis M. Weckstein, M.D.
Director, The Center for Reproductive Medicine and In Vitro Fertilization
San Ramon Regional Medical Center
San Ramon, California

Advisory Panel on Emotional, Psychological, Ethical, and Economic Issues of Infertility

Linda Applegarth, Ed.D.
Mary Lou Ballweg
Gay Becker, Ph.D.
Karen Berkeley, M.S.W.
Marsha Blachman, LCSW
Pam Brett, LCSW
Lynn Brokenshire, MFCC
Judith Calica
Jean Carter, M.D.
Michael Carter, Ph.D.
Janice Chiappone, Ph.D.
Pat Cody
Joan Rice Corbett
James Donahue, Ph.D.
Joan Emery, M.P.H.
Jeanne Fleming, Ph.D.
Janet Fox
Ellen S. Glazer, LICSW
Loni Hart, LCSW
Sherokee Ilse
Janet Kirksey, R.N.
Cecile Terrien Lampton, M.S.
Melanie Lawrence

Karen Lebacqz, Ph.D.
Esther Levine, R.N., N.P.
Charles McCoy, Ph.D.
Carole McGregor, R.N.
Maryl Walling Millard, M.A.
Michael Policar, M.D.
Kris Probasco, LSCSW
Mary Anne Rodgers, J.D.
Margarete Sandelowski, Ph.D.
Constance Hoenk Shapiro, Ph.D.
Derwent A. Suthers
Cecilia T. Valdes, M.D.
Donna Vogel, M.D.
Wendy Wasserman
Sheri Glucoft Wong, LCSW
Susan Wood
Marsha Young, Ph.D.
Joyce Zeitz

Advisory Panel on Nutrition, Fitness, and Alternative Medicines

Julie Baller, M.D.
Peggy Chipkin, R.N., F.N.P.
Adelaide Donnelley, MFCC
Joan Hangarter, D.C.

Kathleen Hill
Christina Pepper, M.A.
Miki Shima, O.M.D.
Gerald Westcott

Advisory Panel on Legal and Psychological Issues of Adoption, Donor Insemination, and Surrogate Motherhood

Philip Adams, J.D.
Suzanne Arms
Annette Baran, M.S.W., LCSW
Jean Benward, LCSW
Martin Brandfon, J.D.
Lynne Fingerman, M.S.W.
Bonnie Gradstein, M.P.H.
Marc Gradstein, J.D.
Beth Hall
Pam Hemphill, M.D.
Sharon Huddle, J.D.
Fay Johnson
Sharon Kaplan-Roszia, M.S.
Andrew Kimbrell, J.D.
Candace Kunz, MFCC
Jeanne Warren Lindsay

Lois Ruskai Melina
Diane Michelsen, M.S.W., J.D.
Mildred Mouw, M.S.W.
Kris Probasco, LSCSW
Barbara Raboy, M.P.H.
Diane Roddy
Mary Rodocker, Ph.D.
Barbara Rohan, J.D.
Jed Somit, J.D.
Gail Steinberg
Shelly Tarnoff, J.D.
Bonnie Taylor
Halcea Valdes, M.S.W.
Anne Marie Whisman
Nancy Whitney, MFCC

General Acknowledgments

Susan Adame
Carlos Alden
Becky Allen
Robert Alpert, M.A.
Teresa Roeder Alpert
Adele R. Amodeo
Jan Antaki
Carolyn Latina Ashman
George Ashman, J.D.
Diane Baker
Josephine Berglund
Pauline Birnbaum
Chris Bliss
Robert Bookman
Linda Brinkman

Gayle Bryant
Linda Burbank
Ken Butigan, M.A.
Susan and Greg Byers
Claire Cade, Ph.D.
Teresa Clark
Carol Cline
Linda Cohen
Carol Comini
Joseph Como
Karen Contreras, R.N.
Gary Cook
Jean Cooley
Barbara Daly
Dandelion

Elizabeth Danner
Doris Davis
Linda Dawson
Susan Dean
Tina De Benedictis
Patricia Ogilvie DeGraw, R.N., B.S.N.
Lynda De Maria
Bill and Norine Dolyniuk
Sandy Duso, R.N., M.B.A.
Joan Emery, M.P.H.
Patty Ensrud, R.N.
Elizabeth Evans, MFCC
Brook Fancher, R.N.
Sharon Foley
Cynthia Forrest
Janica Fox
Normajean Blessin Franco
Carol Ginsburg
Patricia Hanus
Yvonne Harkness
Peggy Harrell, M.Div.
Mary J. Harrington
Nona Hasselbring
Ellen and Barry Hecht
Andrea Heikkinen
Hal Hershey
Esther Jakawich, R.N.
Robin Joseph
Ruth Judy, Ph.D.
Judith Webb Kay, Ph.D.
Patti LaCasse
Diann, Penelope, Mary,
   and Anny Lackey
Cindee Lee
Janie Lee, M.Div.
Vivian Lee
Carol Mangravite
Alex Marquez, D. Pharm.
Rose Cirelli Marquez, D. Pharm.
Karen Martin
Jan Masaoka
Marjorie Casebier McCoy, D.H.L.
Linda McFadden, M.Div.
Jati McKimmie

Shan McSpadden
Jennifer Miller
Marcy Moriconi
Rebecca Mormann
Phil and Judy Mullins
Charlene Nelson
Jim Nishimine, M.D.
Steve Palmer, Ph.D.
Penny Partridge
Dale Petersen
Gail and Bill Peterson
Linda Rampil, M.S.W.
Sandy Ried
Tom Renshaw
Jennifer Roddy
Diana Rogers
Louise Rosenbaum, Ph.D.
Marian Rothschild
Carol Salzano
Denise Nolen Shaffer
Maggie James Shepherd
Doug and Heather Skinner
Barbara Sletten
Kathy Smeland
Denise Smith, R.N.
Eileen Smith
Nancy Benson Smith
Seth Steinberg
Sam Swan
Pat Talbert
Lana Terry
Barbara Thomson
Candy Timoney
Judith Turiel, Ed.D.
Fred and Millie Twining
Georgene Vairo, J.D.
Lynn N. Villagran, M.S.W.
Paulene West
Robert Williams
Donna R. Wilson
Loralee Windsor

Introduction

As OFFSPRING OF LARGE families, my husband and I had always assumed that we were genetically fertile. But when, more than fifteen years ago, we first tried to conceive a baby, we found to our astonishment and frustration that nature refused to cooperate. Although one unsuccessful month, and then year, followed another, we refused to acknowledge the possibility of a fertility problem and postponed seeing a specialist — stubbornly clinging to the hope that pregnancy was just a menstrual cycle away.

I finally made that appointment early in 1977, the initial step of a ten-year journey that would include repeated, frequent, and sometimes complex testing; two lengthy surgeries for endometriosis; several years of drug treatment; three years of primary infertility, closely followed by six years of secondary; and the births, seven years apart, of our two children.

Although the physical ordeal was certainly stressful, and at times debilitating, it was the emotional and psychological trauma of being infertile that terrified and often overwhelmed me. We spent years on the "emotional roller coaster," aptly described by so many infertility veterans: cresting highs of hope with each ovulation and plunging lows of disappointment and despair with the onset of each period, elation after each medical treatment, and frustration and grief as months and then years passed without a pregnancy. Infertility seemed to eclipse every positive aspect of our lives, and we found it difficult to separate the fallout from this chronic crisis from the challenges and stresses of everyday living.

For the first two years of our struggle, we tried to cope with this relentless emotional turmoil and the stress of on-going treatment all by ourselves. Locked in isolation, we began to flounder as individuals and as a couple. Looking back, those helpless, stranded feelings were reminiscent of my first wilderness adventure. On that trip, I was afraid I couldn't complete the unfamiliar, grueling climb and even doubted whether I was on the right path. Sensing my fear, a friend showed me the cairns — stacks of three rocks of graduated size — placed every mile or two along the side of the trail. Left behind by those who had already trudged up the path, they were signs that we were headed in the right direction.

I came to view infertility as a challenge similar to that of the wilderness trek. To scale this metaphorical peak, I needed the cairns of accurate medical information, validation of my feelings, emotional support from others struggling with infertility, and reassurance that one does heal and move forward.

I read everything I could find about the subject and joined the newly formed Northern California chapter of RESOLVE, a nationwide support group for the infertile. Meeting and sharing war stories, fears, joys, disappointments, and victories with other infertile women and men was inspiring, comforting, healing, and empowering. We weren't fighting this alone anymore, and our feelings of isolation and hopelessness began to dissipate. If others could confront this unfair and painful crisis, find the right resolution, and emerge as healthy and fulfilled people, then we could too. Facing and accepting the limitations that infertility imposed on my life during those years allowed me to focus on the talents and gifts that I did possess. The creation of this book was part of that transition.

During this time, I attended several all-day infertility conferences, co-sponsored by RESOLVE of Northern California and Serono Symposia, USA, that offered numerous workshops led by medical, legal, and mental health experts. With the assistance, support, and encouragement of many of these professionals, and that of the National office and Northern California chapter of RESOLVE, I researched and wrote the first edition of *The Infertility Book*. This five-year project involved nearly a hundred concerned women and men, each affected personally or professionally by infertility. They graciously and generously shared their expertise and, through personal, telephone, and written contacts, their sorrow, humor, survival tips, disappointments, and triumphs. Reviewing numerous chapter drafts, sharing dozens of conversations, and reading and discussing poignantly written histories brought moments of insight, clarity, laughter, and tears, and sometimes created healing bridges between us. Meeting and working with these women and men has been, professionally, a tremendous writing and learning experience, and personally, an honor, inspiration, and a joy. I will always be proud of this book and grateful to all who helped with its creation.

Five years and three printings later, I was asked to update the first edition. My initial thought was, "It will probably need a few revisions, but how much could have changed in only five years?" As an empathetic alumna and journalist, I re-entered the world of infertility and found that everything had changed, while nothing had really changed at all.

I learned that the technology of assisted reproduction has advanced at "warp speed" during the past five years, spawning an astonishing and often controversial array of medical options and ethical choices. Similarly, there have been rapid and significant changes in the philosophy and practice of such alternative options as adoption, donor insemination, surrogate motherhood, and child-free living. During this second round of research and interviews, it often felt as if I had journeyed through infertility — a mere six years before — on the original starship *Enterprise*, and had now "beamed up" to meet "the next generation" of medical specialists, adoption professionals, birthparents, and infertility patients.

We are living in an amazing, exciting, bewildering, and sometimes frightening technological and social era. To paraphrase Charles Dickens, this is perhaps the best and the worst of times to be infertile. Today, infertile women and men, those professionals assisting them, and our society at large, must grapple with perplexing and largely unexplored ethical issues: Given the redefined parameters of maternal age, how old is "too old" for medical treatment, pregnancy, or other parenting alternatives? When is it time to stop treatment and pursue another path? At what physical, emotional, marital, and financial cost is pregnancy being pursued? What are the long-term consequences of this technology, and other non-traditional methods of family-building, for the individuals, couples, and children involved? How should these options be regulated or controlled, and who should have access to them? Given these quandries, technology also offers some hope to many infertile women and men who have tried repeatedly and unsuccessfully — often for years — to conceive and who, in previous eras, would have little or no chance of ever birthing a child.

I also saw that, despite these extraordinary changes, the heartaches and challenges of infertility remain the same. The eloquent voices quoted throughout this text speak of a yearning and inner pain that is ageless. Whether one was deemed "barren" a century ago or is infertile today, this experience deeply affects core feelings of identity, self-worth, limitations, life purpose, and mortality. It often brings the fragility of life, the depths of grief, and the healing power of love, communion, and empathy between people into a poignantly sharp focus. And it inevitably necessitates moving forward: confronting, mourning, and accepting the innately unjust and wrenching life crisis of infertility, and with determination and purpose, overcoming it — while trying to keep your body, heart, soul, spirit, and relationship intact.

Technology, for all its promise and wonder, has not provided any emotional shortcuts. Like their predecessors ten, fifty, or a thousand years ago, those infertile today must search for the right path, climb the proverbial mountain, and heal from the wounds of the journey. Before attempting an actual ascent, mountaineers advise carefully studying the terrain, acknowledging the inevitable pitfalls, preparing yourself mentally and physically for the challenge, and never, ever climbing alone. As you consider these highly personal and often life-altering decisions, become your own consumer advocate — read about your medical problems and prospective resolutions, carefully select your specialists, counselors, and adoption professionals, take good care of yourself and your partner, find and reciprocate emotional support with those who understand infertility, and consider — for everyone involved — the lifelong effects of your choices. Make this climb with pride, love, and respect for yourself, each other, the struggle you have undertaken, and the child you hope to parent.

From conception to birth, *The Infertility Book* has been a labor of the heart. And it seems fitting that both editions have been conceived, nurtured, labored through, and birthed by those who have been personally or professionally touched by infertility. It is a tribute to the spirit, creativity, perserverance, and resilience with which they have confronted and surmounted a considerable life challenge. It is offered as a cairn for yours.

❦ *Part One*

The Infertility Experience

One Woman's Story

Donna grew up in the mid-sixties, one of five children in a happy, loving Midwestern family. As the eldest, Donna was given a lot of responsibility for household tasks and child care from an early age. She loved her brothers and sisters and enjoyed the company of children. As a teenager, Donna was also a favorite babysitter with many of the neighborhood kids.

She started menstruating when she was about twelve. Her periods were irregular and she sometimes experienced painful premenstrual cramps. Donna's family doctor examined her but could find no physical problem. He assured her that she would eventually bear as many children as she wanted.

Donna worked hard in high school and was awarded a full scholarship to an Eastern college. From a young age she had dreamed of going to college and having a career in business. She also wanted a loving marriage and several children and hoped to combine the two. She envisioned this life in her late twenties or early thirties. For now she was eager to go away to school and then begin her career.

Donna did well in college and graduated with honors. She soon found an entry-level management position with a large corporation. She advanced quickly and was encouraged by her employer to work toward a master's degree in business administration. She enrolled in a program at a nearby university and met Nick in one of her classes.

Donna and Nick were about the same age, shared many interests, and were very involved with their careers and graduate studies. They dated for several months and decided to marry. During the first three years of their marriage, the couple finished their degrees and saved for a house. Believing they were fertile, they faithfully used contraceptives during this time. They were each about thirty when they moved into their home and decided it was time to get pregnant.

Donna read that it takes most couples six months to a year to conceive. She and Nick decided to stop using birth control and let nature take its course. Each month they hoped for a pregnancy. Donna's periods were still irregular, so they would become excited as five and sometimes six weeks passed between periods. She became so hopeful she denied the telltale signs of cramps and bloating. She requested pregnancy tests on several occasions, but all were negative.

After each anxious wait, Donna's period eventually started. When she realized she was not pregnant yet again, she would cry alone in the bathroom. Nick also felt disappointed each month but was more concerned about Donna's unhappiness and frustration.

Meanwhile Nick and Donna's friends and siblings became pregnant with their first and second children. Donna found herself jealously eyeing pregnant women on the bus. She felt angry that she was infertile and wondered why she was left out. Donna dreaded family gatherings where someone inevitably announced another pregnancy and somebody else always asked Donna what *she* was waiting for. They never approached Nick! She attended a few baby showers but found herself depressed and tearful for days afterward. Before long Donna began to decline invitations to both showers and family occasions.

After a year of unsuccessful attempts at pregnancy, the couple sought help from an infertility specialist. Donna felt frightened that something was wrong with her and ashamed that she had to see a physician at all. Why couldn't she "just get pregnant" like other women?

Their specialist suggested they chart Donna's basal temperature each morning and make love on alternate days around the time of ovulation. A semen analysis was done for Nick with normal results.

As the months progressed, Donna underwent a series of workup tests and became increasingly depressed and frustrated. Her sexual relationship with Nick was also noticeably affected. Their lovemaking never seemed spontaneous anymore and both of them carried a mental picture of her temperature graph. They felt under tremendous pressure and, for the first time, out of control of their lives. They argued more often, especially on the days when Donna thought she was ovulating or her period started. She felt guilty and inadequate and offered to divorce Nick so he could find a fertile woman.

Donna mentioned these problems to her specialist. He told her these were common reactions and recommended that she and Nick join an infertility support group to ease their isolation and pain. Nick was skeptical about the idea but so worried about Donna that he agreed to attend one meeting. They both felt apprehensive and embarrassed when they walked into the room. As the evening progressed, they were amazed and relieved to discover five other couples had similar stories and backgrounds. It was a great relief to hear others complain, laugh, and cry about the same problems. These people were loving, healthy, and well-adjusted, yet they were all experiencing fertility problems. Donna later told Nick that this was the first time in months that she didn't feel weird, abnormal, or out of place.

As the last part of her workup Donna underwent a diagnostic laparoscopy. During this procedure her specialist found endometriosis on the outside of her ovaries and tubes and surgically removed it. Donna and Nick now have a 50 percent chance of conceiving a child. The physician also mentioned several high-tech medical options if surgery is unsuccessful.

This news was both a shock and relief to Donna. She was relieved that a medical reason had been found for their infertility. But she was also shocked and angry that her body was "abnormal" and "diseased" and that her chances for childbearing were only half those of other women.

Donna and Nick have continued meeting with their support group and are discussing the high-tech options as well as adoption, surrogacy, or child-free living if she should not conceive.

Infertility has changed both Donna and Nick. They feel sadder and wiser about life but remain firmly committed to each other. Donna is tired of the emotional and medical stresses of her fertility struggle. She is also frightened that she and Nick may never experience pregnancy and birth. Nick is angry that Donna has had to endure the tests and still faces surgery. He is also weary of his wife's constant unhappiness. They both worry about the high cost of infertility care and wonder why this had to happen to them.

One Man's Story

JIM IS THE SECOND OF THREE SONS, an all-American boy who grew up in Southern California in the early seventies. His parents encouraged their sons to excel in athletics, scouting, and academics. Jim played varsity basketball and ran cross-country in high school and college. His grades were consistently high and he was particularly drawn to electronics. Jim was popular in school, had gone steady with many girls over the years, and was sexually experienced by the time he began college.

Jim never thought much about fatherhood while growing up. Once in college he figured that if he ever married, he would probably want to have a couple of kids. This idea, however, was never as important as getting through school and establishing a career in communications.

A few years after Jim graduated from college, a mutual friend introduced him to Lisa, a high school teacher about his age. They had similar interests, hit it off immediately, and married within a year.

At first neither Jim nor Lisa wanted to have children. They had an active social life and busy careers and traveled a great deal. Lisa took birth control pills for the first six years of their marriage and both assumed pregnancy was just a "few tries away" if they did want a child. After she turned thirty, Lisa mentioned having a baby more often. Jim had also been thinking about fatherhood, and they agreed to quit the Pill.

Many of their siblings and friends were now parents, and at first they were excited about having a child of their own. After six months, however, their excitement had changed to anxious frustration. They had not conceived and it seemed that someone was forever asking, "Aren't you pregnant yet?"

After a year of unsuccessful tries, Lisa's gynecologist suggested they begin an infertility workup. Both Jim and Lisa were dismayed by the suggestion of infertility but agreed to a few simple tests. They wanted to know if there was a problem.

A semen analysis was ordered for Jim. He balked at the idea of masturbating into a jar and having his sperm graded for quality and quantity. He knew his sex life was normal and assumed that his sperm was too. Because Lisa was so insistent, he grudgingly agreed to stop by the lab. With a great deal of embarrassment, he produced the sample and gave the jar to the technician. Then he drove to work and tried to forget the experience.

Lisa's doctor called a few days later and asked them both to come to his office. Jim's sperm count was quite low with poor motility, and the physician thought Jim should see a urologist for further evaluation before Lisa underwent any invasive fertility testing. Jim and Lisa were stunned by the news and couldn't think of much to say. They wrote down the name of the urologist and quickly left the office.

They drove home in silence. Jim's thoughts flickered with images of basketball games, school dances, and past sexual encounters. He remembered sweating out a couple of passionate evenings when no one had bothered about contraceptives. He couldn't believe he wasn't fertile. He wondered if he would eventually become impotent.

When they got home, Lisa tried to talk about the visit but he angrily told her to leave him alone. They agreed to see the urologist the following week and drop the subject until then. They somehow got through the next few days. On a few occasions Lisa tried to touch or hold Jim, but he brushed her away.

They went to the urologist's office at the scheduled time. Lisa was close to tears and Jim was frightened. The doctor interviewed them in his office and then gave Jim a thorough physical examination. He found a varicocele of the left scrotum that he said might be contributing to the problem. He also asked Jim to produce another semen sample so he could personally evaluate it. He suggested Jim and Lisa return in two days to assess the situation.

When they got home, Jim could hardly face Lisa. He was scared, ashamed, and, for the first time in their relationship, felt inadequate. Maybe she would leave him. Lisa was worried about Jim and frightened that she would not bear a child. She tried to console him, suggesting that the urologist might help them. Jim angrily told her to leave him alone and go find a fertile man; she could have a divorce anytime she wanted. It was one of their worst arguments. Lisa left the house in tears and returned late that evening. Jim pretended he was asleep.

On their next visit the urologist confirmed the low sperm count and poor motility problem. With no treatment at all they had roughly a 25 percent chance for a spontaneous pregnancy. With treatment their chances for pregnancy might increase to 30 to 50 percent, providing Lisa did not have any fertility problems. He offered to review the medical and surgical alternatives in detail, now or at a later appointment. He also mentioned the options of donor insemination, adoption, and child-free living and urged the couple to call anytime with questions or concerns. Finally, the physician encouraged them to seek emotional support.

Both Jim and Lisa were devastated by the news. At best they had a 50 percent chance of having a child. In reality their odds were probably less than that. Once they were home, Jim stated that he didn't want to have surgery or adopt and he certainly didn't want another guy's sperm inseminated in Lisa! She was furious with him. She'd certainly undergo surgery or take fertility drugs if *she* had a problem!

Lisa now seemed obsessed with having a baby. Jim reminded her that she had put it off for years. Why was this such a big deal now? Why couldn't she drop the idea and enjoy what life gave them? They could travel, sleep late every weekend, buy a new car.

Another week of hostile, bitter exchanges followed. After yet another horrible argument, Lisa tearfully told Jim she loved him but couldn't go on this way. She thought they needed professional help, as well as emotional support. She suggested they see a therapist experienced in fertility problems, confide in their closest friends and relatives, and check out an infertility support group. Jim, too, wanted to save their marriage. He agreed to this course of action.

Their families had mixed reactions. Lisa's mother and Jim's sister had lost several pregnancies and were sympathetic and supportive. Jim's parents, however, seemed defensive and embarrassed by the news. His "best" friends weren't exactly helpful either. "I'd be happy to stand in for you, buddy!" and "Shooting blanks, huh, Jim?" were a couple of responses. For the first time in his life Jim felt abnormal and sadly alone.

When they attended their first support group meeting, Jim sat in a distant corner of the living room. He couldn't identify with infertile people. Jim didn't say much but listened carefully. Several of the men also had low sperm counts and the couples were experiencing the same marital and self-esteem problems as he and Lisa. Some of the women complained that their husbands "didn't care" about their infertility problem. It dawned on Jim that men have been culturally conditioned to work, compete, provide, and, to a certain extent, hide their emotions. He saw that he wasn't alone and began to look forward to the meetings.

Lisa and Jim also sought counseling from a professional therapist. In weekly sessions they are now clarifying their feelings about having a child and examining the options available to them.

Despite this support, infertility is a difficult burden to shoulder. Jim and Lisa are painfully aware that many other couples conceive easily, some of their friends and relatives continue to offer endless advice, and they still wonder, "Why us?"

CHAPTER 1

Self-Images and Social Pressures

❦ The last straw came at a Christmas party in a home filled with small children. While my husband held an infant, someone loudly remarked, "Oh, doesn't he look so natural holding that baby? He ought to be a daddy."

I walked outside and sat in the dark. Waves of hate washed over me both toward them and myself. Why doesn't my body work right? Why can't people think before they speak? Why do their thoughtless remarks still hurt?

❦ I have always been an avid reader of history. Barrenness has been a curse and stigma in every society I've studied. In my own ethnic heritage it is the worst thing that can happen to a woman. Small wonder I felt the doom of the ages when I learned of my own infertility.

HUMAN BEINGS HAVE BEEN mating and, with varying degrees of success, reproducing for millions of years. Although billions of babies have been born, countless couples have also encountered fertility problems or pregnancy loss throughout the ages. This is because nature has endowed both females and males with delicately balanced, complex reproductive systems. The slightest obstruction, imbalance, or abnormality can disrupt the intricate harmony of the chemical processes necessary for sperm production, ovulation, fertilization, implantation, and a successful pregnancy to occur.

Still we live on a crowded planet, surrounded by fertile humans, fauna, and flora. As a result, many people tend to take fertility for granted, assuming they can plan or control childbearing. Although most couples do achieve a pregnancy within a year of unprotected intercourse, millions of Americans experience fertility problems at any given time.

How many Americans are infertile? Estimates of the number of women and men affected by infertility or pregnancy loss vary considerably. Over the years, many popular books and magazine articles have estimated that as many as 10 million Americans suffer from fertility problems at any given time. This figure, and the often proposed theory that the incidence of infertility is rising, has been questioned by a variety of experts.

In its 1988 compendium of the multifaceted policy issues surrounding this problem, *Infertility: Medical and Social Choices,* the Office of Technology Assessment (OTA) estimated that 2.4 million couples — plus an unknown number of singles and couples who have not sought treatment — are infertile. The report, which is based on data collected in the early 1980s, also cites an increasing fertility problem among younger people (between twenty and twenty-four years of age) primarily because of the incidence of such sexually transmitted diseases as chlamydia and gonorrhea.

More recently, the National Center for Health Statistics released the results of its 1988 National Survey for Family Growth (NSFG). This report — based on data gathered from interviews with about 8,500 women of all races, aged fifteen through forty-four, across the United States — compares the national rates of infertility between 1965 and 1988. Respondents — both childless women and those who had birthed one or more children — were asked if they believed for any reason, medical or otherwise, that they or their mates had an infertility or miscarriage problem. Those who answered affirmatively were counted as "infertile" for purposes of the study. From this data, the NSFG estimated that 2.3 million American couples are infertile at any given time. Single men or women, men who may have lower-than-average sperm counts or motility, and couples who have not yet tried to conceive were not factored into the data.

The researchers concluded that the although incidence of infertility has remained about the same — around 8 percent of all women between fifteen and forty-four years of age, the percentage of women affected by infertility does rise with age. About 20 percent of women and 36 percent of childless couples, between thirty-five and forty-four years of age, reported fertility problems. (On a positive note, the 1976 survey reported a 54 percent infertility rate among childless couples in this age group — 18 percent higher than the 1988 statistics.)

The NSFG also noted a significant increase, between 1976 and 1988, in the *number* of childless women in this age category — from 565,000 to more than 1 million. They concluded that the aging of large numbers of the post-World War II baby boom generation, and their growing tendency to delay childbearing to their mid to late thirties, accounted for this rise.

The OTA statistics also affirmed the biological reality that fertility inexorably declines with age: 13.6 percent of those aged thirty to thirty-four will encounter problems conceiving, as will 24.6 percent of thirty-five to thirty-nine year olds and 27.2 percent of those between forty and forty-four. Miscarriage rates also rise dramatically — from 25 percent to 50 percent in women between the ages of thirty-five and forty-five.

Although the actual numbers are difficult to ascertain, millions of American women and men are touched and deeply affected by fertility problems. Regardless of their age or the contributing causes, these women and men discover that a healthy, full-term pregnancy is an elusive, or even unattainable, goal. Trying to accept, cope with, and resolve this dilemma, as individuals and partners, often permeates every aspect of their lives.

The Social Pressures of Infertility

❦ I measure each month by how pregnant my friend, co-worker, relative is. I then look at how un-pregnant I am. Sometimes it's too painful to tell my husband that someone else is pregnant.

Recently I received a letter from a high school friend. She wrote about her two children and how she was pregnant with her third. She did ask if I had any children. I wrote back saying, "No, but I have had three miscarriages." I wanted her to know what we are really going through. The answer "no" to having any children just doesn't seem enough.

For millenia it was essential for humans to multiply lest the species die out. Although the earth is now a dangerously crowded planet, that value persists and is encountered by both infertile women and men and couples who are voluntarily child-free. The social pressure to bear a child is usually conveyed by family and friends, and these relationships often become awkward or strained.

❦ I think my relationship with my mother has suffered the most. I have felt inadequate and ashamed to discuss my infertility with her. When my younger sister had her babies, I felt myself drift away from all of them. They couldn't understand my feelings and it was less painful to avoid their company.

In a society where few are bold enough to ask your annual income, nearly everyone will inquire about your fertility. If a couple does not produce a child within a "reasonable length of time," their friends and relatives usually ask why. Remarks and questions may range from the subtle ("You two sure would make great parents!") to the guilt-provoking ("I'm just dying to be a grandmother!") to the downright cruel ("What's wrong with you two?" "Just relax, you're trying too hard." "Don't you know how to do it?" "When are you going to stop shooting blanks?").

This external pressure on the infertile couple is further intensified by specific occasions and social situations that celebrate pregnancy, children, and the extended family: holidays, other women's pregnancies, and baby showers.

❦ Christmas was the pinnacle of pain, especially the year our nephew was born on Christmas Eve. Everyone raved about how much he looked like my husband. I'll always remember the way my husband wept in my arms that night. Seven years of his being strong for me finally ended in an emotional release for him.

Throughout the year holidays bring almost monthly reminders of one's infertility. Mother's Day and Father's Day, Halloween, Passover, Easter, Thanksgiving, Hanukkah, and Christmas are largely centered around children. You may have fantasized for years about how to celebrate these occasions with your child.

Christmas and Hanukkah are probably the most difficult holidays for the infertile. Store windows are filled with toys and adorable tots line up to visit Santa. Cards arrive from smiling and perhaps growing families, along with invitations to family reunions and holiday parties. These gatherings usually involve contact with children and infants, and the merriment and refreshments encourage remarks and discussion of your fertility.

And when you long for a baby, jealousy and anger toward pregnant women are natural reactions; it is difficult not to stare at their bulging bellies with frustration. Seeing someone else's body swell with child can hurt deeply.

> ❦ My feelings were very intense and on occasion the thought of being around a pregnant friend would reduce me to hysterical crying.

> ❦ My friends' pregnancies were especially difficult. I respectfully called them, but avoided seeing them. I called when they gave birth, bought gifts, and visited. I unwillingly held one friend's baby because she wanted me to. I didn't want to. I still hadn't gotten over why she was able to have a baby and I lost all of mine. I'm getting better, though. I just try to become numb when someone else tells me they are pregnant. I used to feel guilty about not feeling happy for them; now I just don't feel.

It often seems as if everyone you know is expecting. The pregnancies of close friends and relatives are especially painful and often evoke ambivalent feelings. You may feel genuine happiness for their good fortune yet dread socializing with them, fearing your own reactions as well as pity or insensitivity from others.

> ❦ I wished I would never have to suffer my hysteria after yet another baby shower. Finally, I stopped going. I could no longer deal with my feelings.

These intense feelings are exacerbated by the inevitable baby shower invitations. These gatherings often epitomize an infertile woman's isolation. She must sit in a room filled with women — most of whom are already mothers or perhaps also expecting — and watch an extremely pregnant friend open gifts of cute baby things. Her infertility either goes unnoticed or, perhaps even worse, is acknowledged in pitying glances. Back home she may cry for hours or even days afterward, wondering for the thousandth time, "Why me? What did I do to deserve this?" Her husband is often unable to console her and may experience similar feelings on occasions like Christmas or Father's Day. (Chapter 7 includes suggestions for coping with these social events along with a discussion of the unique pressures encountered by infertile stepparents and single and gay women.)

The Emotional Fallout of Infertility

❦ Infertility is a silent tragedy. How do you explain to someone that you had a rough night because there was no baby to keep you awake, that your house is too clean and there are no toys cluttering the floor? Would anyone understand that you have cried over Pampers commercials?

❦ I never imagined I would have difficulty getting pregnant. I always believed I was fertile and ovulating each month. I had the mucus. I had the Mittelschemertz!! I thought getting pregnant would be a snap. If anything, I thought I would work on trying to plan the sex of our baby. God, have my priorities changed. Sometimes my "desire" for a baby feels like a need.

Last year's holidays were terribly painful and I still cry when I think about those feelings. And we have to start thinking about this year's now. Although lately, I don't need a holiday to cause me to start weeping. In church, when I see a baby, I start to cry. At dinnertime, when it's just my husband and myself, I really feel an emptiness, as if something or someone is missing.

Although millions face this problem, each infertile individual usually feels isolated and alone, largely because this is an invisible affliction. Without asking, we can't tell who has shared our experience and, until recently, infertility has rarely been discussed or acknowledged. Many couples are still reluctant to reveal their problem to friends or relatives.

The 1990s are a particularly painful decade in which to be infertile. The post-World War II baby boomers, many approaching their late thirties and forties, are now producing a boomlet of their own. The current wave of maternity fashions, natural birthing classes, infant fashions and equipment, and breast-feeding debates emphasizes an infertile couple's isolation and loneliness. "I felt I was being excluded from some magic parent's club," one woman remarked. "It was as if everyone had been asked to dance but me."

❦ People frequently tried to blame my infertility on some weakness in myself, something about my attitude — maybe fear, maybe stress, maybe caring too much. I was deeply insulted by the implication that fertile people are somehow superior to the infertile.

Many people are also tempted to find, and offer, a cause for a couple's infertility — be it psychological or physical. "Perhaps you really don't want to be pregnant," or "You exercise too much (or too little)" add to the confusion and guilt the infertile partners already feel. Many temporarily withdraw from the world of fertile acquaintances and children while they confront the powerful feelings raised by this experience.

ALTERED SELF-IMAGES

❦ Everywhere I looked I saw pregnant women. I felt conspicuously infertile. The high following my surgery faded into depression and disgust with my body when I again failed to conceive.

"I'm no good," I'd fume. "It must be a curse. Other women can do it easily. What's wrong with me?"

Many infertile women and men feel disappointed or angry with their bodies. Often premenstrual cramps and fullness bring on tears and intense feelings of failure for a woman, and she may feel her body is defective on these days. Long-term infertility can also make a man feel inadequate and undermine his sense of masculinity.

Understandably sexuality can also be affected. Women and men may feel physically unattractive or associate sex solely with procreation. The goals of pregnancy and pleasure become fused, and the failure to realize the former often affects the latter.

Old childhood insecurities and feelings of inferiority often resurface now. Once again we may feel odd or that we don't belong. Back in high school we may have yearned for blonde hair, a perfect figure, or athletic prowess. Now it is the ability to conceive after six to twelve months of unprotected intercourse. Strong self-images that took years to develop often weaken.

Many psychologists posit that how one confronts and processes any life crisis, including infertility, is influenced by the sense of self-worth and the coping mechanisms developed in childhood. In recent years, a plethora of popular books have been written about the life-long effects of growing up in "dysfunctional" families — those which, to varying degrees, do not establish and nurture a child's sense of security and self-esteem. Jeanne Fleming, Ph.D., a clinical psychologist, observes that an infertility crisis may trigger earlier coping strategies in adults from such dysfunctional backgrounds. Some learned, as children, to block out their feelings and thereby avoid a painful reality. They may fall back on such behavior during an infertility crisis by minimizing or denying its emotional impact. Others, who as children fully absorbed that early pain and fear, may later feel overwhelmed by the emotional fall-out of an infertility problem and allow these intense feelings to reshape their adult self-images. In either case, consultation with a counselor experienced with both infertility and "adult child" issues can help you to separate past issues from the present and to develop a positive self-image and effective coping strategies.

GUILT FEELINGS

❦ It's Thanksgiving and I cry again. Mourning my unborn child, not knowing if he would have my husband's curly hair or my big round eyes. What have I done in my past not to be able to do such a simple thing as make a baby?

❦ I remembered hushed conversations I wasn't supposed to hear as a child. A "barren" woman would be discussed in pitying voices amid speculation of what was wrong with her. As our infertility dragged on, I became more fearful and defensive. I started to think that I was being punished.

Many search for a reason why they are infertile. They wonder if this is punishment for being "bad" and undeserving of happiness or retribution for past "offenses," such as an abortion, a miscarriage greeted with relief, or premarital sex. Religious training can reinforce such thinking; some try to atone for past wrongs and regard painful or embarrassing workup tests and procedures as part of their punishment.

An infertile partner often feels guilty for causing the problem, thinking: "It's all my fault," or "If she was with someone else, she could get pregnant." To compensate for this inadequacy, either or both partners may try to keep the relationship perfect in other ways, or conversely, may seek solace or intimacy from others.

LOSS OF CONTROL

❦ Two days ago my period came again. We tried so hard this month, timing our intimacy to create a new life. We, who try to control everything in our lives so perfectly. Do we try again and again? When do we, or should we, give up? We feel as if our lives are on hold.

For anyone who wishes to plan childbearing, rather than just "let it happen," infertility is a frustrating turn of events. Successful, self-confident individuals and over-achievers can be particularly devastated by this problem. After reaching other goals, they are unable to perform the "simple" biological feat of a successful pregnancy. In reality, of course, fertility is not always easily managed or controlled.

A long-term fertility problem often creates a state of limbo for both partners. They do not know whether they will have the child(ren) they want, how long to pursue treatment, whether adoption or child-free living is an appropriate option, or even if their marriage can withstand this crisis. Women especially may defer career moves or advanced studies until their infertility is resolved. It may also be difficult to make mutual decisions about occupation changes, job relocation, and financial investments during this time.

RESENTMENT

❦ My younger brother and his wife called to say they were expecting a child and it was a "surprise." We had invested many years and dollars in charts, drugs, and surgeries to no avail. It wasn't hard to imagine the pity the rest of the family would direct toward infertile me. It was so unfair.

Media reports of unwanted pregnancies and tragic instances of child abuse are ironic and frustrating realities to the infertile. Eager to parent, they endure any number of medical procedures and untold emotional stress in their desperation to have a child — and often resent those who complain about or neglect parental responsibilities.

Unfortunately the ability to reproduce is not related to goodness or whether one deserves to have a child. Conceiving and bearing a healthy child is largely a matter of luck and genetics. Like other victims of disease or misfortune, the infertile are simply unlucky.

Psychological Stages of Infertility

Infertility is often described as a "life crisis," a time of both internal turmoil and external pressure. Many women and men pass through several psychological stages of confrontation and acceptance. They also experience complex feelings of loss: of the joyous event of "just getting pregnant" without medical testing or treatment, of control over the ability to plan reproduction, and to some extent, one's life. For some, infertility becomes an obsession and a symbol of their failure to meet personal as well as cultural expectations.

Many mental health professionals apply one of two models, or a combination of both, to describe and facilitate the coping process of infertility. The Kübler-Ross/Menning model suggests a finality of psychological acceptance after several stages of denial, anger, and grief. The chronic coping model, developed by Jeanne Fleming, Ph.D. and Kenneth Burry, M.D., likens infertility to a protracted process, and for some people, a lifelong reality.

KÜBLER-ROSS/MENNING MODEL

Elisabeth Kübler-Ross in her landmark work, *On Death and Dying,* identified transitional stages that individuals experience when facing their own death. Barbara Eck Menning, a nurse and founder of RESOLVE (a support organization described at the end of this chapter), has applied Ross's theory to the infertility challenge. Like those confronting death, Menning suggests, the infertile individual or couple passes through similar stages during the struggle for acceptance and resolution. This is not a linear process; each partner will probably move through these stages at a different pace, and either may periodically regress to a previous phase.

✾ Infertile. Not me. Maybe next month I'll get pregnant and this will all have been a bad dream. Seeking help would make the infertility real.

Denial or surprise is a common initial reaction, perhaps after years of avoiding pregnancy, to a diagnosis of infertility. Believing you had been controlling reproduction, you suddenly discover pregnancy is difficult or perhaps impossible to achieve. This denial serves an important psychological purpose. It gives us time to absorb and process distressing news before pursuing a course of action.

Denial gives way to anger or rage toward life in general, at God, the cosmos or fate, or, more specifically, toward your infertile spouse, physician, or fertile friends and coworkers.

❦ **I was busy withdrawing from friends who were having their second children while I was having my second operation. This time major surgery determined and possibly corrected the cause. My chances of conceiving weren't good, but I was ecstatic and once again full of hope. I began to bargain with God for a pregnancy.**

No results. In my subsequent anger I began questioning the existence of God. Was He not listening or just not there? How could I deal with all my anger?

This anger may also be tinged with feelings of envy, frustration, powerlessness, or resentment of this injustice. It may explode outward, often over seemingly minor or trivial matters, surprising you with its intensity. Anger may also be vented inward in the form of depression. You may feel victimized and out of control. Symptoms include apathy, insomnia, lethargy, a marked increase or decrease of appetite, crying spells, anxiety, and feelings of hopelessness or despair. Long-term infertility can become an obsession or the central focus of life.

A period of grief, either for your present infertility or for the baby you will never birth, commonly follows anger or depression.

❦ **I finally let loose. The pain, hurt, and guilt screamed their way out. I was immobilized and cried for three days. As I sobbed in my husband's embrace, I wondered why this was happening to us.**

❦ **My daughter is fourteen months old. I gave birth to her and yet I feel like crying now just remembering the intense pain at thinking I would never become pregnant. Not ever being able to have a baby — or at least experiencing the possibility of that — calls for intense grieving, as if you have lost a child.**

The duration and intensity of mourning depends on whether infertility is long-term or permanent, as well as on individual temperament. Most people report periods of grief lasting several months to a year, although medical treatments and just plain hoping may continue indefinitely. Some carry this pain far into old age and are moved to tears at the mention of their infertility or miscarriage of three or four decades ago.

Our society does not acknowledge infertility as an occasion for mourning, and at first we too may not recognize grief as it occurs. While women often release grief through tears, because of cultural conditioning men often bury pain until it erupts in some other way. In any case going through the motions of everyday life, meeting job responsibilities, and interacting with family and friends can seem an overwhelming burden.

Each individual and couple grieves in a private way — some by crying alone, examining their reactions, or sharing their feelings with close friends, others by writing poetry or creating rituals or rites of passage.

❦ It was hard to overcome my bitterness. I finally understood that bitterness was turning me into a person I didn't want to be. I found it much harder to stay soft in my sorrow, to relax through those hard edges which inevitably formed with each disappointment. I had to make a choice, though, not to be bitter. With my choice, I found a new level of compassion opening up, along with a reluctance to judge or censor.

❦ Sarah and I had dreamed of a biological child for years and had accumulated booties, rattles, and other gifts. After years of medical treatments, we finally decided it was time to pursue adoption. To release our grief, we buried the gifts in the backyard. We feel this ritual marked a passage in our lives and created a place to hold our grief. Now we can search for our adopted child with a new love and enthusiasm.

You must finish the grieving process before acceptance of infertility can occur. While this seems to last forever, it does gradually diminish. You probably won't forget your infertility, but memories will be fleeting rather than daily obsessions.

❦ While I awaited surgery, I slowly began to accept my infertility. This stage was not as bad as waiting for the diagnosis. I began to see myself as unique and special for experiencing something that not everyone does. The pain of infertility, even intractable infertility like mine, can be a stepping stone to greater insight and compassion for the human experience.

Infertility has changed me forever and no one will ever care about it as much as I do. Everyone must resolve it his or her own way. You are alone in this, as at death. Others can support and talk with you, but you yourself must come to terms with it and finally face the fertile world again.

Accepting your infertility is the first step toward resolution. "Resolving" is a complex concept that includes acceptance of infertility and a healing from its losses, followed by a desire to pursue an appropriate option such as adoption, continued medical treatment, or child-free living. At this stage a resurgence of energy and self-esteem usually occurs.

CHRONIC COPING MODEL

❦ Infertility has been a part of my life for nine years now. Some days it weighs more heavily than others. But it's there every day. I haven't really reached acceptance that this has happened to me, but I have learned to live with it.

Jeanne Fleming, Ph.D., and Kenneth Burry, M.D., among other health professionals, suggest that many couples view infertility as a chronic problem. For example, those with mild or moderate fertility problems often have endless hope of achieving a pregnancy during their reproductive years. Others may encounter unexplained or secondary infertility or may embark on a medical or surgical treatment that has a fairly good success rate and creates new hope for pregnancy. But after months or years of continued infertility, some become chronically depressed or immobilized by the problem, like those coping with a handicapped child, troubled marriage, or a loved one who has run away or disappeared. Couples caught in this chronic model often avoid poignant reminders of their infertility, which they describe as a "lifelong reality" they are unable to accept or resolve.

Fleming and Burry suggest that these couples should approach their infertility in two ways:

☐ Decide whether and how they will parent by clarifying their attitudes toward adoption and child-free living;

☐ Develop appropriate ways to cope with their long-term problem.

The latter strategy involves acknowledging each partner's feelings, rebuilding confidence and self-esteem through other goals and achievements, and finding emotional support.

Fleming suggests that this approach leads to a positive change in how you ultimately perceive, value, and take care of yourselves. As you begin to grow again in positive ways, the infertility no longer dominates your identity or sense of self-worth. You can acknowledge infertility as a part of your life experience, while maintaining strong and positive feelings of self-esteem.

Tools for Meeting the Challenge

❦ You can reach out and look for those special people who can say, "I understand. I've been there too." There were times when I clung like a drowning woman to people who let me. And when my head was high enough above water to have some perspective, I tried to be there for those who were sinking.

For years there were few sources of emotional support for the infertile. Fortunately this is no longer true; you need not face this problem alone. Many have found vast relief just hearing someone else verbalize their anger and heartache. Reading about the struggles and triumphs of others, or speaking to them by phone or in support groups, can provide inspiration and a much-needed reality check. Some specialists encourage such dialogue and will, upon request, introduce their patients to others in the same situation.

SUPPORT GROUPS

❧ Talking about infertility has helped us cope, and being part of a support group put infertility into perspective. No one should be afraid of a support group. Sometimes you cry, but there's lots of laughter too!

❧ My infertility forced me to face that I was not the open, non-defensive male I thought I was. Sure I was there for my wife when she had to deal with family and friends asking, "Sooo, are you pregnant yet?" But I was unable to share my own sorrow.

It wasn't until we joined a support group for couples with fertility problems that I was forced to confront the distance I was creating between us through my inability to talk about what was going on with me. It came up around the sixth session of our group. All five of the women said they felt cheated out of the experience of being supportive to their husbands, because they were not being given the opportunity to do so. It was they who cried, and we who comforted. It was they who talked about their irrational anger toward couples with babies and we men who cooly dispensed insights on why their irrationality was rational under the circumstances. And it was they who had to bring us the news of their unwanted menstrual periods month after month.

Within the past year, I have given my wife more than ninety Pergonal injections with an inch-and-a-half long needle, each day after which she has had to go to the doctor's office to have a blood test to closely monitor her estrogen levels. Surely having endured this, along with numerous invasive procedures, two laparoscopies, one major surgery, and a miscarriage, my wife deserves at least some mention of my feelings of pain at not being one month closer to having a new baby in our arms.

Our wives hungered for us to drop our stoic pretenses and trust them with our vulnerable egos. But big boys don't cry. I am learning, though. Just tonight I opened up about how hard this infertility thing is for me as the months and years slip away. And of course, she was there for me. I even let her see a tear. One small step for man, one giant leap for man-kindness.

Robert Bookman

Many people are hesitant about joining an infertility support group. Some even think seeking such help is an admission of emotional instability. Mental health professionals, however, agree that the intense and often overwhelming emotions associated with infertility are a natural reaction to a real crisis.

Support groups are a safe refuge from a fertile world, where one can express feelings and receive empathy and understanding. The groups focus *solely* on the feelings and problems of infertility, so other personal issues are not addressed. This setting can provide valuable coping suggestions and moral support.

While a support group can't guarantee a pregnancy, it can ease some of the pain and isolation of infertility. Many couples find it a useful vehicle to examine their feelings and options for resolutions.

> ❦ One of the women in our group brought her newborn adopted baby to our meeting. It was incredible: We passed the baby around, and for many of us, it was the first time in years we'd been able to hold and touch a baby without terrible pain. It was as if this baby was a symbol not only of what we could ourselves have one day if we wished, but also of all the sorrow we'd gone through. We felt so close to each other that night and went home feeling as if we'd been touched by something really miraculous, having been able to open ourselves up to our feelings instead of shutting down for protection.

A feeling of unity often develops in support groups as couples move toward resolution, and lifelong friends are sometimes made in the process.

PROFESSIONAL COUNSELING

> ❦ After seven years of infertility we decided to consult a therapist. It was the best thing we ever did. With her help we were able to separate the effects of our infertility from other personal and marital problems. We finished our therapy feeling better about ourselves and deeply committed to each other.

Some individuals or couples are reluctant to confide in new acquaintances or feel awkward in a support group. If feelings of depression or inadequacy persist, a consultation with a therapist experienced with fertility issues may be helpful. Such counselors may be psychologists (Ph.D. or Ed.D), licensed clinical social workers (LCSW), or marriage, family, and child counselors (MFCC). They should be knowledgable about the effects of infertility on the individual, couple, and family. RESOLVE chapters (see below) often provide referrals to such counselors, many of whom have personally experienced infertility.

Because infertility often raises old insecurities, it is important to separate the misfortune of this problem from such notions as punishment or inferiority. This is also an opportunity to examine other personal and marital issues and how they are influencing your feelings and behavior, and in the process, develop effective ways to cope and support each other.

RESOLVE

RESOLVE is a nonprofit organization founded by Barbara Eck Menning, a nurse who had personally experienced infertility. Unable to find emotional support, Menning began the first RESOLVE group in Boston in 1973. For many years she devoted her energy to providing medical information, emotional support, and referrals to infertile women and men, as well as to the medical community. Today RESOLVE, Inc., has grown to a national office and more than forty affiliated chapters within the United States — many of which offer monthly meetings, support groups, adoption information, phone counseling, medical referrals, and newsletters — and, with Serono Symposia, USA, cosponsors numerous all-day educational conferences. Throughout this book, the reader is referred to this important ally for both the infertile and concerned health professionals. (See Resources for more information about RESOLVE and the Infertility Awareness Association of Canada [IAAC] — an organization dedicated to support, education, and referrals for the infertile in Canada.)

The infertility struggle, focused both within and without, is a rocky passage with an uncertain outcome. Even if every recommendation is followed to the letter or every suggested treatment is tried, there is no guarantee of a "happy ending" — a healthy, full-term baby. This reality raises a number of complex issues for women and men alike. Do we expect ourselves to produce a biological child at any physical, emotional, or financial cost? How do we assess available medical treatments? Given the dazzling array of high-tech options, when do we say "enough is enough" or "we are too old to undertake parenting"? Are adoption or child-free living acceptable alternatives? How will our extended families react to our choices? How can we keep ourselves and our marriages intact while searching for an appropriate resolution? In their own time, each couple or individual must struggle with these issues and find their own answers.

An infertility experience also provides an opportunity for personal growth and triumph. By confronting the problem, weathering its challenges, and learning to cope as individuals and partners, you can emerge as healthy, loving, and fulfilled people. The following chapters offer information, personal insights, and coping suggestions for this arduous task.

CHAPTER 2

Impact on the Couple

❦ Bill and I have been married for seventeen years and I have never been pregnant. Back in our early marriage I had a very strong desire to have a baby. Nothing ever happened. We decided to go through many procedures including numerous sperm counts, laparoscopy, and donor insemination. It was a tremendous strain on our marriage. I was always depressed, felt like a failure, and hated to be around baby things. I wondered, "Why me? Why am I so different? What's wrong with me?" I felt abandoned by my friends and not understood, even by my husband.

❦ Infertility was a great sorting out of our relationship with two results: we wanted to be married and felt a strong need to be parents. We both agree that, if this is the problem we were dealt in the game of life, we'll take it and run!

A FERTILITY PROBLEM, USUALLY DETECTED within the first decade of marriage, may be a couple's first encounter with a major adversity. For many, infertility appears after other life goals have been carefully planned and successfully realized. Unlike other problems, however, infertility does not always respond to rational planning, thoughtful analysis, or short-term crisis strategy. In fact a couple faces the emotional and physical turmoil of tests, surgeries, or other medical treatments with no guarantee of a healthy, full-term baby.

Many couples who have waited until their thirties and early forties to try for a pregnancy experience fertility problems (see chapter 1 for statistical information). Some have deferred pregnancy until careers or financial stability were established. Others have embarked on second or subsequent marriages and are anxious to become pregnant right away. Marriages in which one mate is considerably older than the other may also encounter difficulties. For all these couples the pressure of a ticking biological clock magnifies the other stresses of infertility.

In addition, the increasing incidence of sexually transmitted diseases (such as chlamydia, which is often symptomless) is affecting the fertility of many women and men in their teens and early twenties. They too may encounter fertility problems when they try to become pregnant, some at a fairly young age.

In any case, just as having too many children too soon can tax a marriage, infertility exacts a heavy toll on a couple's relationship. The impact of this crisis is tempered by the childhood histories and earlier adversities experienced by each partner, their orientation toward pregnancy and parenting, and previously developed coping mechanisms. Nearly every infertile couple will encounter some problem with divergent cultural perspectives and expectations, communication, sexuality, and decision-making — issues that often arise unexpectedly and sometimes simultaneously. Even stable, loving marriages of five or ten years can be strained by these new challenges and dilemmas.

Once these issues are confronted and addressed, this painful period of adjustment and growth can also be an opportunity to enhance and deepen your respect for each other and your commitment as partners and lovers.

Men's and Women's Perspectives on Infertility

Because of their cultural conditioning and perhaps ethnic heritage, women and men often bring very different perspectives to an infertility problem. As pressures build, each mate may be unable to understand the other's reactions. This may trigger frequent arguments, or conversely, cause a couple to drift apart in angry silence. An honest discussion of each partner's point of view and a sincere attempt to understand each other's perspective — though often emotionally difficult and exhausting — can improve communication over time. By acknowledging and understanding their differences, they can once again support each other as they move toward resolution.

In the early 1980s, Dr. Janice Chiappone, a Massachusetts psychologist, studied the responses of several hundred Northern California infertile men and women through personal interviews and questionnaires. She concluded that infertility affects women's lives to a larger extent than men's and has a significantly greater effect on a woman's self-image and feelings about marriage, sexuality, and career.

Chiappone suggests that bearing and raising a child is often intricately tied to a woman's self-concept. Because of cultural conditioning and ethnic background many women define an essential part of their identity through the relationships of marriage and motherhood. Even in the United States, many ethnic cultures grant women status primarily through these achievements. From the time they are little girls, most females are taught that women become mothers through pregnancy. Adoption is rarely mentioned in some cultures and may actually be a stigma. And the choice of a happy and fulfilled child-free lifestyle is seldom discussed with growing girls. Thus when the prospect of biological motherhood is threatened or unattainable, women often feel bitter disappointment, anger, and grief. Conversely, our society largely defines a man's identity through his work or occupation. Although saddened by an inability to sire a child and the subsequent loss of genetic lineage, men usually do not dwell as long on the issue. And, unlike women, men do not lose the physical experience of pregnancy and birth. (In most cases, a man's reaction to a diagnosis of male-factor infertility is significantly different. See discussion below.)

Women may also think and talk more about infertility because they, more than their husbands, receive the questions and comments of curious relatives and friends. Even when the man is the infertile partner, he is seldom asked about the couple's child-free lifestyle. And because of cultural conditioning and expectations, few men volunteer information about their infertility or ask for emotional support.

Finally, a woman often feels more isolated by infertility. Those oriented to the traditional roles of wife and mother, without educational or career accomplishments to offset the absence of children, are often unable to find support from friends and family busy bearing and raising their own children.

Women who have already attained educational or career goals and wish to plan and time their pregnancies are often surprised and feel isolated when a fertility problem occurs. They may encounter several reactions from family and friends, including criticism for waiting too long while pursuing personal goals and comments about their obsession with becoming pregnant should they opt for drug, surgery, or high-tech treatment.

Male-Factor Infertility. Recent research by medical anthropologist Gay Becker, Ph.D., and Robert Nachtigall, M.D., reinforce these findings in couples with female-factor infertility. However, Becker and Nachtigall noted a significant difference in perception toward infertility in men diagnosed with a fertility problem. These men reported feelings of stigma, loss, lowered self-esteem, inadequacy, and failure. Their perspective and self-images closely paralleled those of women toward a fertility problem. The researchers also discovered that women tend to react emotionally in the same way toward the couple's infertility, regardless of whether a physical problem is diagnosed in themselves or their mates.

Clearly, such contrasts in cultural perceptions and individual reactions can strongly affect the couple's communication, sexuality, and decision-making processes during the resolution of their infertility.

Communication

❦ We would often lie awake at night and talk about being childless. I felt terribly guilty that I had the physical problem.

"If he had chosen someone else," I would think, "he would be a father right now."

We went around in terrible circles.

"I know you really want kids and you're not having them with me." I would shakily initiate the argument.

"Yes, I'd like to be a father. But you're more important to me than fatherhood."

"Great choice! Me or your kids. You could have both with someone else."

"I don't want somebody else. I want you."

So it would go. We'd drop the subject for a few weeks and then
it would start all over again, usually when a period marked
another month's failure.

Infertility is often a time of unrelenting pressure and stress for a couple.
Besides meeting the daily challenges of life, they must make important decisions
about fertility testing, medication, possible surgery or other invasive treatment,
or alternatives such as donor insemination, egg donor in vitro fertilization, surrogacy, adoption, or child-free living. It is a time when open and honest communication is essential. Yet their lives — as individuals and as a couple — are
increasingly engulfed by the emotional and physical realities of their infertility.
Their jobs, relationships with friends and relatives, sexuality, emotional health,
energy levels, and sense of physical well-being are often significantly impacted
or impaired.

Often resentments surface and tempers flare under such pressure. Effective
communication and joint decision-making in any of these arenas becomes a
challenge, especially when either or both partners feel guilty, frightened, or
angry. Unfortunately, these emotions often cloud the couple's relationship and
hamper their willingness or ability to communicate.

Guilt may be experienced individually or as a couple. When a medical
problem is found in only one partner, she or he may feel solely responsible for
and guilty about the situation. Miscarriages can also evoke guilt, as can past
abortions, perceived wrongdoings, or transgressions. The advent of the high-
tech era of fertility treatment has resulted in yet another variation of guilt. One
partner may feel guilty that she or he hasn't "done enough" medically. Or one
mate may wish to stop treatment and the other feels guilty about not trying just
one more procedure.

Fear may permeate the marital relationship in several ways. One partner
may be literally terrified of the medical aspects of infertility — tests, injections,
surgery, inseminations, and so forth. Many people, in fact, bring a lifelong fear
of needles, hospitals, or operations to this experience. Other partners may fear
for their mate's safety or well-being during the medical process. Both may worry
about the effects of this experience on their marriage, wondering whether it can
survive this trauma. Infertile partners sometimes fear that their mates will leave
them for someone who can become pregnant or father a child.

Anger may be felt on several levels. Either partner may be angry about the
need to personally undergo testing, surgery, or other forms of treatment, or feel
angry that his or her mate must be subjected to this. Both are often incensed
about the unfairness of the situation, the lack of emotional or financial
resources, and the hardship infertility has placed on their lives.

EXPRESSING FEELINGS

❦ My husband waited until this year even to admit our problem. I
think back to my son's infancy as a happy time of life, one in which I

thought I was normal. After all, I'd had a baby I didn't try to conceive. Little did I know he was to be my first and last. I went through the entire range of feelings from denial to anger to depression and tears. I have been waiting at the point of acceptance for my husband. He faulted me for a lack of faith and effort during these past three years. As a result I have not shared a lot of the pain that I felt. Now my husband is reaching acceptance that we will have no more biological children. I hurt for him because I know how he feels.

❦ It is not part of my experience as a male to talk openly of my feelings about failure. Even after six years — on and off — of dealing with infertility, it is still difficult for me to allow my feelings to surface. I take refuge in numbness. Numbness allows me to deny my pain, anger, and confusion as my hopes are routinely drowned in the wake of my wife's menstrual cycles. This denial system has a deadening effect on joy, love, and hope. By losing contact with my own feelings, I also lose contact with the people to whom I am close. In order to break this cycle of numbness, denial, and alienation, I have had to confront the code of silence with which men traditionally surround themselves when dealing with infertility. For it is our fear of expressing our feelings on this subject that distances us from ourselves and others.

Robert Bookman

The issue of when, how often, and in what manner to vent feelings is a common communication problem. Partners often differ in the way they address and express their emotions, and each may move through the emotional phases of infertility at a different pace — one may reach acceptance while the other feels chronically depressed or angry. Cultural conditioning often surfaces in their behavior: While a man often buries his guilt, fear, frustration, or anger in painful silence, his wife may cry often or vocalize her feelings frequently to her mate, caregivers, counselors, or friends and relatives willing to listen.

Such disparate methods of coping with these powerful feelings often widens the communication gap between the partners. Women often complain that their partners "tune out" when they express their feelings: "He just doesn't care about our infertility!" Many men, on the other hand, feel overwhelmed by endless infertility conversations and tears: "She can't stop talking about it!" Other men, aware of their wives' physical and emotional pain, try to spare them additional grief by holding in their own feelings.

Mental health professionals offer several suggestions for managing the "venting" issue. One is the "twenty-minute rule," which was originally developed by Merle Bombardieri, a clinical social worker and infertility counselor. An agreed-upon time limit, which may actually range from ten to thirty minutes or longer, is equally divided between the partners to air their feelings. Both agree to give the discussion their undivided attention, and after the time is up, not to discuss infertility again until the next scheduled conversation. When and how often to schedule these intense discussions depends on the emotional needs of each partner. Some circumstances — such as hearing about the pregnancy of a friend or sibling, receiving a baby shower invitation or birth announcement, facing another holiday get-together, or realizing that yet another medical treatment has failed — may require frequent sessions for awhile.

This highly structured approach to venting feelings may not work for every couple. In these cases, experts suggest trying to validate and honor feelings and provide support and comfort to each other whenever necessary. Each couple must find the combination of frequency and length of discussion that works for them. Sometimes just a gentle touch or a simple statement, such as, "I know this is so hard to bear; I love you and I'm here," is all your mate may need. Infertility counselors do caution, however, against obsessing too much or dwelling too often on their feelings, and emotionally overwhelming themselves or their mates. Some couples find that joining an infertility support group provides a perspective on their problems and fosters understanding between them (see chapter 1). Others derive solace through speaking with another infertile person or with a trusted friend or relative. Professional counseling with a therapist knowledgable about couples' infertility issues may also be helpful.

However you choose to vent emotion, it is also essential to create time for relaxation and diversion from infertility — both as a couple and as individuals. This is especially important if you are coping with a long-term problem. An occasional break or "vacation" from this stress provides some perspective and the opportunity to reassess your priorities and options, which may indeed change with time.

Sexuality

❦ When my temperature fell a few tenths of a degree and then rose the next day, we would enter "egg night syndrome." There would be a scheduled atmosphere to sex. At first we would joke about command performances, but before long the humor faded.

We would both become anxious. I would expect him to "deliver" and worry he would be too tired or upset to have sex. He would feel the pressure of that expectation and resent being forced to perform. We later realized, after many heated arguments, that as a man and woman, we approached this situation from very different perspectives.

As a woman, I felt I was carrying the medical burden of infertility. I was going for monthly checkups, facing possible surgery, and taking my temperature daily. All he had to do was deliver his sperm at the right time of the month.

He told me he resented my assumption that he could perform at will. The tension increased as the months passed. We found ourselves arguing more often around that time of the cycle.

Infertility's emotional roller coaster of hope and despair will undoubtedly affect a couple's sex life to some degree. Along with the pressure to make love "every other day around ovulation," there is anger and frustration when menstruation marks another month's disappointment. Low self-esteem and feelings of inadequacy and guilt often become tied to sexual performance. In this negative atmosphere past sexual problems may also resurface. At a time when each partner most needs understanding, tenderness, and intimacy, the couple may in fact drift apart, argue more often, and resent each other.

This strain usually intensifies over time. After repeated, methodical attempts to conceive, lovemaking often becomes a scheduled and even mechanical task. It is common to feel self-conscious and obsessed with "successful sex" — ejaculation of semen into the vagina. The couple's orientation changes from pleasure and the expression of loving intimacy to reproduction. Both partners may now focus on the woman as a receptacle for sperm, and her pleasure or sensitivities may be ignored. Similarly the male may be expected to deliver his semen on demand (either in the bedroom or at the lab or doctor's office for tests or inseminations), with scant attention to his needs for tenderness and arousal. Thus there may be little understanding or concern for the sexual feelings of either mate.

If infertility persists, lovemaking may actually become associated with failure, and either partner may feel sexually undesirable or inadequate. That infertility will affect your intimacy seems just as inevitable as the necessity of scheduling lovemaking on your optimal fertile days. There may be a few ways, however, to counteract and alleviate this stress. Experts offer the following suggestions:

☐ Discuss your sexual concerns at a time when you are most relaxed and won't be interrupted. Your infertility poses many obstacles to spontaneous and healthy lovemaking. This is a chance to communicate openly and improve your sexual relationship during a difficult and challenging time.

☐ Consider forgoing temperature charting or predictor kit testing after two or three cycles; or, if you wish to continue, take turns testing or recording temperatures and initiating lovemaking on fertile days. This monitoring often becomes an obsession for many couples. Before long, you may find yourselves making love only on Days 10, 12, and 14 of the cycle, or daily between Days 9 and 17! Some couples, who find that the woman has become the "sex dictator," assign charting or testing tasks to the male. It can be an enormous relief to share this responsibility with your partner, and it may even bring a little excitement back into your sex life!

☐ Think of sex as an expression of love *throughout the month,* rather than associating it solely with reproduction. Be spontaneous as often as possible — especially during "non-fertile" times — and take time to hold, love, and arouse each other. Let your partner know what pleases and excites you.

☐ Be realistic about the effects of infertility on your sex life. Don't expect the earth to move every month around ovulation time or insist on making love if your partner feels especially tired, uncomfortable, or ill. Remember that touching and holding each other are also important expressions of love. Although every infertile couple wants to maximize the chances for a pregnancy each month, genuine respect and consideration of your mate's feelings is also important. Gentleness and understanding, especially in cases of long-term infertility, may prevent sexual problems from surfacing either now or after resolution.

☐ Remember that even long-term infertility is still a brief time window in your sexual relationship. Before you decided to get pregnant, pleasure and loving intimacy was the sole focus of your sexuality. This will again be true after you have resolved your infertility or completed your childbearing.

☐ If permanent infertility is diagnosed, expect a grieving period when partners feel angry, sad, and depressed. For awhile, lovemaking may be associated with sadness, futility, or failure. As both partners heal over time, their vitality and desire for intimacy usually returns. A consultation with an infertility therapist may be of great help during this transition.

Sexual problems are common among infertile couples and usually subside with resolution. If, however, you are concerned about your intimate relationship, ask your specialist for a referral to a therapist familiar with sexual problems associated with infertility. It is important to find the right counselor because the dynamics that infertility creates in an intimate relationship differ significantly from those present in other types of sexual dysfunction. If you are uncomfortable with discussing this matter with your doctor, you might seek a referral from other infertile couples or your local RESOLVE chapter (see Resources).

The Challenge of Decision-Making in the 1990s

❧ Infertile couples these days often feel confused. There are just so many choices and possibilities. Trying to decide among them, while coping with all the stress, is often overwhelming.

❧ In my practice, I rarely see infertile couples who are in agreement on how to resolve their problem. Most often one partner wants to pursue pregnancy much more than the other. Their challenge for decision-making is to find a meeting ground. They must reach within themselves and answer the tough questions: How much do I want this? How much does he or she? Can we manage this — emotionally, financially, ethically? How will the continued quest for pregnancy, or on the other hand, of finally letting go of the dream, affect our relationship?

Effective and responsible joint decision-making has always been a critical issue for infertile couples — one that has been affected, to varying degrees, by their differences in cultural perspectives and ability to communicate their feelings and priorities. Now, as we approach the new millenium, the myriad and often overwhelming array of family-building options — in the high-tech medical, adoption, and child-free arenas — has further complicated decision-making for those struggling with infertility in the 1990s.

In the past, couples tried the recommended procedures or surgeries. If they did not become pregnant, their physicians said, "I'm sorry. We've done everything we could." The closure of their medical options, together with age limits imposed by themselves or adoption agencies, greatly reduced their choices. In a sense, the medical and adoption professionals often set the parameters for their decisions.

All of this has changed. The development and refinement of the Assisted Reproductive Technology (ART) and particularly the advent of egg donor in vitro fertilization, along with significant reforms in the practice of private and agency adoption in the United States, have extended the boundaries for pregnancy and parenthood (see chapters 14 and 17). Pregnancy may indeed be possible for women in their middle to late forties, and even early fifties. Birthmothers can, and do, place their babies with couples of all ages.

For infertile couples, these amazing breakthroughs have also raised several bewildering questions: "When is enough, enough?" and "How old is too old?" For the first time, the couple alone must set their own boundaries and limits. They, instead of their physicians, must now say "Enough, let's move on," or, "We've passed the time for bearing or adopting babies." More than ever, the couple must identify their priorities and goals — as individuals and partners — and make these difficult decisions together.

To begin the decision-making process, it is often helpful to answer a number of key questions:

- ☐ Do you have a diagnosis for female-, male-, or combined-factor infertility?
- ☐ Have you thoroughly educated yourself about any detected problems and the success rates for proposed treatments?
- ☐ Do you have enough emotional support? Would a consultation with an infertility therapist be helpful in facilitating communication and decision-making?
- ☐ Can you afford medical treatment or the expense of adoption? Do you have medical insurance and will it cover proposed treatment? Will you have to use all your savings or borrow money? Do you want to invest all your resources in one option?
- ☐ What other demands do you have in terms of jobs, education, family responsibilities, and other obligations?

After establishing these parameters, each partner's priorities and feelings about infertility might be examined.

How does each view pregnancy and parenting? What is most important about birthing a child or parenting through adoption? Does one mate already have children from another marriage? Has each mate given child-free living fair consideration? Has one or both reached "burn-out" with the medical options? Would one partner prefer one resolution at this point over another? As more high-tech options — using both the couple's and third-party donor gametes — become available, each partner's ethical and moral principles also enter the mix.

As these feelings and priorities are expressed, the couple can weigh them against the first set of questions and perhaps recognize which goals and dreams are indeed attainable — and at what cost.

Couples are rarely in perfect accord about infertility resolution. Although sometimes painful and usually tiring, continuing dialogue is critical in the decision-making process. Ignoring your mate's feelings, or suppressing your own, is not a good idea. Buried resentments may resurface later and jeopardize the relationship. If you reach a stalemate, consider consulting a therapist experienced with infertility issues.

Decision-making is an on-going process, requires lots of time and thought, and usually is not linear. Partners often vacillate or express ambivalence as they consider the options. Infertility therapist Loni Hart, LCSW, advises couples to reflect upon and reclaim the strengths that were present in their relationship before infertility. What foundations can they build upon? Which of the available options fit well with their temperaments and their lives? When this approach is taken, the couple's goals and feelings may change.

Additional guidelines and specific suggestions for decision-making for such complex choices as surgery, donor insemination, Assisted Reproductive Technology (ART), surrogacy, adoption, and child-free living are also offered in chapters in this book.

Taking Responsibility. Once decisions for treatment or resolution have been made, mates may argue over who should take responsibility for the work inherent in these processes. Often the woman feels she is shouldering too much of the struggle: scheduling doctor appointments, studying medical literature, following up on adoption leads, investigating child-free living, and so on. If her spouse assumes a passive role, she may resent spending so much of her time dealing with their problem. The burden is compounded if she is also confronting a medical problem.

Some couples ease this pressure by dividing the tasks and giving each partner some responsibility. For example, one might schedule medical appointments and research relevant literature, while the other mate follows up on adoption leads or contacts counselors or support organizations.

Honoring Your Commitment and Strength as a Couple

❦ February is great! There are no holiday cartoon specials, Halloween goblins, store Santas, Easter baskets, or other painful reminders of what each of us is striving to achieve. Once a year this twenty-eight-day month (the perfect cycle) ushers us from winter into spring. This is a month to celebrate!

Sometimes we are so obsessed with the infertility struggle that we forget ourselves as a couple. Tension begins to rule our relationship and cloud our feelings for each other. February is the month to put our struggles aside for a moment and reflect upon what it is to be a couple again — those two people who met, fell in love, and made a commitment.

Valentine's Day, with its traditional flowers, candy hearts, and cupids symbolizes that love. This day should be enjoyed just for its romance. Let this day be your holiday to reinforce the romance in your marriage.

Have fun, laugh, and enjoy yourselves! Most important, celebrate that the two of you are already a family. May this brief renewal bring added strength to face the future and what it may hold.

Carol Salzano
Former President, RESOLVE of
Northern California

It is tempting to assume, in the midst of an infertility struggle, that "if we could only have a baby, we'd live happily ever after." In reality, fertility in itself does not guarantee a loving, lifelong marriage. The divorce courts are filled with couples who had no problem at all reproducing. And those who have birthed a child after infertility can affirm that marital stress does indeed continue after parenthood.

During this difficult time, it is also easy to forget that first and foremost you are partners and lovers. It was love, respect, and passion that brought you together long before you knew about infertility. You began your family as a couple, and regardless of whether you have children, you hope to greet old age as a twosome.

Like other painful and unfair challenges, an infertility crisis provides an opportunity to reflect on your goals, as a couple and as individuals, and to take pride in your strength, commitment, and accomplishments. You deserve a lot of credit for weathering this together. Honor your determination and courage, treat yourselves to many pleasurable rewards during this trying time, and remember the ancient saying, "This, too, shall pass." If dealt with in a healthy and positive way, the infertility experience can renew and strengthen the bond between you.

CHAPTER 3

The Economics of Infertility

❦ Infertility treatment and the cost of independent adoption have been incredibly expensive. Over twelve years, we've both had complete workups including laparoscopy, donor inseminations, intrauterine inseminations with both natural cycles and ovulation induction, and three in vitro fertilization attempts. Our insurance has covered perhaps $20,000 of these costs. We've paid out about $50,000 ourselves, using all of our savings and taking a hefty second mortgage out on our home. Not all infertility patients are wealthy and many incur considerable debt.

THE DIAGNOSIS AND TREATMENT OF INFERTILITY, as well as the pursuit of adoption, are expensive ventures. Testing, frequent office visits, laboratory procedures, surgery, medication, and Assisted Reproductive Technology (ART) treatment or birthmother expenses can quickly consume thousands of dollars (see Table 3.1).

To finance this struggle, which often lasts several years or longer, many couples and individuals rely on medical insurance coverage. Currently, however, a health care crisis resulting from the continuing economic recession and the spiraling costs of medical care and health insurance premiums, has left, at this printing, 34 million Americans without any medical insurance coverage at all, and millions of others with reduced or shrinking benefits. In response to this crisis, there have been proposals for a national health care plan. At this time, it is unclear whether infertility treatment would be included in such a system, and how it would be prioritized.

Many who are insured are dismayed to find coverage for infertility treatment claims either denied or severely curtailed. Many carriers have specifically excluded in vitro fertilization and other ART procedures, which commonly cost $8,000 to $10,000 per treatment cycle, from their plans while often covering such family-planning procedures as sterilization and abortion. Patients without insurance coverage, or those undergoing excluded procedures, must deplete savings, refinance homes, or find other ways to finance infertility treatment or adoption. For many, even partial responsibility for medical bills creates financial hardship.

TABLE **3.1** Costs of Infertility Tests, Treatments, and Adoption

Procedure	Charges*
Initial Visit, Interview, Physical Exam — Female	$250 plus any lab work ordered
Initial Visit, Interview, Physical Exam — Male	$100 – $150 plus any lab work ordered
Semen Analysis	$75 – $100
Postcoital Test (PCT)	$75
Sperm Antibody Test	$75 – $150
Hysterosalpingogram	$400 – $500 for radiologist and hospital charges
Various Hormonal Blood Tests for Women and Men	$50 per test
Testicular Biopsy	$800 – $2,000 depending on whether performed in physician's office or hospital
Endometrial Biopsy	$250 for physician's and laboratory charges
Sperm Penetration Assay (SPA)	$250 – $400
"Fertility Drug" Treatment with hMG (Pergonal)	$1,500 – $2,500 per cycle for drug and monitoring
Donor Insemination (DI)	$225 per insemination
Laparoscopy plus Laparoscopic Surgery	$8,000 – $8,500 for surgeon, anesthesiologist and outpatient hospital charges
Zygote intrafallopian transfer (ZIFT) Gamete intrafallopian transfer (GIFT)	About $8,000 – $10,000 per attempt
In Vitro Fertilization (IVF)	$8,000 – $10,000 per attempt, depending on procedures and individual program
Frozen Embryo Transfer (FET)	$1,000
Major Surgery for Removal of Tubal Blockages, Adhesions, or Severe Endometriosis	$5,000 or more for surgeon, assistant surgeon, and anesthesiologist charges, plus hospital charges of $7,000 or more, depending on length of stay, time in operating room, medications, etc.
Vasectomy Reversal Variocele Surgery Duct Obstruction Surgery	$2,500 – $6,000 $1,500 – $4,000 $4,000 – $7,000 Male surgery charges for surgeon, assistant surgeon, and anesthesiologist and hospital, depending on length of surgery and type of anesthesia
Independent Adoption**	$2,000 – $10,000, depending on birthmother's and newborn's needs for living, counseling, and medical costs plus $3,000 – $4,000 for attorneys' fees and other legal costs

Procedure	Charges*
Agency Adoption**	Varies from several hundred dollars for some types of public agency adoptions to thousands of dollars for some private agency and international adoptions
Surrogate Arrangements**	From about $12,000 for an arrangement based on the independent adoption model, to $35,000 or more when fees for surrogate and agency services are added

*Costs vary in different locales. These charges are based on an average of 1992 fees of several San Francisco area hospitals, physicians, and laboratories.

**Adoption and surrogate expenses are based on an average of costs incurred by several Northern California couples in 1992. Expenses vary in each situation.

To complicate matters, it's hard to predict how much a medical procedure will cost. Each health care provider or department, such as surgeon, assistant surgeon, and anesthesiologist, or radiology, pharmacy, laboratory, operating room, and recovery room usually submit separate bills and may be unable to estimate costs beforehand. It is also difficult to estimate the duration of surgery, what supplies or drugs will be used, or how long a patient may be hospitalized (although significantly shorter surgical stays of one to three days are now common). And many insurance companies pay a flat, pre-determined, and non-negotiable rate (sometimes called "usual and customary rate" [UCR]) for medical costs. If specialist or hospital charges exceed these fixed rates, patients are often responsible for the difference.

Couples pursuing open adoption face a similar dilemma. They cannot estimate the total cost of the birthmother's or newborn's expenses, or, in many cases, whether the adoption will actually be finalized. Some medical or employer plans will reimburse a portion of adoption expense; others do not.

Infertility and the Medical Insurance Crisis

For a number of years, a certain level of affluence, combined with excellent medical insurance benefits, has been necessary to effectively challenge fertility problems. As costs escalate with inflation and technological advances, and insurance coverage decreases, increasing numbers of Americans are being priced out of infertility treatment or adoption.

In response to this crisis, consumer groups in a number of states have actively pursued legislative insurance reform, arguing that infertility coverage would not significantly increase insurance industry costs. According to the Department of Health and Human Services, Americans spent $643.4 billion on health services in 1990. In 1987 (the latest figures available), the Office of Technology Assessment estimated that $1 billion was spent on infertility diagnosis and treatment costs (of that sum, about $66 million was spent on IVF and other

ART procedures). After adjusting for a 10 percent annual rate of inflation, or even tripling this figure to reflect 1990 costs, infertility expenditures still account for less than 1 percent of total health care costs.

Beginning at the grass-roots level, concerned individuals — often affiliated with local RESOLVE chapters — have obtained hundreds of letters of support, educated and lobbied lawmakers, and testified before legislative committees. It has been a tremendously successful volunteer effort. Between 1985 and 1991, ten states have drafted and passed legislation regarding insurance coverage for infertility treatment — Maryland, Arkansas, Texas, Hawaii, Massachusetts, Connecticut, Rhode Island, California, New York, and Illinois. The parameters of these laws vary considerably between states. Some statutes mandate coverage for infertility treatment in all medical insurance policies, while others require that insurers offer a coverage option to employers purchasing group plans. Some laws encompass all medical policies written in the state, while others cover group plans but exempt individual plans. Some statutes specifically exclude ART procedures; others include them with specific guidelines regarding acceptable diagnoses (such as tubal disease or blockage, endometriosis, DES-related fertility problems, or low sperm count), duration of unexplained infertility before attempting ART (often two to five years), limitations on the number of cycles for first and second pregnancies, and embryo cryopreservation.

Patient-consumer groups, trying to initiate similar legislative reform, are active in a number of other states. RESOLVE's national board has created an advocacy committee that is monitoring these efforts and providing encouragement, advice, and networking between groups. The committee welcomes volunteer assistance and involvement. Contact RESOLVE's national office in Somerville, Massachusetts, for further information (see Resources).

Federal Legislation

There has been increasing interest, at the federal level, in passing legislation reflecting the belief that infertility and contraception research should be a national priority. The Infertility Prevention Act (HR 3461 and S1751) has been incorporated into the Prevention Block Grants (S1944). Under this bill, monies would be available to women's health clinics, community health centers, and family planning clinics to expand screening for, and treatment of, sexually transmitted diseases. This bill has passed the Senate and is now under consideration by the House.

Two other relevant bills were incorporated in The Women's Health Equity Act, introduced by Reps. Patricia Schroeder (D-Col) and Olympia Snowe (R-Me). HR 1021, The Federal Employee Family-Building Act, would require all insurance carriers in the Federal Employee Health Benefits Program to cover infertility and adoption related medical expenses as part of obstetric care. As of March,

1992, HR 1021 has thirty-four co-sponsors in the House and is moving through the committee process.

HR 2651, The Contraceptive and Infertility Research Act of 1991, authorizes $15 million for the development and permanent support of three contraceptive and two infertility research centers. This bill, now included in the NIH (National Institutes of Health) Reauthorization Act, has passed the House and is pending a full Senate vote. In the interim, the NIH is funding, on an annual basis, clinical research programs for specific fertility factors at Tufts University, Boston; University of Pennsylvania; McGee Women's Hospital, Pittsburgh; University of Tennessee, Memphis; and University of California, Davis. Contact the respective Departments of Obstetrics and Gynecology for details about each program's protocol and eligibility requirements.

Low Income and Infertility

❦ There is a widespread belief that only upper-middle-class, professional people have fertility problems. This is simply not true.

Many low-income people who do not have medical insurance come to our clinic seeking fertility treatment. They desperately want to have a child, but are without financial resources. I think this segment of the infertility population is largely ignored and forgotten.

> Michael Policar, M.D.
> Medical Director,
> Planned Parenthood of New York City

The media tend to portray the typical infertile couple as white, in their thirties, and college-educated. Although a number of patients certainly fit this category, many couples with lower incomes or from diverse ethnic backgrounds also suffer from fertility problems. Few have savings accounts or other sources of cash; many do not have medical insurance coverage.

These patients often encounter secondary infertility. Many have had one or more children in their teens or early twenties, and then confront fertility problems later in their lives. Like other infertile women and men, they may suffer fertility impairment from previous miscarriages or abortions, tubal disease from sexually transmitted diseases, and endometriosis.

Federal and State Funded Infertility Services

Title X of the Public Health Services Act, passed by Congress in 1969, created funding for the Family Planning Services program. Over the years, family planning clinics have applied for Title X grants to provide patient education, contraception, and infertility counseling and diagnosis.

Initially, funding was used to develop basic family planning programs that focused primarily on contraception. Infertility counseling and education were slowly added as the government recognized the growing need for fertility services. At least one infertility program was funded in each of ten federal public health regions, and guidelines for infertility patient diagnosis and care were established:

- [ ] Level 1: A minimum infertility workup that includes an interview, examination, appropriate lab work, patient education, counseling and appropriate referral.
- [ ] Level 2: Semen analysis, assessment of ovulatory function (by BBT chart or endometrial biopsy), and postcoital test.
- [ ] Level 3: More sophisticated and complex testing and treatment.

In the past, some states have also provided funding for infertility services (workup tests up to, but usually not including laparoscopy, and some medications) to eligible low-income patients. Funding may also be available to train nurse practitioners in basic infertility testing under a physician's supervision.

Unfortunately, both federal and state funding for family planning programs has been drastically reduced over the past ten years. To compensate for this loss of revenue, some clinics have either eliminated infertility services, or reduced them to the minimum Level 1 required by law. There are a few family planning clinics, however, that continue to offer infertility services (often either Level 1 or 2) on a sliding-scale or no-fee basis. City, county, or state health departments may be able to refer you to one within your area. Also check the telephone book's Yellow Pages for family planning programs and prenatal clinics; they may provide referrals to infertility programs, physicians, and hospitals that provide care on a sliding-fee scale.

Support and Advocacy for All Infertile People

Infertility takes a considerable emotional, physical, psychological, and economic toll on those who experience it, whether they are medically insured or not, low-income or affluent, twenty or forty years of age. Many people — whether or not they have personally experienced fertility problems — believe that accurate patient-consumer information, compassionate emotional support, competent medical care, and reputable adoption resources should be available to all infertile women and men. Turning these goals into reality involves determined volunteer work by those concerned with this issue.

Federal and state legislators can be educated and lobbied about the needs of all infertile people, and urged to work for medical insurance reform legislation and increased state and federal funding for infertility research centers and clinics. Employers can be encouraged to provide "flex-time" for medical treatment needs, insurance policies that provide infertility coverage, matching grants for medical or adoption costs, and family-leave benefits for all parents. And infertile women and men can meet together to trade ideas for coping with the high costs of medical treatment and adoption, challenging insurance claim denials, and initiating and completing legislative reform. Local RESOLVE chapters often offer literature and sponsor workshops about these issues. Speaking out about infertility and working for change will benefit both those presently struggling with this life crisis and those who follow.

CHAPTER 4

The Doctor-Patient Relationship

❦ I have the greatest confidence in my doctor. Without his knowledge and kindness, I would not have felt this way. I went into surgery knowing that if anyone could help me, he could.

❦ Our meeting with the doctor about donor insemination was very impersonal. A lot of notes were made about my husband's physical characteristics, the procedure itself was discussed, and we were asked when we wanted to start. Just like that! I asked if there was counseling available to sort through our feelings. He actually laughed and said couples had no business in his clinic if they had doubts. He wasn't allowing at all for any normal apprehensions.

❦ Many people say to me, "You must be so happy when your infertility patients get pregnant!" Sure, I share their excitement, but my heart is really with those patients who try all the treatments and don't get pregnant.

As THESE QUOTES SUGGEST, the doctor-patient relationship is often a personal and sensitive one. We look to our physicians for competent medical care, understanding, and compassion, and we hope they will come to know and respect us. Some patients return to the same internist or family practitioner for many years, and close bonds often develop between them.

Because physicians are highly educated, have prominent social status, and often appear harried or rushed, many patients are also intimidated or awed by them. We may feel nervous, tongue-tied, or uncomfortable in their presence. Some of us find it difficult to ask questions, express concerns, or discuss a suggested treatment during office visits or phone conversations.

Infertility patients approach their specialists with these feelings, as well as with hope and apprehension. Each couple wants to have a child and depends on the doctor to help them achieve this life goal. Although they worry that testing or perhaps surgery will be necessary, they also fear that pregnancy won't occur even after these or other high-tech procedures. Patients who have unsuccessfully seen other physicians often bring a demoralized attitude to the initial interview.

The specialist senses their expectations and unhappiness and is frustrated when patients do not respond to treatment. Many physicians also have difficulty acknowledging uncertainty, ambiguity, or failure in both the diagnosis and treatment of infertility. It is difficult, and for many doctors disheartening, to face an eager and emotionally vulnerable patient and say, "We just don't know why," or "The odds of this treatment working are pretty low."

It is easy to see how resentments, misunderstandings, conflicts, and hurt feelings can surface on both sides. From the outset, the doctor-patient relationship is loaded with high physical, emotional, psychological, and financial stakes.

Underlying this relationship is the challenge that infertility patients take responsibility for their own health care. This approach requires careful selection of a competent specialist and continuous self-education about medical problems and proposed treatment. In addition, a commitment from both physician and patient to open communication, realistic expectations, sensitivity to the other's perspective, and an attitude of mutual respect and trust can enhance and strengthen the doctor-patient relationship.

Choosing an Infertility Specialist

🍃 We wasted months with our gynecologist. He wanted to stick with basal body temperature charts, clomiphene, and simple tests. At no time did he suggest a laparoscopy.

We finally had enough and decided to see an infertility specialist. We had to wait quite awhile for an appointment, but it was worth it. We've often joked that it was like the difference between a Vega and a Bentley. Our specialist was thorough and concerned. He gave us hope without being condescending or glib. After he found massive pelvic adhesions caused by chronic appendicitis, he recommended surgery to increase our chances for pregnancy. At last we had a diagnosis and something to do about it.

All licensed physicians have completed four years of medical school and passed board-approved examinations. After a year of internship, some choose a specialty such as obstetrics and gynecology (ob/gyn). Specializing in a specific area of medicine requires a three- to four-year residency to obtain additional knowledge and clinical experience.

Although infertility has been a recognized subspecialty of gynecology since 1974, not all ob/gyns are adequately educated or trained in infertility diagnosis and treatment. Many medical students receive only one course or perhaps several relevant lectures while in medical school and little surgical or clinical infertility training during their residencies.

WHAT IS AN INFERTILITY SPECIALIST?

Infertility specialists are physicians who have received additional education, training, and experience in the diagnosis and treatment of infertility beyond the ob/gyn residency. Some have completed a two-year clinical fellowship in Reproductive Endocrinology. Others acquire knowledge and training through seminars and other continuing medical education. They devote all or part of their practice to fertility problems, keep abreast of current technological developments in the field, and perform infertility surgery and complex testing on a regular basis. These specialists are best qualified to diagnose and treat all aspects of female infertility. Most male factor and immunological infertility patients are referred to an andrologist — a urologist who specializes in male reproductive problems.

WHEN SHOULD I SEE A SPECIALIST?

Many couples regret wasting months or even years of precious time with well-intentioned internists or gynecologists who were not qualified to diagnose or treat infertility. Consider a consultation with an infertility specialist if:

- ☐ You have not become pregnant after a year of unprotected intercourse (if you are approaching forty years of age or older, many specialists advise a consultation after six months).
- ☐ You have suffered two or more miscarriages (see chapter 13 for further discussion of repeated pregnancy loss).
- ☐ Your infertility is affecting your marital relationship or either partner's self-esteem.

HOW DO I FIND A SPECIALIST?

Your gynecologist or internist may be able to refer you to an infertility specialist in your area. Some couples seek recommendations from infertile friends and relatives, hospital or community referral services, and local medical associations. The American Fertility Society, the RESOLVE National Office (see Resources), and many local RESOLVE chapters also maintain updated listings of infertility specialists and Assisted Reproductive Technology (ART) programs. RESOLVE recommends that an infertility specialist should have at least half of his or her practice devoted to infertility.

WHAT ARE THE QUALITIES OF A GOOD SPECIALIST?

You may want to interview several specialists before selecting one. This is an intense and sensitive relationship in which you will discuss personal aspects of your health, feelings, and sexuality and make important decisions about testing, treatment, and perhaps surgery or other invasive, high-tech options.

Everyone wants a competent doctor who is experienced in infertility diagnosis and treatment and trained in the current medical technology. Your specialist should also be aware of the powerful emotional and psychological dynamics of infertility that can affect the doctor-patient relationship. Misunderstandings can be minimized or avoided through continuing dialogue with a sensitive and emotionally supportive specialist. Other important qualities to look for during your first few contacts include:

- ☐ A willingness and availability to answer your questions during office visits and by telephone (as time allows).
- ☐ Arrangements with other infertility specialists to cover for vacations, days off, evenings, or weekends.
- ☐ A professional and personal rapport with you as a patient and with you both as a couple.
- ☐ The desire to work with both of you on the course of the workup and possible treatments.
- ☐ A friendly, sensitive staff with whom you feel comfortable discussing your concerns. Some practices also include nurse practitioners and counselors on their staff who help with patient treatment, education, or emotional support.
- ☐ An honest discussion of fees before testing, surgery, or other costly procedures, and an arrangement for payment that is acceptable to all.
- ☐ An efficiently run office where you are seen within a reasonable time of your scheduled appointment.

Educating Yourself About Infertility

❦ I think all infertility patients should be thoroughly acquainted with their problem and its management. This requires learning as much as possible through reading and discussion. Good infertility specialists know they must take appropriate time to talk with their patients. However, we doctors are frequently hurried and it may sometimes be necessary for the patient to initiate questions.

❦ My way of "coping" has been to seek information on the rate of healthy births resulting from a treatment in women my age, with similar problems, performed by the practitioner I am considering as well as on side effects (immediate and long term, for the women and offspring) of the treatment. I look for comparisons to less invasive or to no treatment at all. If possible, the sources for my information extend beyond drug manufacturers who will profit from expanded use of a treatment. When I consult the medical literature, I pay particular attention to disagreement revealed among professionals about an intervention, which helps me know what questions to ask.

Learning about the medical, as well as the emotional, issues of your infertility often restores a sense of control. This knowledge can ease fears about proposed tests, treatments, or surgery and provide reassurance about the intensity of your feelings. Your reading, however, will not make you a medical expert. Your specialist has spent years studying these problems and their treatments; the purpose of your research is not to outsmart or second-guess the specialist, but to provide a base of knowledge that, along with your doctor's recommendations, can help you make informed decisions.

A word of warning is necessary. Reading about health problems, particularly in medical journals, can be unnerving or frightening. In fact, medical students often suffer from sympathetic hypochrondria when they study certain problems! As a lay reader you may also interpret medical data incorrectly. For example, some articles report the results of only one study rather than a comprehensive overview. If you are confused or alarmed by what you have read, discuss your concerns with your doctor.

GETTING STARTED

Ask your specialist for recommendations of relevant books and journal articles, and check local bookstores for the latest titles on infertility. The public library also offers a wealth of resources. Consult the card catalog, accessed by computer in many libraries, and the *Reader's Guide to Periodical Literature* (under the subject heading Infertility or specific medical complaints, such as Pelvic Inflammatory Disease) for books and magazine articles for the lay reader. Some libraries also carry the *Index to Health Periodicals*, a more specialized guide to medical literature. Each reference you locate will probably recommend other readings on the same subject.

Fact sheets on specific medical problems are available from RESOLVE. There are also several medical research services that, for a fee, will send you detailed information on a specific topic. One of these is Planetree Health Resource Center, which also has a medical library and bookstore (see Resources). Your doctor, pharmacist, nurses, and other health care providers may also be helpful.

USING THE MEDICAL LIBRARY

You can find more specialized, technical books and journal articles — written by and for physicians, nurses, and other health care professionals — in a medical library. These libraries are found in some universities and most nursing and medical schools and are usually open to the public.

The card catalog, which is also accessed by computer in many medical libraries, lists books by author, title, and subject. Articles specific to your interest can be found by using *Index Medicus,* an annually compiled index that lists articles published in all national and some international medical journals by author and subject. Recent issues are usually shelved alphabetically by journal title. Older editions may be bound and stored, or available on microfilm, which can be scanned by computer. If you need help, ask the reference librarian.

You can read about specific drugs in the *Physicians' Desk Reference* (PDR) and the *Medical Letter.* The PDR is an annual publication that compiles information from the manufacturers about indications for, and all reported side effects of, various drugs. Designed for use by physicians, the PDR contains a lot of medical jargon, lists hundreds of rare side effects as well as common ones, and may be difficult or even disturbing reading. The *Medical Letter is* a periodical that evaluates various drugs on the market and also lists references to appropriate journal articles and other readings.

The *Hospital Formulary* and *Essential Guide to Prescription Drugs* are other sources of information about prescription drugs. Each is written for pharmacists and physicians and may be difficult for the average reader to understand. It may be easier to consult several good books about prescription drugs, written by physicians and pharmacists for the lay reader, which are often available in libraries and bookstores.

The Infertility Patient's Perspective

❦ I remember the first time I saw the sign on the door: "Joe Jones, M.D., Obstetrics, Gynecology, Infertility." I felt my heart and spirits sink. I hated admitting I was infertile and that I needed medical help to get pregnant.

I wanted to get out of that role as soon as possible and become a pregnant patient. But my infertility dragged on even though we progressed quickly through the workup and surgery.

I kept at it, though, going monthly for postcoital tests and pelvic exams while I took clomiphene. I soon associated my frequent office visits with failure, inadequacy, and depression.

My doctor's moods also varied with each visit. Sometimes I sensed that he was optimistic about my chances; other times I felt he was also depressed and didn't really know what to say to me.

I remember one occasion when he called me and reported a positive test result. I sensed that he was relieved, and for once, I felt hope because something was normal. I said to him, "Now do you think I'll get pregnant?"

His attitude changed immediately. He became very serious and said, "We make no guarantees here about pregnancy. It's very important for you understand that."

My elation disappeared and I again felt infertile.

All transitions can be unsettling and even frightening. Infertility is an especially unhappy and difficult one. During this "time window" of our lives, we are struggling with the reality that we cannot easily conceive or birth a child. It is a sad time and one we wish to end quickly. Regardless of our commitment or diligence, however, there is no guarantee of a pregnancy.

By the time most patients see a specialist they are already frightened, anxious, and perhaps desperate. Some are ashamed to be seeing an infertility doctor at all. Many fear they will never get pregnant, whether they have been trying for several months or years. They are all reacting to a myriad of stresses and may not have found adequate emotional support. On top of all this, few begin the workup with much medical knowledge. In fact, this may be their first experience with a physical problem that requires treatment.

ATTITUDE TOWARD THE SPECIALIST

Every infertility patient hopes this will be a short-term relationship. Patients want the specialist to restore their fertility so they can become pregnant. As the workup and treatment progress, this perspective can result in several attitudes toward the physician.

Some patients are awed by doctors and view them as all-knowing miracle workers. They often expect the doctor to take total responsibility for their health care and fear giving offense by complaining, airing their feelings, or being "a nuisance." Some patients are afraid that if they are too pushy, their specialist won't see them anymore. DI (donor sperm insemination) patients often feel especially dependent on the doctor. Their specialist may be the only person aware of their insemination treatments and may select the donor who will be their child's biological father.

Other patients look toward their specialist for emotional support. Because the doctor must maintain a certain amount of professional and personal distance, such patients are often disappointed. Some patients complain that their specialists are cold or unfeeling about their emotional pain and feel frustrated or let down after office visits or phone conversations.

Still other patients take a cold, rather callous view of their physicians. They may resent the specialist's emotional detachment, high fees, bedside manner, or fertility symbolized by the pictures of his or her children in the office. Some regard physicians like professional athletes, showing interest only in the specialist's statistics of pregnancy successes. This may be their one chance for a child and they fear selecting a physician with a low success rate.

In any case every infertility patient wants, and perhaps expects, to become pregnant despite medical problems, prognosis, or age. Many become disillusioned, impatient, and angry if this does not occur within a few months of treatment. That it may take several years for a successful pregnancy to occur (if at all) can be hard to accept. As time passes, it is a challenge to maintain a positive attitude toward both the specialist and the course of treatment.

The Physician's Perspective

❦ It's often discouraging for me to practice this form of medicine. I know my patients want only one thing from me: fertility. But I also know the numbers: less than half will have a successful pregnancy.

This is hard to accept for all of us. The joy of working with these couples is that they're the best patients in the world and follow your instructions to the letter. If I tell my patients that the latest infertility cure is to stand on your head on the sidewalk at high noon, they'll only ask, "Should I put a towel on the ground or just place my forehead directly on the cement?"

It's heartbreaking for me when they don't succeed.

Infertility specialists are responsible for the care and treatment of many patients. They often work closely, for months at a time, with the patient or couple. As a rule these model patients are diligent, dependable, and cooperative. They usually keep their appointments; follow instructions exactly; undergo necessary tests; take their medications as ordered; and, if asked, chart their daily basal temperature for months on end! Specialists develop an emotional attachment to many of their patients.

Emotionally, infertility is one of the more difficult medical specialties to practice. It is a heartbreaking reality that only about half these patients will become pregnant. In fact many specialists actually have a lower success rate — perhaps 30 to 40 percent. This is because the more fertile patients often become pregnant while under the care of their gynecologists. The cases referred to a specialist are usually more difficult and have smaller chances for success. The physician may keenly feel the couple's successes and failures, along with their disappointment when fertility remains an elusive goal. It can be difficult for both physician and patient to decide whether to try yet another option or end treatment.

Despite their commitment and sympathy, however, physicians must maintain a professional distance from each patient. Otherwise it would be impossible to see a dozen or more new and returning patients each day, perform surgery several times a week, and meet the demands and needs of their own families.

BEDSIDE MANNER

Each physician develops his or her own bedside manner — a personalized way of conveying expertise, reassurance, and sympathy to patients. Some doctors use a frank and honest approach both in explaining medical problems and in expressing their own feelings. Others are more reserved, preferring a more formal doctor-patient relationship with little show of emotion. Patients' reactions to their physicians also differ widely. Some like a gentle, reassuring manner; others prefer to hear the straight facts and skip any show of emotion.

Many doctors are cautious about expressing feelings or confidences, aware that patients often discuss physicians and their personalities with friends and acquaintances. It is also difficult to judge how much encouragement or hope to hold out to a patient. Even among patients with a favorable prognosis, many do not become pregnant.

Nurses and Other Health Care Professionals

❦ No one can remove the pain of infertility, but by providing a warm, caring atmosphere, trust can usually be established. If patients feel that all areas of testing and treatment have been explored, they are more receptive to an alternative resolution to their infertility. The couple facing the problem of infertility may have many negative feelings about themselves and their relationship. Health professionals working with these couples need to be aware of this emotional trauma and assist the couple attempting to cope with it. All of this requires an investment of time that reaps rewards many times over — the success and satisfaction of helping a couple conquer their battle with infertility at whatever level they can.

Esther Levine, RN, FNP

❦ Few patients realize how many demands are placed on the nursing staff. One nurse will often have three or four patients who need attention, help, or medications at the same time. Our patients also tend to express their anger and resentment about the hospital, their illness, or life in general to us rather than to their doctors. I try my best to be cheerful, efficient, and reassuring to my patients. But I can only be in one place at a time, and I have good and bad days like everybody else.

It hurts when patients are rude or critical, although I know that being hospitalized is traumatic and unsettling. I also wonder what happens to patients after they are discharged. Few call back or write to let me know how they're doing. When someone does, it means a lot.

During infertility testing and treatment patients see a number of health care providers such as nurses, lab technicians, and medical assistants. Some of these are short-term relationships that nonetheless influence your medical experience. In other instances, both nurses and nurse practitioners maintain close contact with infertility patients over the course of their workup and treatment. They may perform basic testing and sonograms, call with test results, or answer questions in the office or by phone. They often provide the humor and warmth that gets a patient through a frightening or difficult procedure. Many patients rely on these professionals for both information and emotional support. Surgical and in vitro fertilization program nurses also provide invaluable care and support for their patients.

Through the course of a day or night these providers are responsible for the care of many people. They realize that patients, either in the doctor's office or a hospital setting, are often tense and unhappy. Still it is painful when patients treat them in an insensitive manner or consider their work and feelings unimportant. They may also be frustrated if their contact with the patient is brief. Unlike the physician, they do not always know how patients fare after testing or surgery.

Some patients are not aware of the many demands on the care provider's time and emotions. Often a nurse's hurried manner or tense body language is misinterpreted as a lack of concern toward the patient. It is comforting when nurses take the time to explain a medical procedure or offer reassurance and a kind word.

There are times when nurses or technicians are insensitive or unkind, or patients are unnecessarily rude or short-tempered. When problems occur, either party should try an honest statement of feelings and expectations. If this does not work, a patient might discuss the problem with her or his physician. Nurses can air their feelings with their supervisors and physicians.

Building a Relationship of Mutual Respect and Trust

❦ It is only through the development of an honest, respectful, and informed relationship that the needs of infertility patients can be met. I think most of my colleagues are aware of this and appreciate active patient participation. It is also important to realize that sometimes specific answers are not available, and both doctor and patient must live with less-than-optimal information. Even in these cases your doctor should be able to put the clinical situation into perspective so you can make appropriate decisions regarding management of your infertility problem.

❦ For months I thought I was just another patient to my specialist. During my treatment, I've gone through many emotions over dozens of visits: anger, hope, frustration, fear, depression, gratitude. At first I figured he really didn't care how depressed I was, how often I left his office and cried for hours. After I told him how I felt (months later), he admitted that he too was sad and depressed by my continuing fertility problems but didn't know how to express that.

We both changed over time, after lots of conversations. I came to expect less, he to give more. All told he has spent long hours talking to me and, in surgery, trying to heal my body. After my surgery, he was at the hospital day and night, monitoring my progress. He even had the lab call him at home during the night with my blood test results. He tried everything medically possible to enable me to get pregnant. And finally he offered me emotional support.

I'll never forget all he did for me. I wish I knew the words to tell him of my gratitude and how very, very special he is.

Given the different perspectives of specialist and patient, and the highly charged issues of infertility, it is not surprising that misunderstandings can and do arise. There aren't any pat answers or suggestions for the ideal doctor-patient relationship. Depending on the length and intensity of your treatment and the personalities involved, stressful and unhappy moments can occur in even the best situation. The following suggestions are offered as a base for building a partnership of mutual respect and trust that can withstand the stresses of infertility.

CLEAR OBJECTIVES AND TEAMWORK

Optimally, the couple and specialist clarify the goals for diagnosis and treatment early in the workup. After some education about the suspected problem, the couple must decide which treatments are acceptable. If they cannot agree on how much or how long to investigate their infertility, a consultation with a therapist experienced with fertility issues may be helpful.

The couple should keep their specialist apprised of their wishes and objectives. After the workup is completed, the physician will make recommendations for treatment. Together they can weigh the chances of success, expense, and risk of each suggested procedure and plan an appropriate course of action.

HONEST, OPEN COMMUNICATION

Patients often complain that their physicians do not take the time to answer their questions or explain medical problems adequately. Even after several conversations some patients do not fully understand their medical problem or why a certain treatment has been recommended. Others are distressed when the doctor does not return their calls within a few hours. This can be especially frustrating if a patient is waiting for a test result or has a specific worry.

On the other hand, physicians often observe that some patients do not ask questions or voice their concerns during office visits but want to spend an hour or so on the phone later that day. Doctors also feel that many patients take out their frustration with infertility on them, and do not acknowledge their competent medical care.

Both specialist and patient should feel comfortable in stating expectations and concerns as they arise. Because it is easy to forget details when you are nervous or sense the doctor is rushed, it may be helpful to write down questions before office visits. Ask your physician to simplify any medical language you do not understand and attend visits with your mate whenever possible. Your partner often catches information or suggestions that you have missed and may remember questions you meant to ask.

If a misunderstanding occurs, try to discuss the situation as soon as possible. An honest exchange of feelings, with sensitivity to each other's perspective, often results in a workable compromise. However, personality clashes do occur. A patient may be put off by a physician's impersonal bedside manner. The specialist, on the other hand, may sense resentment or hostility in the patient's attitude. Sometimes each party can bend a little and change his or her approach. This would certainly be the most desirable outcome, particularly if both doctor and patient have invested a lot of time, testing, and resources in the relationship. If a compromise cannot be reached, it may be best to see another specialist. In that case, be sure to obtain a copy of your medical records, including test and surgery reports.

REALISTIC EXPECTATIONS ON BOTH SIDES

Infertility patients often enter this relationship with unrealistic expectations. Many assume that the specialist will:

- ☐ Immediately determine the cause of their infertility and fix the problem expertly .nd quickly.
- ☐ Be cheerful, supportive, and optimistic during each office visit and phone conversation.
- ☐ Be available at their convenience for discussions or procedures.

Many also expect a pregnancy a month or two after beginning treatment. When any or all of these hopes are not realized, patients often feel disappointed, misled, or angry.

Most specialists find it difficult to meet their patients, as well as their own, high expectations. They must also balance each patient's demands for information, reassurance, and emotional support against the needs and impatience of those sitting in the waiting room. Every specialist sees a wide spectrum of fertility problems among his or her patients. Some have a fairly good chance for pregnancy, while others are faced with a poor prognosis. Yet each patient probably feels 100 percent infertile, depressed, and emotionally vulnerable.

Infertility patients, often in emotional pain, sometimes become self-centered, panicky, and extremely demanding of the specialist's time and energy. Some expect their physicians to be available at all hours for questions or treatment and a few even request a copy of his or her schedule for months ahead! Many physicians feel guilty about taking vacations or time off, fearing that they won't "be there" for their patients. Others fear they will be unfairly blamed when treatment is unsuccessful.

Physicians can also hold unrealistic expectations. Many expect their patients to:

- ☐ Listen stoically to a poor prognosis.
- ☐ Suppress their physical and emotional pain even during stressful tests or surgeries.
- ☐ Organize their thoughts and ask intelligent questions regardless of their state of mind.
- ☐ Expect no emotional support.
- ☐ Follow their expert advice without question.

To build a positive relationship both doctor and patient might strive toward reasonable goals. The patient may expect the specialist to perform a competent and timely workup and provide expert advice on appropriate treatments, risks, costs, and success rates. Lengthy waits should be minimized, and when an emergency occurs, an appointment should be rescheduled as soon as possible. The specialist may reasonably expect that patients will take responsibility for health care and self-education (to some degree) about the problem and proposed treatments, initiate discussion, and speak up when concerned or confused.

Ideally, over the course of this relationship both doctor and patient learn to respect each other's strengths and limitations. Both can recognize that there is no guarantee of a pregnancy, and although the specialist can provide medical expertise and some emotional support, the couple alone must make the decisions, undergo the treatments, and resolve their situation. Whatever warmth, caring, and encouragement the specialist can bring to the relationship helps the couple face their reality. Whether or not a pregnancy occurs, they have all done their best.

CHAPTER 5

Surgery

❦ I have had laparoscopies and major surgeries. With each experience, I've learned a lot about myself and those around me. Each time I thought, "I can't possibly go through with this," but I did. And each time, those in my life gave me their love, flowers, poems, and homemade soup to heal me.

I don't think I've ever felt such absolute terror as when I waited outside the operating room. I know I've never felt such happiness and relief when I awoke from the anesthesia, and thought, "It's so good to be alive."

I've felt hatred and disgust with my body because fertility surgery was necessary. I've also felt pride and love, for the strength of my legs and the force of my will, as I got up from the bed and took those first painful, shuffling, independent steps.

I think surgery is one of the ultimate physical, emotional, and spiritual experiences, perhaps like going into combat. You are depending on your body to survive, counting on your heart and mind to hold you together, and trusting in God that it will all be worthwhile.

MANY INFERTILITY PATIENTS UNDERGO some type of surgery. Laparoscopy, a minor surgical procedure performed under general anesthesia, is often utilized as a diagnostic tool at the end of the female workup. In recent years, laparoscopy has also been adapted for pelvic surgery. In many cases, adhesions, tubal blockages, endometriosis, uterine (fibroid) tumors, ectopic pregnancies, and ovarian cysts can be treated or removed through the laparoscope — procedures, which just a few years ago, required major surgery. This technological advance has greatly reduced the trauma, stress, and expense of surgery for many patients.

Although most fertility surgery is performed on women, some men also undergo surgery for testicular biopsy, varicocele, or vasectomy reversal. Laparoscopic surgery is also being adapted for treatment of some male reproductive problems, such as varicocele surgery (see chapter 15).

Currently, major surgery (laparotomy) is still recommended, for a variety of reasons, for up to 20 percent of women opting for pelvic surgery. This procedure usually involves an incision of two to four inches through the abdominal wall, an operation of several hours performed under general anesthesia, one to three or more days of inpatient hospitalization, and three or more weeks of limited activity and convalescence. Laparotomies are also performed for Caesarean births, usually with spinal or epidural anesthesia.

Although this chapter is written largely from the female perspective, the reactions and feelings surgery evokes are universal to all patients. For many, minor or major surgery is a traumatic event in a physical, emotional, and psychological sense. Nearly everyone regards an upcoming operation with apprehension, acknowledging that this is a risk: Serious complications can result from even minor surgery or local anesthesia.

Infertility surgery also raises unique hopes and fears. In most cases, patients' lives or health are not threatened, yet they risk elective surgery in hopes of increasing the chances for pregnancy. At the same time, surgery on the reproductive organs elicits an almost primal, visceral reaction that closely touches sexual identity and self-image. This surgery may be critical to one's future ability to reproduce, and many pin their hopes and dreams of producing a biological child on the success of this attempt. Although the long-term emotional, physical, and financial costs are high, nearly all fantasize that this effort will lead to a pregnancy.

This chapter examines some of the physical, emotional, and psychological dynamics of minor and major surgery and offers personal insights and coping suggestions.

Deciding on Surgery

❦ I put off having a laparoscopy for more than a year. I hadn't been in a hospital since I was a child and didn't know what to expect. I guess I was afraid of the unknown.

But at some point, I wanted to know what was wrong and whether it could be treated. I was getting older and still wasn't pregnant. And we both knew we couldn't go on this way — month after month of tension and sadness. I gathered my courage and said, "O.K., I'm ready. Let's schedule the laparoscopy. Maybe we'll get some answers."

❦ A laparoscopy revealed a tubal abscess. My specialist recommended major surgery to remove it and repair both tubal and ovarian damage. Although I was frightened and dismayed at the prospect of a major incision and hospitalization, I was also excited that perhaps this step would restore our fertility. My husband and I discussed it, and with his support, I decided to go ahead.

For many women and men, the decision to undergo any type of surgery is a difficult one, whether it is indicated for a life-threatening condition, or, instead, "elective" — not necessary to sustain one's health or well-being. Most fertility surgery is elective and patients consider this option to improve their chances for pregnancy.

Either minor or major surgery carries the risks associated with both the procedures and, most often, general anesthesia. Both also involve some loss of time from work and normal activities. Major surgery, which may be recommended under some circumstances, is a significant commitment in terms of time, disability, and emotional stress. Surgery is also a costly undertaking, and even if covered by medical insurance, patients may be responsible for substantial portions of their physicians' and hospital bills.

Working with a competent and emotionally supportive infertility specialist is of utmost importance (see chapter 4). Once a specific problem has been identified, you and your mate can work closely with your physician to weigh the advantages, drawbacks, and pregnancy rates of the recommended surgery. There may be a number of issues relevant to this decision:

☐ Do both partners wish to pursue fertility treatment to this extent? How does the partner considering the surgery feel about undergoing the procedure?

☐ How much will the proposed surgery increase our chances for pregnancy?

☐ Can the surgery be performed through the laparoscope, or would major surgery be necessary? If so, are we prepared for the physical and emotional stress of that procedure and the subsequent convalescence?

☐ How much will this cost? Will any of the charges be covered by medical insurance? Can we afford our share of the bills?

☐ Would Assisted Reproductive Technology (ART) offer better pregnancy rates than microsurgery? (See chapter 14.)

☐ Do we want to invest our emotional, physical, and financial resources in surgery? Would adoption or child-free living be more appropriate?

☐ Do we have a "contingency" plan if the surgery is not successful?

Partners often differ in their feelings about these issues. It is important to take time to carefully consider each mate's feelings and priorities before reaching a decision. (Chapter 2 further explores decision-making issues for infertile couples.) It may also be helpful to speak with other patients who have had the type of surgery you are considering, or those who have resolved their infertility in other ways. Your specialist or local RESOLVE chapter (see Resources) can usually refer you to others willing to discuss their medical, adoption, or child-free experiences.

You may also want (and many insurance companies request) a second opinion from another infertility specialist. Most physicians will respect your decision to obtain another opinion before consenting to surgery.

PREOPERATIVE HOPES AND FEARS

❦ I daydreamed about a successful outcome. I saw myself walking in the sunshine with a big, very pregnant belly. It would all be worthwhile.

❦ I feared the surgery. The idea of my reproductive organs being operated on was terrifying. I was also confused and angry that my body was ill. I had a hard time sleeping at night and often lay awake thinking and worrying. What if something went wrong? I'd never get pregnant.

Most patients approach fertility surgery with hope, faith, and excitement, and fantasize about being one of the lucky successes. It is natural to feel positive and hopeful as one prepares for surgery. It would be hard to go through with it without that boost. At the same time, surgical patients may feel apprehensive as the date of their operation approaches. A number of powerful emotions may surface and patients sometimes:

- ☐ Feel confused, angry, or frightened because surgery may be necessary to restore or improve their fertility and wonder, "Why me? Why can't I just get pregnant like most other women?"
- ☐ Feel vulnerable about their fertility or perhaps their sexuality. The intensity of these feelings is compounded by the knowledge that surgery is a gamble. Many women and men remark that if they only *knew* this effort would result in a pregnancy, they would not hesitate to try. The reality is that there is no surgery or treatment that can guarantee a subsequent, successful pregnancy.
- ☐ Fear that something will go wrong during the anesthesia or surgery and result in complications or even death.
- ☐ Worry they will not "behave properly" during the hospital stay, that they might cry, lose control, or reveal embarrassing secrets while semi-conscious.
- ☐ Worry about the effect of the surgery on their marriages and whether their mates will be understanding and helpful during the surgery, and if necessary, convalescence.

These worries may lead to preoperative symptoms such as sleeping problems, irritability, obsession with the decision, crying, or anxiety. The following coping suggestions may be helpful:

- ☐ Make a list of your worries. Keep paper and pencil handy around the house, in your purse or pocket, and near your bed. Jot down concerns as they occur to you. Fears often surface during late night and early morning hours when you try to sleep. Rather than fighting insomnia, switch on the light and write down your thoughts. Then try reordering them by magnitude, with number one being your greatest fear. Let the paper hold your worries until morning.
- ☐ Take positive, assertive steps to alleviate some of these fears. Start by reviewing your list with your specialist, who may be able to provide reassuring answers, emotional support, and perhaps referrals to hospital staff who can answer your questions.

☐ Speak with someone who has had surgery at your hospital. Former patients can acquaint you with current hospital routines and quality of care.

☐ Prepare yourself for the surgery. Chapter 7 discusses the importance of physical and emotional fitness when coping with infertility. This is doubly important before surgery. Regular exercise, proper nutrition, and relaxation exercises build strength and stamina, release tension, and optimize your chances for a successful surgery and speedy convalescence.

☐ A day or two before surgery, you will have a preoperative appointment with your specialist to ensure that you are in good physical health, and without any medical problems that may affect the surgery. This appointment is also a good time to discuss your concerns. If you have more questions afterward, call your doctor.

Laparoscopy and Laparoscopic Surgery

❦ Although many physicians refer to laparoscopy as a simple or "minor" procedure, many women fear it as much as a major operation. And they are in some ways similar. You still are in the hospital, asked to sign consent forms that list possible serious complications, wheeled into an operating room, given general anesthesia, and wake up in recovery. It takes a great deal of courage to undergo any kind of surgery.

❦ I've had a number of surgeries for endometriosis over the years. There is no comparison between laparoscopic and major surgery. It's wonderful to be out of the hospital on the same day and back to your routine in just a few days. I also can tell the difference between laser and electro-cautery surgery in terms of pain afterward. I had much less pain after the laser was used. My advice to women who need pelvic surgery is to persist until you find a specialist who is skilled in these techniques.

A diagnostic laparoscopy, often performed at the end of the workup, is usually a quick and uncomplicated outpatient procedure. The specialist can view the reproductive organs, and possibly diagnose pelvic problems such as adhesions, tubal abnormalities, or endometriosis. In many cases, laparoscopic surgery, which may require several hours of operating time, may be done at the same time to correct such problems. In other cases, initial or additional laparoscopic surgery is scheduled at a later date.

In any event, your physician and the hospital will contact you in advance about pre-operative examinations, preliminary lab work, and admission procedures. Most hospitals have a special care unit for same-day surgery, where patients report several hours before the procedure. After signing any necessary consent forms, you will be given a locker for your clothing, and a hospital gown and paper coverings for your head and feet. Your mate or a friend can usually wait with you until an operating room is available.

Before you enter surgery, an anesthesiologist will discuss risks and complications with you and answer any questions. (You can also speak with one of the anesthesiologists several days before your surgery by leaving a message at the hospital.) In some cases, the anesthesiologist will begin a mild, intravenous sedative before you enter surgery. Other patients, particularly those who will be discharged the same day, may not receive any medication until they are brought into the operating room.

THE OPERATING ROOM

❦ They gave me a sedative an hour or so before the surgery. Andrew watched them wheel me toward the elevator. He told me later that there were tears in his eyes and a giant lump in his throat when I waved goodbye to him. I don't remember it.

I remember only glimpses, sounds, feelings: the elevator doors opening as my bed was wheeled in; the cool, white tile of the operating room, the feel of cold metal instruments being placed on my body; a steady, rhythmic beating.

"Is that my heart?" I asked no one in particular.

"Yes," said a distant voice. Nothing is familiar.

"Cathy?"

Ah, at last. It's my doctor's voice. My wonderful, wonderful doctor.

"Hiiii," I smiled and he laughed.

I thought of a joke: "I hope you're more coherent than I am." But I can't make my mouth say the words.

I felt, rather than saw, lots of motion. People began to surround me and I fell into a deep sleep.

The operating room is a cool, tiled, sterile, and brightly lit room filled with equipment. The instruments and machines are there to assist your respiration, monitor your vital signs, and if needed, protect your life. The coolness and sterility are necessary to prevent infection. Nevertheless an operating room may be a frightening, sobering sight for many patients.

There will be many gowned and masked people in the room, including your specialist, the anesthesiology team, and several surgical nurses. They will greet, reassure, and perhaps joke with you as you are gently moved onto the operating table. Things may seem unreal or dreamlike. The surgical team members then begin their work, placing monitoring devices on your chest, and preparing you for surgery.

Anesthesia. In most cases, either general or regional anesthesia is used for fertility surgery. General anesthesia, most often used during laparoscopy and major surgery, is actually a mixture of different drugs administered throughout the surgery to induce unconsciousness, relax the muscles, numb the areas of the brain that feel pain, and keep you asleep. An initial injection of a drug such as propofol induces immediate unconsciousness for a short period of time. Once you are asleep, a tube is inserted down your windpipe. Nitrous oxide and oxygen gas is then administered through this tube to keep you unconscious and assist your breathing during the surgery. Your blood pressure and heart and respiration rates are slowly lowered to appropriate levels for the surgery and maintained throughout the procedure. Afterward, you will have no memory of the surgery.

The development of newer drugs has greatly reduced the side effects previously associated with general anesthesia. Most patients do have a sore or raspy throat afterward from the breathing tube. Less commonly, vomiting, nausea, or continued drowsiness may occur for a day or two after surgery. Very rarely (in about 1 out of 10,000 to 20,000 of patients, of all ages and states of health, receiving general anesthesia), severe complications such as paralysis or death may result from this type of anesthesia. The risk to younger patients in good health is probably much less.

Sometimes regional anesthesia such as a spinal or epidural, where the patient remains conscious, may be used. With a spinal, the anesthetic is injected into the spinal fluid and produces numbness in a general area of the body, such as above or below the waist. For some types of fertility surgery or Caesarean births, the lower half of the body from the chest to the toes is numbed. An epidural, similar to spinal anesthesia, is injected into the air spaces of the spinal column. The nerve endings leading to the legs and pelvic area are numbed. Some patients have headaches for a day or two after spinal anesthesia. Few patients experience side effects after an epidural.

Once anesthesia is administered, the surgery begins.

Surgery. During the surgery, a laparoscope (which resembles a thin telescope with a light at the end) is inserted through a tiny incision in the navel. Other small incisions, between one-quarter and one-half inch, in the lower abdomen and perhaps internally through the abdominal wall, may also be made if videolaserlaparoscopy or pelviscopy procedures are utilized to repair, correct, or remove endometriosis, ovarian cysts, tubal abscesses or blockages, adhesions, or in males, varicoceles. (See chapters 10 and 15 for further discussion.)

RECOVERY AND DISCHARGE

❦ I heard someone calling my name from far away. I had to travel many miles to reach that voice. It seemed I had been away for the longest time, and it was hard to come back.

The voice became louder. Now I could speak myself and answer, "Yes, I'm here."

After surgery you are taken to Recovery for several hours to regain partial consciousness. Nurses will continuously monitor your recovery, checking your blood pressure, heart rate, and pulse every fifteen minutes. Your anesthesiologist and specialist will also visit you in the recovery area and speak to you briefly. You are then taken back to the same-day surgery unit to rest until you are alert and ready for discharge. Your physician will probably review the laparoscopy and any surgery performed with either you or your mate, and leave instructions for post-operative care and activity.

In most cases, patients are admitted and released from the hospital on the same day and usually recover in two to three days. During this time, many feel abdominal tenderness and a sore throat from the anesthesia. Analgesics may be prescribed for cramps and gas discomfort. Most women and men recover from laparoscopic surgery fairly quickly and resume normal activities within a few days. The tiny incision across the navel heals quickly.

Hearing About Your Surgery and Fertility Prognosis

❦ "Only about 50 percent of women who have endometriosis go on to have children," my doctor said, watching me closely.

"Why?"

"No one knows."

I stopped listening and looked at my husband, waiting for him to say something.

He didn't. He just looked back at me.

"I don't like those odds." I couldn't think of anything else to say. I was really thinking how worthless I was, how infertile, how barren.

The silence lay between us.

"Well, if that's the way it is," I mumbled.

Inside, I thought, "Hell, I've beat tougher odds than this. I still think I can do it." I didn't dare say it. I didn't think anyone would believe, let alone encourage, me.

That night I lay awake a long time and kept thinking about that 50 percent chance. What are numbers? You just don't get 50 percent pregnant. How do you translate statistics into feelings? It would be easier to get through this if I knew it would eventually lead to a pregnancy. But I don't.

I couldn't think of anyone to talk it over with. My roommate had two kids; the nurses just smiled and plumped my pillows; my mother wanted to be a grandmother; my doctor told me there are no guarantees. And I could hardly face my husband.

After awakening from surgery, most patients are eager to hear about the operation. In the hospital, or shortly after you get home, your doctor will review the surgery and perhaps give you a prognosis for a future pregnancy, often in terms of a percentage.

You may be relieved to hear positive news that brings hope for a biological child. Depending on the nature and degree of the problem, your chances for pregnancy may be fairly good—perhaps 60 percent or greater. The problem may even have been minor and easily corrected. On the other hand, you may be surprised or stunned by a poor prognosis. You may hear discouraging statistics, perhaps in the 10 to 30 percent range, or that your fertility problems were worse than anyone anticipated.

It is frightening to discuss surgery in any case, and feelings of confusion, anger, and fear are natural. Patients feel especially vulnerable after fertility surgery, and a poor prognosis can be overwhelming. This is a time to seek support from your mate, family, friends, and others coping with infertility, as well as information and advice from your specialist.

Evaluating Your Hospital Stay

As a patient and consumer of medical services, it is important to provide feedback to hospital administrators and your specialist about the overall quality of your care. Consider writing a letter, after either your out-patient or in-patient hospitalization, on both the positive and the negative aspects of your experience. It is unfortunate that few people praise the many positive contributions of hospital staff, though most are quick to complain about questionable or poor health care. A letter of commendation will give deserved thanks and recognition to these dedicated, hard-working health care providers.

If you are dissatisfied with your experience, write a letter to the chairperson of the hospital's board of directors. You can obtain his or her name and address from the hospital switchboard. Be concise and thorough in your assessment of the problem, and try to give some suggestions about what could be done to improve the situation in the future. A copy of your letter will be forwarded to the appropriate hospital personnel. Most health care providers appreciate constructive criticism, and changes may be made that will benefit future surgery patients.

Major Surgery

Major surgery usually involves an abdominal incision of several inches (laparotomy) and an inpatient hospital stay of several days. When a laparoscopy has been performed prior to this procedure, many specialists prefer to schedule major surgery four to six weeks later. In some cases, laparotomy may be recommended for tubal repair, some types of endometriosis, removal of severe adhesions or uterine tumors, and hysterectomy. (Some specialists now perform tubal ligation reversals with major surgery on an out-patient basis. Initial recovery time is fairly quick and most women resume a full schedule within a few weeks. See chapter 10 for further discussion.)

As with outpatient surgery, you will receive a packet of preregistration materials several weeks before your scheduled laparotomy. The enclosed forms ask about insurance coverage, room preference, and relevant health concerns for the anesthesiologist and nursing staff.

For companionship, you may wish to stay in a semiprivate room (two beds). If you are on a floor for gynecological postsurgical care, you may find an empathetic roommate with a similar history and experience. Other patients prefer a private room for solitude and privacy. Many hospitals also allow a spouse or friend to "room-in" and will provide a cot for overnight stays. Some patients work out a schedule in advance with friends and relatives for each day of their hospital stay to provide assistance, emotional support, and companionship. Most medical insurance policies cover only the cost of a semiprivate room and require that you make up the difference for a private one, usually an additional $50 to $60 per day.

PREPARING FOR YOUR HOSPITAL STAY

Thoughtful and careful advance planning can ease the stress of a hospital stay. These suggestions are offered by patients who have had major surgery:

- ☐ Pack your suitcase a few days in advance. You will need several nightgowns or pajama sets, underwear, socks, bathrobe, slippers, and jogging pants, caftans, or other loose-fitting clothes.
- ☐ Do not bring jewelry, money, stereo equipment, televisions, or other valuables. Unfortunately theft is as much a problem in hospitals as it is in the rest of the world.
- ☐ Add warmth and color to your room by packing some happy reminders of home, such as photographs of loved ones, favorite books, or a familiar afghan or blanket.
- ☐ Bring stationery, notecards, and your journal. Surgery is often a powerful experience, and you may want to write to friends or jot some thoughts down. If you don't have a journal, consider keeping one for this experience. Ask the nurses to insert your IV needle on your nonwriting hand or wrist. Also pack a few books or magazines.
- ☐ Bring your address and telephone book. Most hospitals provide a telephone by each bed, and you can usually make as many local calls as you wish. Long distance or toll calls can be charged either to your home phone or credit calling card.

CHECKING INTO THE HOSPITAL

Many patients are admitted to the hospital the morning of their scheduled surgery. The admissions office is usually the first stop, where your paperwork will be reviewed, money due for private rooms or noncovered services collected, and luggage tagged with your name and room number.

A hospital volunteer may accompany you to either the laboratory or your hospital room. Blood work and other lab tests may be performed now, although many hospitals schedule preliminary lab work a few days before admission. When you reach your floor, a nurse will greet you and show you to your room. Most hospital rooms have a closet, drawers, television, and phone for each patient, as well as a bathroom with a shower.

Before surgery, you will also be asked to sign consent forms that list in detail the possible complications of anesthesia and surgery. Although the odds of such occurrences are quite small, these forms are often frightening to read. Discuss any concerns with your specialist or anesthesiologist. They will both visit before the surgery to reassure you and answer questions. Most specialists offer their patients a sedative or sleeping pill to help them relax before surgery.

PREPARATIONS FOR SURGERY

❧ I felt like a little girl again going to have my tonsils out — a little afraid and a little happy because the doctor would make me all better. The surgery prep nurse shaved me from under my breasts down to my thighs. Most of my pubic hair was gone. Little by little my pride was going too. I started to feel that my control of the situation was quickly fading.

Before pelvic surgery, most patients are partially shaved from the navel to the pubic area to ensure a sterile surgical area. (The hair does grow back quickly.) Most surgeons also recommend an enema to clear the bowels and help prevent abdominal cramping or complications during and after surgery. Since most patients are now admitted the morning of surgery, you may be asked to give yourself an enema at home.

SURGERY AND RECOVERY

An orderly will take you to surgery on a wheeled bed. Most hospitals have a family waiting area closeby where your mate, relatives, or friends can stay while you are in surgery.

Many anesthesiologists will phone their surgical patients a day or two before the scheduled operation to reassure them and answer any questions. Similarly, most physicians and hospitals encourage patients to phone the anesthesiology department in advance of their surgery if they have any concerns or questions. When you are brought down to the surgery area, the anesthesiologist may start a mild, intravenous sedative. When your specialist is ready, you will be brought into the operating room and the anesthesiologist will begin or increase your medication until you fall asleep. (See previous section for a discussion of the operating room and anesthesia.)

After surgery you are brought to the recovery room to regain partial consciousness, although you may not have a clear memory of it. The recovery room nurses will check you frequently to note your progress. One nurse will call your name and stay with you until you respond. Your anesthesiologist and surgeon will also check on you and perhaps speak with you briefly. You are then brought back to your room to regain full consciousness. Your mate, friends, or family can stay with you here.

The hours following surgery are usually foggy, surreal ones. You will doze on and off for several hours as the anesthesia slowly recedes. You will also be given pain medications, which often make you groggy. When you are fully awake, it will be surprising how much time has elapsed since your surgery. It may be hard to believe you were "gone" for so long.

A catheter (a slender plastic tube) will be inserted in your urethra during surgery. While you are unconscious and immobile, your urine passes through this tube into a plastic pouch. If inserted properly it should not cause any pain. When you are awake and able to move, the catheter is removed. This is usually a quick procedure but may cause some mild discomfort.

GETTING BACK ON YOUR FEET

❦ It was painful and difficult to sit up, even with the hospital bed adjusted to the highest position. It felt as if a metal band had been wrapped around my belly and was being tightened mercilessly. I put my feet on the floor. A nurse helped me stand up. I felt weak and wanted to crawl back in bed.

"C'mon," she coaxed, "you're doing great."

❦ When I was in the recovery room, a voice came from far away and said, "Cough, dear." When I did, the pain was worse than I had ever imagined. It felt as if a fistful of burning matches had been dropped on my abdomen. The voice came to me once more and said, "Cough again, dear," and I was so drugged that I did.

Later in the day I discovered that with fluids constantly dripping in through the IV, I had to urinate frequently. When I asked for a bedpan the nurses said it was time to walk to the bathroom. I couldn't believe they were serious. They were, and I passed out half way there. The bad part was that in order to get back to bed I had to walk there! What amazed me was how much easier it was the second time. By the third trip it was a relative snap.

Most patients are urged to walk immediately after regaining full consciousness. Although it is stiff and painful to move, you can shuffle along slowly and you will be encouraged to walk the short distance to the bathroom. A bedpan will be unnecessary, although sitting on the toilet usually causes noticeable pain around your incision at first.

There may be a measuring cup attached to the toilet bowl to catch and measure your urine. This is sometimes done for a day or two to compare the fluids leaving the body with the amounts entering intravenously. Because the pre-operative enema has cleansed your bowels, it will be three or four days before you have a bowel movement.

During surgery you will be placed on intravenous (IV) fluids to provide hydration and nutrients. The fluids flow from a bottle or bag suspended from a wheeled pole about six feet high called an IV stand. Plastic tubing, with valves to control flow, is attached to the bottle. A needle at the end of the tubing is inserted into an arm vein near your wrist and securely taped in place. For many infertility surgeries, an IV hookup may be used for a day or two to administer medications that ease pain and inhibit scarring and infection. You can push the IV stand ahead of you when you walk.

Pain. Although patients' reactions to pain vary tremendously, most find the pain is severe for a few days after pelvic surgery, and then diminishes each day afterward. You are given pain medication immediately after surgery, and your specialist may leave orders with your nurse for periodic injections for the next several days. Some hospitals also have "patient-controlled analgesia" — automatic devices that allow the patient to obtain controlled doses of pain-relieving medication through the IV as needed.

Each person has a different tolerance for pain, and everyone reacts differently to drugs. After the first day or two after surgery, you can decide how much medication you need and how often to request it. It does take awhile for the drugs to work, so allow enough time to let them take effect.

Vital Signs Monitoring. While you are hospitalized, your vital signs (temperature, blood pressure, and pulse) will be checked every four hours to ensure that you don't develop an infection or other post-operative complication. This necessary procedure prevents you from sleeping more than several hours at a stretch and adds to your fatigue.

Physician's Rounds. Your specialist will visit you on morning rounds each day and perhaps in the evening after office hours. In addition, he or she will be in contact with your nurses to check your progress. Your anesthesiologist will also visit after surgery to ensure that you aren't having any reactions to the anesthesia.

SECOND DAY

Reality sets in as you begin your second day. The full impact of surgery is hitting your body, and it may feel like you've gone ten rounds with a prize-fighter. It hurts to cough, laugh, walk, or even talk. To keep your lungs clear of fluids you must periodically roll onto your side and cough. To regain your strength and reactivate your metabolism, you should walk every few hours. Both these movements will be uncomfortable or painful. The tubes used during general anesthesia often cause a sore throat and hoarseness for a day or two. You have also lost sleep as nurses check vital signs and change IV medications.

For the first day or two after pelvic surgery you will be served a "clear" diet of fruit juice, broth, and gelatin. Although this is bland and unexciting cuisine, it is important to restart the digestive process gently after surgery. Eating rich foods too soon can result in painful intestinal cramps, and many patients who have pelvic surgery experience severe gas pains, which subside as the air remaining in the abdomen passes out.

After a day or two most patients can tolerate solid food. Your menu will be changed to a "soft" diet of oatmeal, boiled eggs, custards, cottage cheese, and similar foods. Between the third and fifth day after surgery, a full diet of meats, starches, fruits, vegetables, beverages, and desserts is introduced. By that time you're ready for hearty fare!

Some patients may be discharged on the day of major surgery or the morning afterward. In these cases, you will be given instructions for diet and activity, and encouraged to get plenty of rest at home. Whether you are at home or in the hospital, the week following major surgery can be tiring and emotionally difficult.

THIRD DAY

❦ I noted a marked decrease in my incisional pain. It was easier, though still painful, to move, cough, or laugh. I took oral pain medicine, rather than injections. Less relenting were my feelings. Though I could be distracted from them by visitors or staff, I cried when alone in my room, feeling an almost cosmic sadness and vulnerability. Yet I was relieved that everyone seemed to think I would be able to have a baby. Though painful, I resumed a lot of my normal activities: eating, grooming, getting up, and walking around. I found the pain to be worse at night. As much as I needed rest and sleep, I did not sleep well, despite the medications.

By the third day, you will be accustomed to the hospital routines of shift changes, vital signs checks, mealtimes, visiting hours, and the quiet nights when the hospital sleeps. Many patients, however, report an emotional crash of tears and depression around this time. Around-the-clock monitoring has taken its toll and adds to overall exhaustion. Expect this letdown and remember it won't last forever. Curl up with a favorite book, call a loved one, or just cry. Above all love yourself for your courage, strength, and spirit.

VISITORS AND PHONE CALLS

❦ I wanted to speak with my grandfather on the phone. "Are you all right?" he asked. He doesn't ask me if I'll be able to have children now as so many others do. I feel better as I talk to him. He always makes me feel special and loved for who I am. Our conversation was good medicine. I felt stronger.

Love and laughter are among the strongest healing medicines. Both during your hospitalization, and later at home, you will need lots of reassurance and emotional support. Surround yourself, physically and emotionally, with caring people. Ask those who make you feel happy and loved to visit or call.

Listen to your body as well as your heart. Do you need solitude, company, or rest? Patients' moods and strength vary each day after surgery. You may feel terrible today but stronger and eager for visitors tomorrow. Pace yourself on the number of visitors and calls and be honest with others about your wishes. Remember that you are in control: You can request the hospital switchboard to hold your calls for any part of your stay.

BODY IMAGES AFTER SURGERY

❦ I was both fascinated and saddened by my incision. It was graphic proof I had been cut open and forever changed. Just as I felt different inside, my body would always look different outside.

Major pelvic surgery requires a "bikini" incision, of two to four inches across the lower abdomen below the pubic hairline. After surgery the incision will be covered by a large bandage or dressing taped across your abdomen. When this dressing is removed on the second or third day, you will see your incision: a bright red, straight, narrow line. It fades with time but will always be visible. The incision is secured both underneath with sutures and on the surface with either knotted stitches of a fine material that resembles fishing line, or "staples," surgical clips that are easily and painlessly inserted and removed. These temporary stitches will be removed in the next day or two. Your abdomen will be puffy and bloated regardless of your previous fitness. It will be some time before your figure returns to its previous shape.

Starting today, you can probably take a shower and shampoo your hair. A nurse will wrap protective plastic around your abdomen to keep the incision dry. Although you are given plenty of hospital gowns, most patients quickly tire of them. Today you can change into more attractive and comfortable clothing. Many patients find that a hot shower and change of attire lift their spirits considerably. It is satisfying to return to daily grooming routines and again do things for yourself.

Many patients are taken off the IV by now. If intravenous medication is still occasionally needed, a "heparin lock" may be used. This device consists of a needle with a plug or "port" attached. The needle is inserted in a vein near the wrist and the device is securely taped in place. Whenever needed an IV or hypodermic needle can be inserted into the plug to administer medication. You will now have more mobility and can walk without the encumbrance of an IV stand.

FOURTH OR FINAL DAY

❦ The fourth day was easier physically. I took fewer pain medications. The feeling of being physically wounded lessened, but I still felt very fragile. I was also aware of healing and realized how far I'd progressed since the surgery.

Over the next few days you will often be asked whether you have had a bowel movement or passed gas. These events indicate your intestines and bowels are again functioning normally. By now, many patients are no longer self-conscious with such personal questions in the hospital setting, although others still feel embarrassed.

Most patients are released between the third and fifth days after major surgery, but each recovers at her or his own pace. Your specialist will review and discuss your progress daily.

Post-op Instructions. On the day of your release, your physician will have specific instructions for gradual resumption of physical and sexual activity. Among other things, you will be advised to get plenty of rest, sleep, and nutritious foods, given a prescription for pain medication, and asked to schedule a follow-up visit three to four weeks later.

Every surgeon is concerned about the patient's first few weeks after discharge. And many patients do underestimate their weakened condition and push themselves too hard — behavior that can result in exhaustion or complications. A laparotomy involves cutting and suturing through several layers of skin, muscle, and connective tissue. It will take three to six weeks for these layers to heal fully. Be careful not to strain your incision by lifting even fairly light objects, climbing more than a few stairs, or even pushing a vacuum cleaner.

CONVALESCENCE

❧ **Coming home was bittersweet. I cried as I walked through each room, touching familiar things. It was good to be home and I felt safe again, but I had so many intense, contradictory feelings! I wanted to be taken care of, pampered, and cuddled. I felt wounded, weak, and helpless yet proud of myself, changed, and different from everyone else. I was stronger and much older than I had been just a week ago.**

Your homecoming may be an emotional one. In less than a week, you have experienced a great deal of physical and emotional stress. Hospital routine often lingers and may take several days to fade. For a few nights, you may wake up routinely for vital signs checks. Your feelings of weakness and dependency may also continue for awhile.

Since major surgeries require a convalescence of three to six weeks, make arrangements with your employer for a six-week leave of absence. Return early only if both you and your specialist agree this is wise.

The first week should be completely devoted to the rest needed for healing from the surgery, regaining strength, and making up for lost sleep. Take both a morning and an afternoon nap, get plenty of sleep each night, and keep visitors and calls to a minimum. You will probably feel weak, and walking will still be slow and stiff. The pain should subside by the end of this week, although you can continue taking the prescribed medication. Pamper yourself with warm baths, good novels, hearty, nourishing meals, and other treats.

The second week is usually an easier one. Your strength should be steadily returning, although rest is still important. Try to take at least one nap each day and get a good night's sleep. You may now want to encourage visiting from friends and family to pass the time and lift your spirits.

By the third week most recovering patients feel much better and some become restless or even a bit stir-crazy. "Confinement" (between hospital and home) is nearly a month old, and many people are now eager to get back into the world. If you feel up to it and your specialist agrees, start taking short walks or outings. Ask a friend to accompany you and try not to overdo any activity.

During the fourth week, you will visit your specialist for a post-operative checkup. He or she will examine your incision to ensure that it is healing properly, note your general progress, and perhaps order a blood count to check for anemia. If all is well, your convalescence will draw to a close. Your specialist may still want you to refrain from full physical and sexual activity for another week or two. You may want to discuss the next stage of your infertility treatment or perhaps schedule another appointment in a month or two for this purpose.

Over the next several weeks, your energy and strength should slowly return. Your body, mind, and spirit, however, have been sorely taxed. Many post-operative patients tire easily for several months after major surgery, and it may take awhile to resume a busy lifestyle. One woman found it took several months before she could again complete a fifty-minute aerobic and toning exercise routine. Try to be patient with your healing and note the strong and steady progress you have already made.

THE EFFECT OF YOUR SURGERY ON YOUR LOVED ONES

❦ Everything seemed to look and taste gray. I would return to the desk every ten minutes and ask for news, but the answer was always the same. The operation was still in progress and nothing beyond that was known. Time seemed to stand still and I felt trapped in an existential hell where time had no meaning.

All kinds of fears began to prey upon my mind. The surgery was only supposed to take an hour. By the time the third hour had come and gone with no word, I feared that cancer had been discovered and her doctor was trying to remove it to save her life.

Fertility surgery is performed either during out-patient laparoscopic surgery or, less frequently, during major surgery following a diagnostic laparoscopy. Your specialist can only guess at how long the surgery might take, and operations commonly run longer than their estimated time. There may also be a wait until an operating room becomes available, or some other delay before surgery begins.

For the groggy or unconscious patient, the actual time in surgery is a blur. It is an eternity, however, for your mate, family, and friends. Time drags until they hear that the operation is over and you are all right. Afterward your specialist may meet with your mate to discuss the procedure and prognosis. Your partner then carries that weight until you are alert and ready to hear it.

Whether for one day or four, your absence will be keenly felt at home and your countless daily efforts sorely missed. Once you are back home, you may still be partially disabled. All told the household may be in turmoil for days or several weeks. Try to remember how difficult this is for your family. Expect everyone to feel exhausted and stressed out before this is over.

Children. Couples experiencing secondary infertility, or those with a stepchild, are often concerned about the effect a parent's surgery will have on their children. (See chapter 6 for a discussion of secondary infertility.) A toddler will only vaguely understand that you will be having an "operation." Children from two to five years old are noticeably affected by your absence, any disability, and the disruption of household routine. Older children are better able to understand your surgery, but still may fear for your well-being.

It is important to be calm and reassuring with any child. All kids worry about their parents' health and the stability of their family life. One pediatrician advised a mother to compare her surgery to repairing the car:

> ❦ When our car is not working right, we take it to the garage to be fixed by a mechanic who understands about car problems. I have a problem with my body. My doctor, who understands about such things, is going to fix my problem at the hospital. I will be fine and can come home the same day [or in a few days]. I'll have to rest a little more for just a few days [or for awhile] after that.

Arrange loving, stable care for your child while you are in the hospital and for as long as you need afterward. Grandparents can fill this role nicely, and close family friends or relatives are also great baby-sitters.

If you are having major surgery, decide on how much visitation, if any, is appropriate. You may prefer to wait until intraveneous medications are stopped because some children are frightened by this sight. Older children can usually cope with hospital atmosphere and will be relieved to see you.

Many hospitals encourage family visits and allow children on most floors. Some provide a visiting lounge on the floor, furnished with comfortable sofas, chairs, and pictures. Ask in advance about your hospital's policies and visiting hours for kids. You can, of course, chat on the phone every day. You may want to call your child in the morning to tell him or her of your progress and then again in the evening to say goodnight.

SUGGESTIONS FOR HELPING YOUR FAMILY COPE

The key to helping your family cope with your surgery is to take good care of yourself. Your outlook and attitude will affect everyone else in the family. Chapter 7 offers many suggestions for maintaining good health. In addition, the following hints are offered:

☐ Plan ahead! Arrange in advance for help while you are hospitalized to relieve your mate. Friends and relatives will offer their assistance. Ask them to help with household tasks, shopping, errands, chauffering, meal preparation, and if needed, childcare, for several weeks after surgery.

☐ Leave your home neat, clean, and organized. Together with your mate make sure the housework and laundry is done, bills paid to date, and freezer and cupboards stocked before you leave. You may want to pre-pare and freeze a dozen or more dinners. A few weeks before the sur-gery, make double batches of any soups, stews, casseroles, or pasta dishes you normally cook and freeze half. This will be a great help dur-ing the first two weeks of convalescence.

□ Fix up your bedroom for a comfortable, enjoyable recovery. You will be spending lots of time resting in your bedroom after surgery. If there isn't a phone there, make sure the nearest one has a cord long enough to reach. You may also want to set up a portable television or radio. One woman even put a cooler in her room and filled it with juices and ice water, so she wouldn't have to go downstairs for a drink! Also stock up on lots of good books and magazines.

□ If your car has a stick shift, plan to borrow one with an automatic transmission for a few weeks. Most specialists prefer that you not drive a car with a manual transmission for several weeks after major surgery because it places additional strain on your legs and pelvis.

□ Have realistic expectations of yourself and your family. Your hospital-ization and convalescence will be a difficult, stressful time. If possible, your mate might arrange a week of leave after your surgery to care for you and supervise the household routine. Otherwise be sure to arrange enough help so you can have complete rest during the important first week of convalescence.

EMOTIONAL AFTERMATH OF SURGERY

For many patients, surgery is a powerful event, a time of transition and intense feelings. Afterward many experience a wide spectrum of emotions, ranging from relief, exhilaration, and triumph to apprehension, sadness, and depression. Some feel significantly different, changed, or older.

In the days following surgery, it is not unusual to find yourself cheerful or sociable in the morning and tearful or withdrawn a few hours later. Some patients become depressed once they are home. The hospital experience is over and their repressed emotions now surface in a safe and loving environment.

This emotional aftermath may remain for sometime, and some patients retain feelings about this experience throughout their lives. Others look back at their surgery as a turning point, a time when infertility came into focus and was confronted with positive, determined action. Whatever their resolution, sur-gery was another important phase of their journey.

CHAPTER 6

Secondary Infertility

🐾 Our son Joshua, almost four and a half, was unplanned, unexpected, and conceived while I used a diaphragm. When he was a year old, we tried to conceive again. At first we discovered a luteal phase defect after I stopped nursing him. Recently I had surgery to remove the endometriosis that stole my fertility in one short year.

🐾 We conceived our daughter Shauna very easily. Wanting more children, we stopped using contraceptives when she was a year old. Years passed without a pregnancy. We were shocked that we could have a fertility problem. We underwent some testing, but nothing was ever detected. Our whole family was affected and saddened by the infertility. I grieved alot and, during this time, learned how to accept failure and let go of obsessing about what I couldn't achieve. Finally, nine long years later, I conceived our son. We had nearly given up hope.

SECONDARY INFERTILITY IS THE INABILITY to conceive and birth another child after one or more successful pregnancies. This problem, which accounts for roughly half of all fertility complaints, affects an estimated 1.4 million American couples and an unknown number of single women.

Women and men of all ages are affected by secondary infertility. Some bear a child early in their lives, perhaps in their teens or twenties. In some cases, couples divorce or birthmothers release a child to adoption. Later in life, they may form a new relationship and have difficulty getting pregnant again.

Many couples who have deferred childbearing into their thirties and forties also experience secondary infertility. Some delay pregnancy for personal, educational, or career reasons while others embark later on first or subsequent marriages. They may easily conceive a child in their late thirties or early forties and then have difficulty conceiving again. In some tragic cases, couples may lose a child through illness or accident, and after grieving this loss, try unsuccessfully to bear another child.

Although similar to primary (first-time) infertility in some respects, this problem raises its own distinctive issues. Ironically a couple's first pregnancy may have been achieved without difficulty, or even accidentally while using contraception. Previously inexperienced with fertility problems, they are often incredulous when the conception of another child proves elusive. They were, after all, quite fertile before. A diagnosis of secondary infertility can lead to unsettling changes of identity and self-image.

Other couples are sadly familiar with infertility. Their only child may have been the miraculous result of years of frustrating tests, drug therapies, surgeries, or high-tech treatments. Lucky once, they decide to challenge infertility a second time. They love being parents and, despite the familiar miseries that lie ahead, are willing to try again. Those painful infertile feelings, which recede somewhat with the triumph of a first pregnancy, usually resurface with surprising intensity.

> ❦ So it began again — thermometers, fertility drugs, exams. After six months and no pregnancy, the old feelings arose again. Even worse, we knew what was ahead. My poor body screamed, "Please, no more!" Feelings of inferiority washed over me with surprising force, magnified by the second pregnancies of our baby-sitting co-op members — those fertile ladies I so gratefully befriended after Jenny's birth.

Their first infertility experience has also consumed a great amount of time, energy, and money.

All secondarily infertile couples have spent several exhausting years parenting a small child(ren). Regardless of their previous path to parenthood, they now face the unique and at times enervating challenges of secondary infertility.

Neither Fertile nor Infertile

> ❦ After eighteen months I finally conceded. Something was terribly wrong — again. Who could I talk to? My fertile friends? They were pregnant again within six months of trying. My infertile friends? I am humbled by the courage of those unable to conceive or carry to term and too ashamed to complain about my problem. After all, I did have one successful pregnancy. I feel all at once greedy, selfish, inadequate, and isolated. I decline invitations to baby showers yet again.

One woman describes secondary infertility as "neither fish nor fowl." Indeed many people find this problem a contradiction in a couple with one biological child. With one success visible in their firstborn, friends and relatives have difficulty accepting the couple's subsequent infertility and its attendant pain and anguish. They reason that if pregnancy happened once, it will easily occur again. Many couples are similarly astonished to receive a diagnosis of secondary infertility, particularly if their first pregnancy was easily achieved, and surprised by the intensity of their feelings.

Those struggling with primary infertility usually offer little sympathy. They often resent couples who have successfully birthed a child, have little patience with their fertility complaints, and believe their own pain would disappear if only they could bear one child. They may not welcome the presence of those experiencing secondary infertility in support groups or workshops.

Regardless of how many children they have already birthed, victims of secondary infertility often feel anguish when their fertility is impaired and grieve for their babies not yet born. Both fertile couples and those with primary infertility find this pain difficult to comprehend. Each group may view one success as enough, leaving the secondary infertile couple isolated and without support.

Social Pressures

❦ Well-meaning people advise, "Don't wait too long to have another" because "one is so lonely." Maybe they didn't hear me say I was infertile? Maybe they don't believe me?

Often I've found myself apologizing for being the mother of an only child.

Those with secondary infertility usually encounter tremendous social pressure to enlarge their family. Although there are increasing numbers of one-child families, sometimes intentionally so, many people still believe that a threesome is not a complete family and that parents have an obligation to provide a sibling for their firstborn. Some observers also assume that marital discord or unhappiness with their only child are the motivations for a one-child family. Parents of "onlys" often find themselves defending their decision or, if infertile, explaining and perhaps apologizing for their one-child family.

The secondarily infertile also hear the same ubiquitous and insensitive remarks as those with primary infertility: "Just relax"; "I had a friend who . . ."; "Take a vacation!"; "How about a test tube baby?"; and variations on this theme. Along with advice on how to conceive, there is often curiosity about the ease or difficulty of their first pregnancy. Secondary infertility also prompts its own unique comments such as, "Be grateful for the one you have!"; "Relax! If you had one, you'll have another!"; and "What are you waiting for? Give this child a brother or sister!"

In recent years, the concept of what constitutes a family has significantly changed in our society. Many people now recognize that families do not need two parents, or three, four, five, or more members to be real or complete. There are families of varying sizes in this world, some biologically related and others not. Child-free couples are most certainly families of two.

When asked why you have only one child, consider a direct reply such as: "We would like more, but we have a medical problem." This will usually stop the questions. Your honesty may also encourage others to discuss their own challenges and create opportunities to share support and empathy. With strangers or insensitive acquaintances, however, complete honesty may not be appropriate. If someone indicates your child and asks, "Just the one?" a simple answer of "Yes" is all that is necessary.

The Infertile Family

❦ Having had no problem whatsoever conceiving our son, my husband and I wanted another child right away. We were twenty-four and twenty-five years old at that time.

After about a year I saw an infertility specialist and underwent the whole workup. My tubes were severely damaged from an old infection I never knew existed. At that time he performed surgery, opening the ends of the tubes. Six months later, still no baby. During that time, my husband and I divorced. While this wasn't our only problem, I'm sure the feeling I could never have another baby made me quicker to leave him.

❦ I experienced the entire range of emotions that come with infertility. In some of my blacker moments, I even forgot I had a child because he forced me to deal with fertile people. We cannot escape the fertile world. Our son looks forward to Christmas parties with relatives. He attends a nursery school where almost monthly someone else becomes pregnant and I envy her excited glow.

THE COUPLE

Secondary infertility often affects communication, sexuality, and stability in even the most secure marriages. One or both partners may be grieving for the child(ren) they cannot bear right now. In some cases, one mate may be content with a one-child family, while the other wants to pursue pregnancy, and if necessary, treatment. Tears, depression, moodiness, irritability, arguments over conflicting goals, and sadness affect both the marriage and the atmosphere in the home.

This stress and tension is compounded when medical treatment is undertaken. Already parents, these couples must juggle appointments, tests, medications, injections, carefully timed lovemaking, inseminations, or treatments with the tiring and ceaseless responsibilities of raising young children — a marital challenge in itself! When combined, the pressures inherent in both infertility treatment and parenthood can seem formidable, if not overwhelming.

Financial concerns often add another worry. Infertility testing, medications, surgery, high-tech procedures, and counseling costs add up quickly. (See chapter 3 for a discussion of the economics of infertility.) In addition to these expenses, the couple is already incurring the considerable cost of raising a child. An endless stream of pediatrician, dentist, child care, clothing, nursery school, and dance, music, or athletic lesson bills arrive almost monthly in the mail.

While coping with all of these stresses, the couple must function in a fertile world. Unlike those coping with primary infertility, they cannot avoid child-oriented activities or events. Having one child has immersed them in a milieu of playgroups, nursery schools, birthday parties, baby showers, and holiday gatherings. Reluctant to discuss their problem with others, infertile parents often feel isolated and find these events awkward, while their child is usually eager to attend parties that include kids. Although saddened by their present infertility, many parents note this enthusiasm and, for their child's sake, try to appear cheerful at these gatherings. Their emotions are often pulled in two directions.

THE FAMILY

❦ **Although seeing the pregnant nursery school moms was hard, I found it more difficult to be alone with my three year old. These moments were so poignant and painful because I realized this might be the only chance I'd have to nurture and love a small child. Outings, such as picnics or a trip to the zoo, should have been pleasurable, but often hurt.**

I realized that it was important to go anyway — for both our sakes. I didn't want to regret, after she was grown, that I had wasted these opportunities. There was one sure fact about all this: She would never be young again and once these years passed, we couldn't get them back.

Karen Berkeley, MSW, a secondary infertility support group leader who has personally experienced this problem, notes that these parents are trying to raise a child while grieving the loss of those they cannot conceive. As their child(ren) grows out of toddlerhood, they often panic at the thought of never having another baby. Some become preoccupied with sadness or even guilt for not providing a sibling for their child. Involvement, and in some cases obsession, with medical treatment or natural attempts at pregnancy can eclipse the joy and poignancy of the present moment with the child they do have.

Berkeley suggests that parents, even as they long for another infant, treasure and enjoy this time with their child(ren). Though some situations bring secondary infertility into sharp and painful relief, they are also precious and irretrievable moments for you and your child. There are myriad opportunities to create lasting memories. It is the daily "being there" — physically and emotionally — with young children that forges the strong foundation of trust and respect so crucial to weathering their adolescent years.

Overprotectiveness. Sensing that their child is literally irreplaceable, parents may become extremely protective of an only child and unusually fearful that he or she may be hurt or killed. These feelings may ease somewhat after grief for lost fertility subsides, although many couples — previously infertile or not — share similar fears as they pass their reproductive years. "Letting go" as a child grows and seeks independence is difficult for many parents.

THE CHILD

❦ **Moms in my groups sometimes note that their children express, in one way or another, the feeling that their parents' sadness and tears mean that he or she is not enough. Mommy and Daddy need another baby to really be happy.**

Children, sensitive to parents' feelings and moods, are often affected by a parent's infertility but cannot fully understand why.

Many kids will blame themselves for the sadness and worry that he or she is not a "good enough child," that "Mommy and Daddy can't be happy with just me," or that "I'm doing something wrong." Keeping in touch with your child's feelings is important. Children need reassurance that grief and sadness do subside and, most important, that they are in no way responsible for their parents' unhappiness. Some parents find that explaining their feelings in a positive and loving way makes a difference in their child's reaction to the problem:

> ❦ You have been so wonderful and so much fun that we would like to have another baby. We're just sad because it's taking a long time for this to happen. At the same time, we're also really happy because we have you.

Children may also be frightened if complex testing, surgery, or high-tech procedures are undertaken, and confuse their parents' sadness or grief about infertility with the medical treatments themselves. Fears for their parent's physical well-being and the security of the family may be compounded if extra assistance, perhaps from unfamiliar helpers, is needed with housework, errands, and child care. Trying to maintain some normalcy, patiently answering questions with age-appropriate information and explanations, and providing lots of reassurance and love helps children cope. (See chapter 5 for further suggestions if surgery or bed rest are necessary.)

A Sibling or Not?

> ❦ There were times when I felt guilty for feeling so obsessed with getting pregnant. Maybe I should have been thankful for having one beautiful, healthy baby when there are couples who have none. But I felt the same feelings childless women have when they see "pregos" or a newborn, and I also felt incredibly guilty for my son, who will never have siblings.

Social pressure aside, many parents want their child to have one or more siblings. When infertility prevents an addition to their family, guilt or a sense of failure often result. These feelings are compounded when children, around the age of three, ask why they do not have siblings like their friends.

It is usually wise to be honest with children, in discussions appropriate to their ages, about fertility problems. Explain that you are sorry that you cannot have another baby just now, but you are still a family.

> ❦ We'd all love to have a little brother or sister for you. Maybe we'll have another baby some time, and maybe we won't. Whatever happens, we're lucky to have you. We love each other and are a wonderful family of three.

Some couples initiate adoption proceedings to enlarge their families. In such cases, it is helpful to gather information and guidance about "blended families" of both biological and adopted children. An honest discussion about adoption can also ease your child's worries during the waiting period and the first few months after your new child's placement. (See chapter 17.)

If pregnancy is not likely or possible and adoption is not the right choice for you, try "extending" your family with close friends or relatives, as well as compatible others with "onlys."

Coping as a Family

❦ We've learned patience and acceptance because of it. My son amazes me with his awareness of what is going on. He has never asked why he has no sisters or brothers; he knows because we discuss it. As for Joshua, he's only four; the best is yet to come!

It is difficult, but important, not to let infertility dominate your lives. Try to take advantage of the flexibility of a family of three and set aside time for fun and enjoyment. Perhaps this is the year for that first trip to Disneyland or a camping trip in the mountains. In time you will decide whether to be content with one child, pursue further medical treatment, or adopt. It helps to share your sadness as a family, while maintaining a positive attitude that you will persevere and triumph together.

CHAPTER 7

Taking Care of Yourself

❦ The first three and a half years of my treatment were aimed at inducing ovulation. For the last year and a half prior to conception, however, I was ovulating regularly and all other tests on my husband and myself were normal. In thinking back on that time, I realized what was different:

I was getting regular aerobic exercise twice weekly for one hour.

I had weekly massages.

I incorporated the use of "positive visualization."

I gave up my longtime addiction to chocolate and coffee after hearing about the connection between caffeine and fibrocystic breast disease. I thought this couldn't hurt, since I had cystic ovaries.

I was living a healthier life in general. At the time I became pregnant, I had come closer to accepting that it would never happen. Previously it had been an all-consuming obsession, a stage in infertility I feel is hard to overcome. I believe in a holistic approach to infertility treatment, including stress awareness and reduction, nutritious diet, regular aerobic exercise, and a foundation of hope (along with the moments of despair) if pregnancy is indeed possible. Because infertility is a very stressful life crisis no matter how it is resolved, taking care of one's self physically and emotionally can benefit everyone.

IT IS COMMON TO EQUATE INFERTILITY with disease or poor health. Although organic problems may be detected in either partner, infertility itself is not always an indication of disease, illness, or weakness. Other signs of physical well-being, such as a strong cardiovascular or nervous system, a normal hormonal balance, or overall strength and stamina often exist in the presence of infertility.

The physical, emotional, psychological, and social pressures of infertility, however, often affect our well-being and influence our lifestyle. Through anger or depression, we may punish ourselves with sleepless nights, infrequent or nonexistent exercise, or indulgence in empty-calorie, fattening junk foods. Over time these habits can take a toll, creating a syndrome of depression and poor health.

Both women and men can avoid this pitfall by taking good care of themselves physically, emotionally, mentally, and spiritually. Such a lifestyle fosters a healthy self-image. Infertility then becomes a personal challenge to tackle as a strong, determined, and healthy person, rather than a weak and passive victim of life.

Fostering Physical Well-Being: Diet and Exercise

A healthy, nutritious diet is essential throughout your life. During times of extended stress it is especially important to provide the carbohydrates, protein, vitamins, and minerals that your body needs to maintain optimal physical and emotional well-being.

If you are trying to conceive during infertility testing, think about nourishing your baby during early gestation. Several critical weeks of fetal development may pass before pregnancy is confirmed. Even if you are unable to become pregnant right away, good nutrition now is an investment toward a safe pregnancy, a healthy baby, and a stronger parent later. Many experts recommend preparing your body for a full year before trying to conceive.

WHAT IS A HEALTHY DIET?

Over the past decade, there has been extensive research and debate among nutritional and medical experts about what constitutes a "healthy" diet. Their findings indicate that a diet high in complex, whole grain carbohydrates and fresh vegetables and fruits and low in fats, salt, sugar, and refined foods optimizes health and deters many types of disease. Because foods differ in nutritional content, a wide variety should be eaten to achieve a balanced diet.

Americans, especially, tend to eat too much protein and not enough complex carbohydrates. Only about three or four ounces of protein are needed daily to maintain good health. This can be obtained through animal products, such as meats, fish, eggs, milk and cheese, or plant sources such as soy or vegetarian protein combinations that contain complementary amino acids (such as beans and corn or nuts and grains). If you eat animal protein, try to select those with a lower fat content—lean cuts of beef, skinless poultry, and fish. Whenever possible, choose meats that have been raised without hormones or other feed additives.

Eating a wide variety of complex carbohydrates—grains, legumes, vegetables and fruits—is the key to good nutrition. Whole grains, which retain the nutritious outer husk or bran, are preferable to white rice and refined wheat products. The outer shell of the grain, which is discarded during the milling process, contains essential vitamins and minerals and roughage to move food quickly through the body. Brown rice, oats, barley, rye, millet, whole wheat and triticale—eaten by themselves or in the form of breads, pastas, and cereals—are delicious and life-sustaining whole grains. Complementary vegetable proteins are easily found in beans, peas, nuts, and seeds.

Vegetables and fruits, preferably grown without pesticides, provide a variety of essential nutrients. Dark, leafy greens, yellow or orange vegetables, and fruits such as citrus, berries, and melons are especially nutritious. Include chard, collard greens, kale, parsley, peppers, squash, spinach, bok choy, cabbage, broccoli, Romaine lettuce, beets, potatoes, tomatoes, yams, corn, carrots, cantaloupe, berries, apples, oranges, pineapples, bananas, and any other favorites in your weekly menus. If you have the time and an amenable climate, growing your own produce is a healthy and rewarding hobby. Working with the earth and harvesting a seasonal bounty is a comforting and healing process for many who feel infertile.

Once hard to find, there is also a wide assortment of organic foods available in some supermarkets and rural or urban farmers' markets. Some grocery chains participate in monitoring programs that randomly sample produce for pesticide residues. In order to be labeled organic, a farmer's soil must test pesticide-free for at least three consecutive years. Eating fresh and untreated produce, whenever possible, enhances your own health, safeguards the well-being of those who grow and harvest our food, and protects our ecosystem from the deleterious effects of harmful chemicals.

FAT, SALT, SUGAR, AND THE AMERICAN DIET

It is best to either reduce or, over time, eliminate fatty, salty, sugary, and highly processed foods from your diet. They are loaded with empty calories, high in fat or sodium, and low in essential nutrients. Unfortunately, many Americans find it difficult to give up their high-fat favorites: chips and dip, cookies, pizza, candy bars, and cheeseburgers and French fries. Some also associate sentimental, comforting, or soothing memories with certain foods and crave them when upset, angry, or sad. Many of us consume up to 40 percent of our daily calories in fats—the equivalent of a cube of butter or margarine per day! Only a tablespoon of any type of fat—oil, butter, cheese, margarine, milk or meat fat—is required to maintain good health. Our bodies will manufacture any more that is needed. Ideally, fats of any sort—animal or vegetable—should make up only 20 to 30 percent of daily caloric intake.

A high-fat diet may contribute to such health problems as high blood pressure, obesity, heart disease, and certain types of cancer. Red meats, many dairy products, tropical oils such as palm and coconut, and many commercially baked goods and fried fast foods are also high in saturated fats (those which are solid at room temperature) and, along with genetic disposition, contribute to increased cholesterol levels.

Cholesterol is a fatty substance that is naturally present in all animal cells. We ingest cholesterol by eating saturated fats and our livers also manufacture it. Medical experts are increasingly concerned about the correlation of high amounts of cholesterol with heart disease. Both the level of blood cholesterol (ideally less than 200 milligrams per 100 milliliters of blood) and the amount of low-density lipoprotein (LPL) and high-density lipoprotein (HDL) are important predictors of cardiovascular health. HDL, which is thought to actually cleanse the blood vessel walls, is considered "good" cholesterol and can be increased through a low-fat diet and a regular aerobic exercise program. LDL, on the other hand, contributes to cholesterol accumulation in the blood vessel walls, which increases the risk of heart attacks and stroke. LDL levels increase with a high-fat diet, smoking, and obesity.

The average cholesterol count of Japanese who adhere to their traditional low-fat diet of rice, vegetables, and seafood is about 165. If they adopt a higher-fat, Western diet, their levels rise to those of Americans—often to 220 and higher. Interestingly, breast cancer rates among Japanese women also rise significantly when a Western diet is adopted.

Medical experts recommend that every adult have their cholesterol level tested. A count below 200 and a cholesterol/HDL ratio of 3.5 to 1 is encouraged. Fortunately, a change of diet, regular exercise, and weight loss often lower cholesterol levels naturally without medication. And for every 1 percent drop in cholesterol, there is a 2 percent decrease in the risk of heart disease.

Also, try to limit foods high in refined (white) sugar or sucrose. Besides contributing to tooth decay and perhaps diabetes and hypoglycemia, sucrose creates an artificial "high." Unlike complex carbohydrate sugars, which are absorbed slowly by the body, sucrose enters the bloodstream almost immediately. The body must then produce excessive amounts of insulin to process it, which over time exhausts the pancreas. After the sucrose is burned off, the blood-sugar level plunges and creates a feeling of letdown or depression.

Many of us consume refined sugar products all day long, driving our pancreas ever harder to process all those doughnuts, candy bars, sodas, cookies, and other sweets. In addition, many prepared foods such as catsup, mayonnaise, salad dressing, snack crackers, granola bars, and cereals contain excessive amounts of sucrose in the form of corn sweeteners. Try substituting fresh fruit, which contains fructose, for refined sugar products. Read labels carefully before buying any product, and try to eat as much fresh, unprocessed food as possible.

Americans consume a largely refined grain and high-fat diet, and have one of the highest rates of colon cancer in the world, and spend millions of dollars on drugs to alleviate constipation. Daily bowel movements will occur naturally with a regular exercise program and a diet that includes whole grains. If you feel the urge to snack, try popcorn or fresh fruit instead of candy, potato chips, or other empty-calorie junk foods.

WEIGHT CONTROL

Many Americans are obsessed with weight loss and constantly seek the miracle diet or consume pills to shed unwanted pounds. Nutritionally unbalanced or "crash" diets, which strain the metabolism and nervous system, are detrimental to both emotional and physical health. Diet pills are harmful drugs, stimulants that affect the body's chemical balance. Weight can usually be controlled naturally with regular exercise and a nutritious, low-fat diet. (A gram of fat contains nine calories as opposed to four calories per gram of protein or car-bohydrate.)

Caffeine, alcohol, artificial sweeteners, nicotine, and other drugs are also harmful to the body. They deplete vitamins, may cause numerous health problems, and should be avoided if you are trying to conceive.

EXERCISE

❦ For me exercise was a positive counterpart to the negative self-images of infertility. Although my body would not easily conceive, it did respond beautifully to a daily workout. I felt and looked better physically at thirty-four than I did at twenty-one.

Many experts believe that engaging in regular aerobic exercise is as critical to our health and well-being as consuming a nutritious diet. Such exercise strengthens the cardiovascular system, tones muscles, and sheds fat. Exercise is also a great outlet for tension and an antidote to the physical and emotional demands of a stressful world. For these reasons, you may wish to consider a life-time commitment to regular aerobic exercise—appropriate to your age, stamina, and overall health.

Many people are unsure of what aerobic exercise is, or how it differs from the calisthenics of their high school or college days. *Aerobic* combines the Greek words for *air* and *life* and is defined as "living or thriving on oxygen." Essentially, aerobic exercise is a consistent, uninterrupted workout that demands steady exertion of the body's muscles and cardiovascular system for thirty to forty minutes. Full deep breaths, which nourish and sustain the working muscles with oxygen, are inhaled and then expelled in a *comfortable* breathing pattern. You are not out of breath and should be able to carry on a conversation. Jogging, jumping rope, walking, swimming, dancing, "step aerobics," stair climbing, rowing, cross-country skiing, and bicycling are all popular aerobic exercises.

Before starting an aerobics program ask your physician whether you should have a complete physical examination and review any medical conditions such as obesity, heart problems, or injuries. Long-distance running, for example, can exacerbate knee, foot, and shin injuries.

If you have a sound heart and good overall health and are not seriously overweight, you should be able to *gradually* master an aerobic routine of thirty to forty minutes duration over a few *months*. Don't try to do the entire routine the first few times. If you feel out of breath while exercising, slow to a walk and finish your time. Don't stop suddenly and "surprise" your heart!

Always begin an aerobic workout with an eight to ten minute warm-up to slowly and gently stretch your muscles and gradually elevate your core body temperature. Ease into the aerobics segment, gradually increasing your heart rate to its "target working zone." This number, which varies with each individual, is usually computed by subtracting your age from 220 and multiplying this number by .60 and .80. Thus, for a thirty-five-year-old:

$$220 - 35 = 185 \text{ X } .60 = 111$$
$$= 185 \text{ X } .80 = 148$$

Ideally, he or she will sustain a working heart rate of between 111 and 148 beats per minute during the entire aerobics routine. As we age, the working rate decreases; the target zone for a forty year old is between 108 and 144. (A pregnant woman, regardless of her age, is advised to keep her heart rate below 140 beats per minute and, throughout her pregnancy, to consult regularly with her obstetrician regarding the advisability, duration, and frequency of exercise.)

To compute your heart rate during a workout, find your pulse at the wrist or carotid artery (at the side of your neck midway between your earlobe and chin), count the beats for six seconds and multiply by ten.

Fitness experts caution that "perceived working rate" is an equally important measurement. This is a subjective gauge of how you *feel* during the workout. Imagine a scale of one to ten, with one representing no perceived effort at all and ten signifying exhaustion. Ideally, you would rate your perceived workout in the middle—at a five or six. It is important to listen to your body and modify (or if you feel ill, skip) your routine accordingly.

After you have completed the aerobics portion of the work-out, give your heart a chance to slow down gradually over several minutes. While walking or cycling slowly, you can take a "sixty second recovery" pulse rate and compare that number with your peak working rate. Your heart rate should decrease twenty to thirty beats per minute within sixty seconds. If it doesn't, lower your working rate until you find your ideal activity level. Working beyond your endurance capabilities can stress your body and defeat the benefits of exercise. Similarly, repeatedly working under your potential does little to build stamina.

You should find your endurance and strength increasing with time. To avoid repeatedly taxing the same muscle groups, experts advise alternating aerobic activities. For example, if you walk or jog on Monday, Wednesday, and Friday, try bicycling or swimming on Tuesday and Thursday. *To maintain fitness, a minimum of three and a maximum of five aerobic workout sessions per week are recommended.*

An additional twenty to thirty minutes of stretching and toning work on your arms, abdomen, thighs, hips, calves, and buttocks is also recommended during each exercise session. Finish the workout with eight to ten minutes of slow and thorough stretching to cool down and relax the muscles. After exercising, and throughout the day, be sure to drink plenty of good-quality water.

Whenever you exercise, be gentle with your body. Modify your workout if you have any muscle, spinal, leg, foot, or neck problems. Trained instructors can suggest alternate positions for exercises that are painful or uncomfortable. Many gyms also offer classes in low- or non-impact aerobics, which minimize the pounding movements on the legs and feet.

Choose an aerobic activity you enjoy. This is one area of your life that you can control! If you would rather exercise alone, design your own program.

There are several resources for the individual exerciser. Personal fitness trainers can help you plan an aerobics and conditioning program. Physicians specializing in sports and fitness medicine can also provide advice and treat many exercise-related problems. Fitness-oriented magazines often review and recommend good aerobic exercise books and videotapes.

Make exercise a special part of your day. This is a time to renew your body and mind, strengthen your heart and lungs, shore up damaged self-esteem, and vent a lot of nervous energy! This conditioning is also an important asset for the arduous and demanding job of pregnancy, birth, and early parenting if you should conceive, the physically exhausting first year of parenting if you adopt, and the stresses of everyday life if you remain child-free.

Alternative Medicines:
Regaining Balance Through Natural Healing

Some women and men have, either solely or in conjunction with medical treatment, utilized alternative medicines such as acupressure or acupuncture and herbal treatment, chiropractic, and homeopathy. Although each of these modalities varies in theory and approach, all share the philosophy that when balance is restored the body can heal itself. They strive to create an environment where natural functions, like ovulation, spermatogenesis, or conception, can be restored. The history and symptoms presented by the patient are closely observed and specialized treatments are recommended to alleviate discomfort and promote healing.

ACUPRESSURE, ACUPUNCTURE, AND HERBS

❦ When working with infertility patients, I first advise a workup with a specialist to determine whether there are physical problems that require medical attention. I also request blood tests for hormonal levels and any infections or viruses. Then I design a one-year program of acupuncture and herbal therapy, synchronized with their medical treatment.

I see the unhappiness of infertility in both the faces and bodies of my patients. It affects them profoundly, tensing and twisting their muscles. Acupuncture and herbs can help, both physically and emotionally, to restore harmony and balance to the body. But patients must also work toward a consistent lifestyle of adequate rest and sleep, regular meals that include a high complex carbohydrate and low-fat diet, at least thirty minutes of brisk walking daily to enhance blood circulation, and stress reduction. There is no magic or fast solution to infertility. Patients can, however, enhance their health and utilize both Eastern and Western medicine to improve their chances for conception and a healthy pregnancy.

Acupressure is an ancient Eastern healing technique that applies gentle pressure to key energy points or "meridians" to restore balance within the body. Acupuncture, in which slender disposable needles are inserted in specific areas of the body, similarly strives to restore natural health and functions such as menstrual regularity and normal sperm production.

At the initial consultation, the practitioner asks for a medical and health history and notes the patient's manner and appearance. Any complaints such as illness, pain, lethargy, fatigue, or depression are noted. In addition to specific pressure or needle applications, Chinese herbs may be recommended to revitalize the system, cleanse the body of toxins, and improve blood circulation—especially in the lower abdomen.

These methods attempt to stimulate the pituitary and hypothalamus toward hormonal production and balance, creating an environment where ovulation and conception can naturally occur. For some patients, this type of treatment may be as effective in inducing ovulation as some types of fertility drug therapy. One practitioner estimated the cost of a three- to six-month course of treatment at about $1,000.

CHIROPRACTIC

❦ I have seen many women with pinched nerves or subluxations in the neck or lumbar (lower back) region of the spine who were experiencing menstrual and ovulation difficulties. Chiropractic adjustment helped restore normal cycles without drugs.

Practitioners differ in philosophy and approach. I urge patients with reproductive problems to find a chiropractor who has expertise in this area. I also emphasize that the body must have time to heal and prepare for conception. Although we can work toward restoring balance, pregnancy may not occur right away. We have to respect the innate intelligence of our bodies.

Chiropractic treatment involves manual adjustment of the spinal column, rather than drugs or surgery, to relieve nerve pressure that can result in back and neck pain, menstrual cramps and irregularities, and tension headaches.

According to chiropractic theory the nervous, endocrine, and muscular systems are closely aligned and strongly affect each other. A pinched nerve or misaligned vertebra may create a wide range of symptoms and influence normal bodily functions such as hormone production, ovulation, and menstruation. Once vertebrae are in alignment and nerve pressure is alleviated, the body begins to heal and function normally again.

The patient usually is evaluated and examined at an initial consultation. Health history and any present complaints are noted. Many chiropractors recommend at least one set of spinal X-rays to determine misalignments or other problems. Others will forgo X-rays and devise a treatment plan after manually examining the neck and spine. Number and frequency of visits vary with each individual. Some undertake a two- to three-month program of intense treatment (two to three weekly adjustments), followed by a "maintenance program" of monthly or bi-monthly check-ups. Cost of initial consultation, examination, and X-rays is about $175. Office visits for adjustments run about $35.

HOMEOPATHY

❦ I had worked for a number of years as a nurse but had become increasingly concerned about the side effects of prescribed medications on patients. I became interested in homeopathy and now work exclusively in this field. I think homeopathic medicine can be beneficial for those with unexplained infertility, ovulatory problems, tubal scarring if it is not too severe, and threatened miscarriage.

Homeopathy, which is a form of natural medicine developed by Samuel Hahnemann more than a century ago, attempts to rebalance the vital forces and energy of the body so it can again function naturally. Homeopathy theorizes that stress, illness, and possibly inherited weaknesses can cause imbalances and symptoms of disease. Minute doses of natural substances, which are sometimes toxic in large quantities, are used to strengthen the body's defenses and alleviate symptoms. The practitioner selects specific substances based on the patient's health history and current symptoms.

During the initial interview (about an hour and a half), the practitioner takes a thorough history and recommends appropriate medicines. Evaluation and follow-up appointments are usually scheduled four to six weeks later and, if appropriate, continued for up to a year. Cost for the first consultation usually runs between $225 and $300. Follow-up visits are about $65 and medicines cost about $20 per month.

If you decide to try acupuncture, chiropractic, or homeopathy, exercise the same care and caution as in choosing any health care professional. All fields have their share of unethical or incompetent practitioners. It is best to be an educated and cautious consumer: Read up on the treatment you are considering, obtain recommendations and referrals from other patients and health professionals, and interview several practitioners and compare their charges. Also ask your insurance company about coverage for alternative medical treatment. Some plans will cover part or all of the fees.

Many practitioners of alternative medicines suggest a medical consultation and perhaps some preliminary infertility testing before recommending treatment. Some work closely with medical specialists, coordinating treatment plans. It is important to ascertain whether there is a physical problem in either mate, such as scarred or blocked Fallopian tubes or a duct obstruction, which might impede or prevent pregnancy.

Some infertile women and men who utilize one of these alternatives, either alone or in addition to medical treatment, report a resumption of ovulation, an increased sperm count, a greater sense of well-being, or success in conceiving.

Do these methods offer genuine hope to the infertile? Would those pregnancies have occurred anyway? No one knows.

Medical specialists are the first to admit how little we really know about infertility. It is important to remember, though, that no person or method can guarantee a pregnancy. In our anxiety to become pregnant, it is easy to pin all hope on standard or alternative health treatments. If we can keep a perspective that there are no guarantees or cure-alls, these options, along with stress reduction and relaxation techniques, can ease the inevitable pressures of an infertility challenge.

Maintaining Emotional Health— Reducing and Coping with Stress

❦ I conceived four months after stopping clomiphene therapy. I was ovulating with it for a year and a half before. I'm not sure exactly how or why I got pregnant after five years, but I believe that weekly massage helped relax my body and perhaps affected my hormonal problems. I don't mean to imply that people should "just relax" and they'll get pregnant. But if a hormonal problem is involved, perhaps relaxation techniques could help bring your body back to balance.

Many women and men utilize techniques such as massage, meditation, and visualization to reduce the stress of infertility. They find that massage releases tension that has concentrated in certain areas of their bodies. Others state that quiet periods of meditation put worries into perspective and calm the spirit. Increasing evidence shows that visualization of a healthy, healing body is effective in treating many diseases, including cancer. Several good books about these techniques are listed in the Bibliography.

The social pressures of infertility, exemplified by the comments of others, the pregnancies of friends and relatives, and the occasions that celebrate children are, at times, unavoidable. These often painful situations may also threaten or undermine emotional health. There are ways, however, to soften their impact on your self-esteem and marital relationship, and in this way, further reduce the stress of your infertility. The following coping suggestions have worked for other infertile women and men and perhaps may help you through an awkward or difficult time.

THOUGHTLESS OR INSENSITIVE REMARKS
FROM RELATIVES, FRIENDS, AND ACQUAINTANCES:

☐ Consider discussing your infertility with those you trust, perhaps a sibling, cousin, or grandparent with whom you have been close. Confiding in someone you love and trust can ease your tension and give them a positive way to help.

☐ Be selective in whom you confide. Not everyone will understand your feelings or treat you in a sensitive, caring manner. Sometimes temporary physical or emotional distance from insensitive or thoughtless people is helpful.

☐ Together, decide what is private information about your infertility, and what each of you is comfortable sharing with others. Discuss ways to handle comments and support each other when such situations occur.

At parties or gatherings, you might stay close to each other and handle questions or comments together. Women often find that they are approached when they are alone or with a group of other females and "put on the spot" with remarks about the couple's fertility.

Some partners put their arms around each other, smile, and say, "We're working on it!" Others kindly but firmly state they would rather not discuss the subject. Some couples prefer to use humor with each other and curious relatives.

☐ Share the following letter, reprinted from Ann Landers' column, to persistent friends or relatives. It may both ease your discomfort and help them better understand the realities of infertility.

Dear Ann Landers:

Please print this list of requests for relatives and friends of infertile couples. It could save a lot of tears:

1. Please don't call every month and ask if I'm pregnant. If I were, I'd be so excited I'd shout it from the housetops.

2. When your kids misbehave, don't ask me if I want them—or worse yet, if I would like to buy them. I'd pay anything for a couple of kids—well-behaved or not.

3. At the next baby shower, don't say to me, "You'll be next." I've been disappointed so many times that I have a terrible feeling that I will never get pregnant. It's all I can do to look at baby clothes without crying.

4. Don't make us feel guilty when we buy some luxury by telling us you can't afford such things because your kids cost so much to raise. We'd gladly give up all the extras to have children like yours.

5. Don't put us down for considering adoption and say you couldn't honestly love someone else's child. The minute that adopted baby is in my arms, he will be the same as my very own.

Ann, please find space to print this. There are thousands of childless couples who have to put up with these insensitive and hurtful remarks every day.

(continued)

P.S. My husband and I have spent five years and thousands of dollars on tests that have shown no reason for our infertility. We are now waiting to hear from one of many adoption agencies.

—MAYBE SOMEDAY

DEAR MAYBE: Let me know when you get pregnant or a good news call from an agency. I'll rejoice with you!

☐ In a private setting, ask well-meaning family and friends not to bring up the subject again. Explain what a difficult time this is and ask for their support. They may think their interest is a form of caring and concern. Being honest about your reactions to their remarks will help them understand your feelings.

Other well-meaning relatives and friends may not know what to say to you, fearing they will hurt your feelings. Both cases provide an opportunity to let them know what helps and what hurts. This benefits everyone, including yourselves. Instead of feeling victimized, you can take charge and let others know what you need during this time.

OTHER WOMEN'S PREGNANCIES

Coping with the pregnancies of other women, especially those you know and love, is often painful for both sides. Your mixed feelings of envy and happiness are natural and understandable; in turn, your pregnant friend may fear her success will jeopardize your friendship. She may also feel ambivalent about her pregnancy if it was unplanned, or anxious if she has previously miscarried or been infertile.

There are also mixed feelings when infertile friends become pregnant or adopt. Because this experience has bonded you, it is natural to feel abandoned or alienated when they become parents.

These suggestions may be helpful:

☐ Try to have an open exchange of feelings—although envy as well as happiness often surfaces—about how the pregnancy is affecting your relationship.

❧ During this period one of my pregnant friends took the time to call and spend time with me. She shared her pregnancy with me in a compassionate, sensitive way. The more I wanted to withdraw and hate myself, the more she stayed with me. Another pregnant friend did not, and we are now casual acquaintances. Because of the caring of my one friend, I am able to share joy in other people's pregnancies and babies. I know that their ability to have or not have babies will never make me either fertile or infertile.

☐ Record your feelings. One infertile woman kept a journal of her feelings during her best friend's pregnancy. Her attitude slowly changed toward her friend and the unborn child. The newborn, once a source of pain, became a treasured and precious baby to her.

☐ If an honest expression of your feelings will be either ineffective or inappropriate, decide how much, if any, contact with pregnant acquaintances you want. As you heal and move toward resolution, this jealousy usually subsides. You can again share a pregnant friend's happiness, aware that parents do not have idyllic lives and may sometimes envy you!

☐ If you want to, decline baby shower invitations and simply send a gift. You are entitled to your feelings and no apology or explanation is necessary. After resolving their infertility, some women feel comfortable attending baby showers and may even host one for a pregnant friend.

SURVIVING THE HOLIDAYS

Holidays, those seasonal reminders of one's infertility, are often difficult to live with. You can, though, soften the "holiday blues" in some specific ways:

☐ Accept that holidays are often awkward, stressful occasions for everyone, and especially for an infertile couple. Instead of denying sadness or anger, set aside time to express your thoughts to trusted friends or a counselor.

☐ Choose which holiday events to attend and stay only as long as you feel comfortable. You may want to schedule several "escape events" that you know will be enjoyable. For example, some infertility support groups plan child-free festivities during the holidays to laugh, celebrate, and commiserate.

☐ You are already a family of two. Why wait to create your own traditions? Perhaps you can go skiing during Christmas, or plan a romantic getaway on Mother's Day or Father's Day to renew your commitment.

☐ Seek others who find holidays difficult. Perhaps you have neighbors who live far from relatives and would welcome company during Christmas or Hanukkah. Seniors are also often alone on holidays, and hospitals, nursing homes, and churches welcome volunteer help then.

SPECIAL COPING SUGGESTIONS FOR STEPPARENTS

In this era of widespread divorce and remarriage, many women and men are creating "blended families" composed of newly married partners and children from previous unions. The stepparent role, a difficult one in many cases, can intensify the emotional stress of infertility. The partner without a biological child is often pressured by his or her family to produce "a child of your own," and many couples want to have at least one child together. In any event your partner was once fertile with his or her ex-husband or wife. You are not—at least for the present. Jealousy, anger, and a sense of inadequacy toward your mate and his former partner are natural reactions.

❦ When I began my infertility treatment, I was already a stepmother to three- and seven-year-old daughters who lived with us. While most of the time I felt more fortunate than other infertiles in that I had an opportunity to be a mother, the times that their biological mother visited heightened my pain. I was essentially ignored by the girls. This seemed to emphasize my lack of fertility — reminding me that I was not their "real mother."

You can soften these feelings by acknowledging that even though your partner did reproduce with someone else, he or she still grieves for the infertility of your union. Mourning together for your unborn baby is an important process.

Although stepchildren cannot replace a child of your flesh, a close and loving relationship with them enables you to experience a different, but nonetheless important, kind of parenting.

❦ Seven years later, the three-year-old who is now ten, still lives with us, and feels as much mine as my year-old daughter whom I carried inside me for nine months.

SPECIAL COPING SUGGESTIONS
FOR SINGLE WOMEN AND LESBIAN COUPLES

❦ I could not find a specialist who was willing to administer donor insemination to an unmarried woman. Everyone who hears I am single and infertile criticizes me for my desire to parent a child alone.

❦ I went through several years of unsuccessful inseminations. It was so difficult to find emotional support. Most people think lesbians have no business being mothers anyway, and even among the gay community there are those who are opposed to pregnancy or uneducated about infertility. So I felt alone and very frustrated with my infertility.

A growing number of single women, who hear the reproductive clock ticking in their thirties and forties, are choosing to have a child through donor insemination. This decision is often criticized by friends and relatives, and a single woman must constantly justify why she wants and deserves to be a parent. She may also be refused treatment by disapproving physicians or clinics. If she encounters a fertility problem or a pregnancy loss, her experience is usually not acknowledged as the "real problem" that a married woman might suffer. Single women also hear all the tactless infertility comments, plus a few others: "You're not getting pregnant because there is no man in your life," or "Just get married and then you'll get pregnant!"

A single woman does not have to contend with a resistant or uncooperative partner and can make unilateral decisions. At the same time, no one else has a vested interest in her fertility and she lacks a support system to provide empathy and interest. This isolation, along with the negative reactions of others, often leads her to suppress her emotions and inhibits the process of resolving her infertility.

Infertility also occurs among lesbian couples who wish one partner (or both) to bear a child. Well-meaning friends often suggest that the other (presumably fertile) partner simply bear the child, thus negating the pain and grief of the infertile woman. Like single women, lesbian couples are also often criticized for their wish to parent. Since most infertility and adoption literature and support is geared toward middle-class, heterosexual, married couples, it is difficult for single and/or gay women to find peer support. Times are slowly changing, though, and more is being written about all infertile women. In addition, some women's health clinics and other referral agencies facilitate or encourage support networks.

Fostering a Positive Attitude

❦ I recognized that I had gained the strength through all this to handle pregnancy or childlessness. I think a great deal of my earlier motivation was my fear of not having children and being labeled a barren and therefore useless woman.

Now I knew that I had proven myself to the only person who mattered—me. I had gone all the way with the medical options, had faced the challenges, and done my best. I realized that it wasn't necessary to have a baby to prove my worth or value as a woman. Pregnancy would be a welcome gift, not a mandatory condition for my survival. Either way I would go on.

I tried to plant positive seeds in the relationships and projects with which I was involved. I kept busy and, when I was depressed, reminded myself that it was normal to feel low about infertility. Even fertile people get the blues; they're part of living.

Together with physical and emotional well-being, a positive mental outlook enables you to face infertility with determination and strength. The importance of psychological and emotional support cannot be overemphasized. To laugh, cry, and talk with another infertile woman or man provides the reality check to get you through a tough day. Keeping a journal during this experience is therapeutic and provides a valuable perspective on a challenging time.

During your infertility, it is also important to keep in contact with children. They provide a very different and often refreshing world view. One woman suggests clocking some "baby hours" with the infant of an understanding friend or relative. This may ease your ache for a baby and provides a welcome respite for weary parents. The wails and constant demands of an infant or toddler also bring parenting into a realistic perspective. If caring for babies is too painful, try including your friends' or siblings' older children in some of your activities. The ages of seven to twelve are golden years when kids require little physical care and are delightful, fun-loving companions.

Humor is also an essential part of mental health and an invaluable ally during an infertility struggle. Without the ability to laugh at adversity it would be difficult to face any problem. Infertility has its share of absurdities, enabling us to laugh as well as cry.

> ❦ Misery not only loves company but also develops a sense of humor. It's extremely comforting to know that other husbands besides mine practically pack their bags when their wives get their periods. My husband isn't the only one who gets chided by friends for "shooting blanks" or for not "figuring out how to do it yet." I don't even feel so strange anymore for having made love once when I had strep throat and poison oak and he had a broken leg, simply because it was "that time of the month."

Think about the "props" of infertility: thermometers, BBT charts or ovulation predictor kits, drugs, syringes, postcoital tests. Or the awkward situations: four close friends who call the same day with news of their pregnancies; a nagging grandmother-in-waiting who looks at you and sighs a lot; and the out-of-town visitors who show up on your fertile night. When all else fails, many find someone who understands and trade infertility humor.

Others find solace and hope through professional or spiritual counseling. They use these sessions to confront anger, grief, and sadness, clarify goals, and perhaps search for meaning in the experience. Often, over time a renewed sense of purpose and direction may be gained.

Enhancing physical, emotional, mental, and spiritual health can lead to a path of healing and personal growth. After assessing your situation and pursuing an appropriate resolution, you can again take control of life by channeling your health and energy into fulfilling and attainable pursuits.

Part Two

Diagnosis, Causes, and Treatments of Infertility

PROLOGUE

Human Reproduction

KNOWLEDGE OF THE ANATOMICAL and hormonal aspects of human reproduction is critical to a patient's understanding of the diagnosis, causes, and treatments of infertility. A basic and highly simplified discussion of the female and male reproductive systems, as well as the miraculous processes of ovulation, spermatogenesis, and conception, follows.

The endocrine system, composed of a group of glands that secrete essential chemicals called *hormones* directly into the bloodstream, plays a critical role in orchestrating all body processes, including human reproduction. The endocrine glands — the thyroid, parathyroid, adrenals, pancreas, pituitary, hypothalamus, testes, and ovaries — ideally work in unison to maintain health. Hormones such as thyroxin, adrenalin, and insulin (secreted by the thyroid, adrenals, and pancreas) influence various metabolic processes.

Endocrinology, the study of this intricate system, has become an important part of infertility treatment. Scientific advances in the past decade now enable measurement of subtle hormonal changes and treatment for many abnormalities. More couples with infertility problems caused by hormonal imbalances can now be helped.

The synchronized interaction of the hypothalamus, pituitary, and sex glands direct sperm production, ovulation, and early pregnancy. This is accomplished by the "sex" hormones estrogen, progesterone, prolactin, and testosterone, which are produced in both men and women.

The *hypothalamus* plays a critical, if not fully understood, role in directing hormonal activities. Located under the cerebral cortex of the brain, this important gland controls many functions, including appetite and body temperature. The hypothalamus receives signals from the brain, and has the crucial function of translating these messages to other reproductive organs.

In response to chemical and electrical messages, the hypothalamus secretes gonadotropin-releasing hormone (GnRH) into miniscule blood vessels that travel to the pituitary gland. Communication between the hypothalamus and pituitary is necessary for ovulation or sperm production (spermatogenesis) to occur. It is known that extreme stress can disrupt hypothalamic activity, which may temporarily stop its signals to the pituitary and cause menstrual irregularities or even cessation of menses. (This reaction, however, is more common in adolescents and not considered a likely cause of infertility.)

The *pituitary* gland also plays a crucial role in male and female reproduction. Less than half an inch in diameter, it is located at the base of the brain, between the eyes. This tiny gland synthesizes and stores several hormones necessary for normal functioning of the ovaries and testes.

The Female

Unlike the male's, a woman's reproductive organs are contained entirely within her body (see illustration). The *vagina*, the passage between the vulva and the uterus, is between three and five inches long. It is a muscular organ that normally has a fairly acidic environment with a pH of about 4.5. The penis is enclosed within the vagina during intercourse and ejaculates semen into it during male orgasm.

The *cervix* is the narrow base of the uterus, which connects it to the vagina. Its tiny opening, the *os*, allows semen to enter and menstrual fluid to depart.

The Female Reproductive System

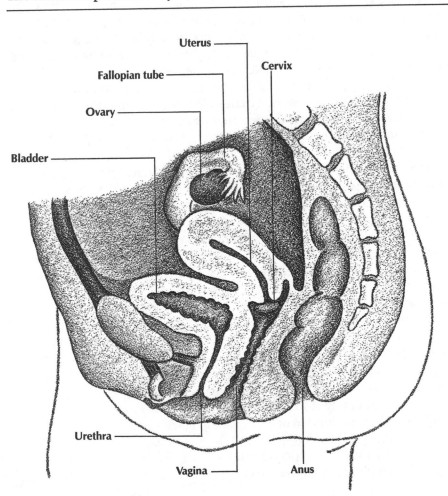

The cervix contains many tiny glands that secrete different types of mucus throughout the menstrual cycle.

The *uterus* (also called the *womb*) is a pear-shaped, muscular organ lined with endometrial cells and can stretch to many times its normal size to accommodate a growing fetus.

The *Fallopian* tubes (or oviducts), each about four inches long, are attached to the uterus at the narrow end of each tube. Their wide, trumpet-like openings hover near each ovary. Tentacle-like projections called fimbria protrude from the ends of the tube, surround the ovary, and retrieve the egg. The tiny inside passage of the tube—a mere 1/70 inch in diameter—is lined with cells that secrete lubricating fluids, as well as hairlike cilia that beat more than 1,000 times per minute. The cilia and lubricants propel the egg toward the uterus.

The almond-sized ovaries are attached by stalks to the uterus. These female sex glands, which ideally release at least one mature egg (ova) each menstrual cycle, also produce estrogen and progesterone hormones.

THE MENSTRUAL CYCLE

A female infant is born with one to two million immature ovarian follicles called *oocytes*. Many oocytes distegrate throughout childhood during the *atretic* process. When menstruation begins *(menarche)*, most girls have about 400,000 ova. Although the atretic process continues throughout life, most women retain enough viable follicles to ovulate about 400 eggs during their reproductive years.

At around nine years of age, the hypothalamus "wakes up" in young girls, initially secreting gonadotropin-releasing hormone (GnRH) only at night. Activity gradually increases until GnRH is released about every ninety minutes around the clock. The ovaries and pituitary react to this signal, release other hormones, and the first menstrual period occurs.

Ideally the hormonal cycle that results in ovulation and menses continues throughout a woman's reproductive years. For most women it is only occasionally interrupted by pregnancy, lactation, or the use of oral contraceptives.

The length of the menstrual cycle varies with each woman. Most have cycles of twenty-six to thirty-four days, with twenty-eight days being the average. In fact, the word *menstrual* is derived from the Latin word *mensis* meaning "month." Although other mammals have ovarian cycles, only humans and some apes menstruate.

It is thought that the most fertile eggs are ovulated in a woman's teens and twenties. During these years, she has about a 30 percent chance of becoming pregnant during any given menstrual cycle. After that, female fertility markedly decreases with age. As she reaches her late thirties and forties, her chance for pregnancy during any given cycle decreases to about 8 percent.

Between the ages of forty-five and fifty-five, a woman simply runs out of viable oocytes to ovulate and begins a gradual cessation of fertility, commonly termed the *climacteric* (technically, menopause refers only to the last menstrual period.) The ovaries, however, continue to secrete low levels of hormones for the rest of her life.

PHASES OF THE MENSTRUAL CYCLE

Although the length of the cycle varies with each woman, a twenty-eight-day cycle is used as an example in this section. Each menstrual cycle is normally composed of four distinct hormonal phases:

1. *The proliferative phase.* This begins with the first day of menstrual bleeding (Cycle Day 1) if pregnancy has not occurred during the previous cycle. Around Day 5 the brain reports low estrogen levels to the hypothalamus, which releases GnRH hormone to the pituitary gland through tiny connecting blood vessels. The pituitary gland reacts to this signal and secretes large quantities of follicle-stimulating hormone (FSH) and smaller amounts of leutinizing hormone (LH).

Responding to increased FSH levels, about 1,000 oocytes begin to develop within each ovary. Through Day 8 the developing follicles continue to absorb FSH and produce more estrogen. One fluid-filled follicle, among the first to develop and usually the largest of both ovaries, soon becomes dominant. In response to the increasing estrogen levels, the pituitary slows FSH production. The smaller follicles cannot absorb enough FSH to maintain themselves and they die off. The dominant follicle absorbs all available FSH and continues estrogen production.

During this phase increasing estrogen levels cause the endometrial lining to thicken. Between Days 11 and 13, hundreds of cervical mucus glands secrete a clear, stringy, "sperm-friendly" mucus and the os dilates slightly.

2. *Ovulation.* Within the ovary, the dominant oocyte (called the Graafian follicle) has fully matured in its sac. The egg is surrounded by two layers: the innermost zona pellucida, surrounded by the cumulus oophorus, which gives the ovum a cloudlike appearance. The ovum's chromosome count has been reduced to twenty-three. When fertilization occurs, the sperm will contribute another twenty-three chromosomes, giving the embryo the normal human chromosome count of forty-six.

By Day 13 estrogen has been maintained at peak levels for forty-eight hours. This prompts the hypothalamus to increase GnRH production, which signals the pituitary to release a surge of LH hormone. When the LH surge has been maintained for about twenty-four hours, the wall of the follicle disintegrates and the surface ruptures. The miracle of ovulation occurs as a fertile ovum, only 1/150 inch in diameter, is released from the ovary.

The egg floats away and is retrieved by the tentacle-like fimbria of the Fallopian tube hovering near the ovary. The fimbria grasps the cumulus layer and propels the egg down the tube.

3. *The luteal or secretory phase.* Responding to the LH surge, the ruptured follicle sac undergoes a "leutinizing process." Its cells enlarge and absorb a yellow pigment called lutein, which the body manufactures from cholesterol. It is now

called the corpus luteum, a Latin phrase meaning "yellow body," and has the critical job of producing a great deal of progesterone and smaller amounts of estrogen for ten to fourteen days. Successful implantation and early pregnancy depend on this perfectly balanced hormonal production.

During the luteal phase, the progesterone surge will trigger other important changes:

☐ LH production in the pituitary will be suppressed.

☐ Basal body temperature will slightly elevate, the basis for "documenting" ovulation through basal body temperature charting.

☐ The endometrium will change to a "secretory state." Its lining will soften and prepare for implantation and nourishment of a fertilized embryo. The character of these post-ovulatory endometrial cells differs markedly from those of the proliferative phase.

☐ The cervical mucus glands shift back to producing thick, opaque secretions, and the cervical opening (os) shrinks. These changes discourage the entry of sperm or other foreign matter.

If pregnancy does not occur within about fourteen days after ovulation, the corpus luteum ceases its hormonal production and disintegrates.

4. *Menstruation.* The endometrium responds to the decreasing progesterone level and releases chemicals called prostaglandins. Uterine contractions and perhaps cramps result, menstruation begins, and the endometrial lining is shed. Bleeding, which varies from light to heavy among women, usually lasts from three to seven days. Most women lose only about two ounces of blood. During menstruation, the brain senses lowered estrogen levels and signals the hypothalamus to secrete GnRH to begin a new cycle.

The Male

The male reproductive organs, pituitary, and hypothalamus compose an intricate and complex system that ideally manufactures, stores, and ejaculates millions of sperm. As with female reproduction, hormonal, environmental, or physical factors can easily upset this balance and cause male fertility problems.

A boy begins the sexual maturation process of puberty at around twelve years of age. Over the next three years, his body manufactures large amounts of male testosterone hormone, which dramatically increases his sex drive, stimulates body hair growth, deepens his voice, and, together with other hormones, produces mature, fertile sperm.

In addition to testosterone, mature males produce other hormones common to both men and women, such as FSH, LH, prolactin, and estrogen. These hormones are secreted on a continuous basis; thus a man does not have a "cycle" comparable to ovulation, and sperm are constantly regenerated throughout his lifetime. Although sperm counts may decrease with age, men do not experience a cessation of fertility comparable to female menopause.

THE MALE REPRODUCTIVE SYSTEM

Unlike the female's, a male's reproductive organs are housed outside the body in the scrotum — a pouch with several inner linings and an outer layer. It has two chambers and hangs behind the penis and away from the body (see illustration).

Each chamber contains a testicle, blood vessels, nerves, and a spermatic cord that transports the sperm. Since sperm production is inhibited by body temperature, this ideal external location keeps the testicles cool (about 94°F).

Each testicle is about two inches long and an inch in diameter and weighs about an ounce. Its primary function is to produce sperm and the testosterone hormone. Each testicle contains convoluted *seminiferous* tubules, which would measure several hundred yards if uncoiled. Within these tubules are the immature sperm cells, which are sensitive to fevers, viruses, and other illnesses. For this reason sperm production may be slowed or halted during sickness.

The *Leydig cells,* located throughout the testes, produce testosterone hormone, which is emptied into the veins and carried into the bloodstream. These cells are not as heat sensitive as sperm cells, so a man's sex drive, voice, or hair growth are usually not affected by illness or fertility problems.

The Male Reproductive System

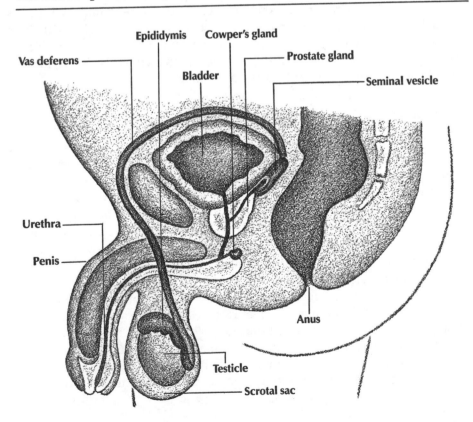

Each testicle is connected to a long, complex, and convoluted system of ducts, which are critical to sperm maturation and transport. The *epididymis,* the first section of this duct system, is only about 1/125 inch in diameter and occupies about an inch of space in a tightly coiled "C" shape. Unwound it would measure nearly twenty feet.

The epididymis is connected to a *vas deferens,* two sturdy ducts that enter the body on either side of the abdomen. Each vas moves up through the groin and the anal canal, behind the bladder, through the prostate gland, and into the urethra. This is the duct that is cut during male sterilization (vasectomy).

The *prostate gland* lies in front of the seminal vesicles and surrounds the urethra. It is about an inch and a half in diameter and generates much of the milky, alkaline seminal fluid. This gland sometimes enlarges later in life, which may cause problems with urination.

The *seminal vesicle* enters the vas deferens through the prostate gland. This duct contributes several important substances to the semen.

SPERMATOGENESIS

A fertile, mature sperm is called a *spermatozoon* and measures about 1/500 inch long. It is a microscopic, wiggly cell that consists of a head, middle section, and tail.

The head of the sperm measures about five microns (one micron = one millionth of a meter). It contains the father's genetic information in a set of twenty-

Detail of Sperm

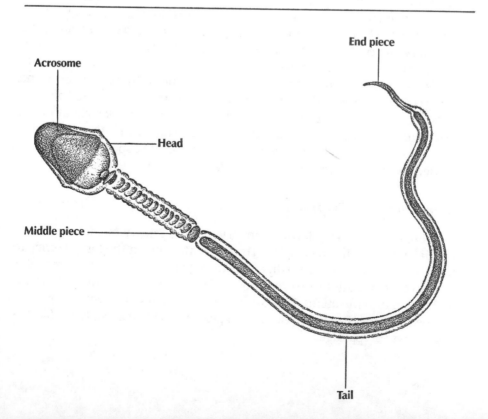

three chromosomes, as well as important enzymes, which are enclosed in a cap called the *acrosome.*

The middle section is quite small but serves an important purpose. It is ringed with bands of mitochondria, which act as "battery packs" to provide continuous energy for the sperm's long journey to the Fallopian tube.

The tail is the longest section, measuring between thirty and fifty microns. It should constantly flagellate, propelling itself toward the ovum at about 1/8 inch per minute.

Spermatogenesis, the process of sperm manufacture and transport, is coordinated by hormones produced by the testes, hypothalamus, and pituitary gland. The hypothalamus initiates this process by releasing GnRH hormone to the pituitary, which in turn secretes FSH and LH, also known as interstitial cell stimulating hormone (ICSH). Testosterone is produced in response to these hormones, the germ cells within the testes begin to mature and develop tails, and the sperm are released into the epididymis. At this stage they are unable to swim or fertilize an egg. They are moved through the epididymis through rhythmic contractions (peristalsis). During this process, which takes ten to fourteen days, they become both motile and fertile.

The sperm next enter the vas deferens and are again advanced by muscular contraction. During this journey, the prostate gland contributes enzymes, magnesium, phosphates, and zinc to the semen. The seminal vesicles add prostaglandins and fructose sugars, which provide fuel to sustain motility. All these substances help the semen coagulate upon ejaculation and then reliquify five to twenty-five minutes afterward in the vagina.

The combination of seminal fluid (98 percent) and sperm (2 percent) make up the semen. A third of this fluid is stored in the last portion of the epididymis; the rest awaits orgasm within the vas deferens. When the male is sexually excited, the semen enters the urethra, a tube that runs through the penis, and is ejaculated into the vagina during orgasm. Because the urethra also carries urine, during erection the body cleverly engages a muscle that blocks urine flow.

The entire process of sperm production and transport takes about ninety days. Although mature sperm die if not ejaculated within a month, the continuous release of FSH and LH hormones results in constant sperm regeneration. The new sperm are transported to the vas deferens to replace the old.

Conception and Pregnancy

Minutes after ejaculation, the semen jells into a thick, white substance that soon reliquifies within the vagina. The sperm then begin the long journey to the Fallopian tubes, a distance that is nearly 3,000 times their length and takes between thirty minutes and several hours. They must first pass through the cervical mucus into the uterus. Even with "friendly" midcycle mucus, only about 400 sperm — out of an initial ejaculate of perhaps 60 to 100,000,000 million — will survive this passage.

Journey of Egg and Sperm and Their Union

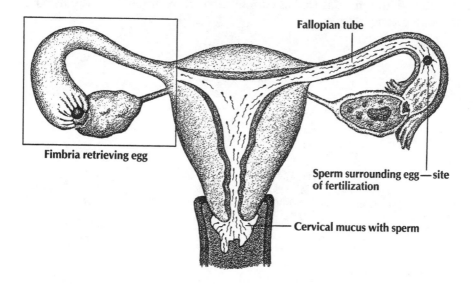

Fallopian tube

Fimbria retrieving egg

Sperm surrounding egg—site of fertilization

Cervical mucus with sperm

Uterine contractions and their own motility (1/8 inch per minute) propel the sperm to the top of the uterus, where some enter the right Fallopian tube and others the left. They are stored in cavities in the Fallopian tubes and are slowly released a few at a time. More will be lost as they swim through the tubes searching for an ovum. Fewer than 200 will reach the egg as it floats down the Fallopian tube.

During this journey the sperm gradually go through capacitation, a mysterious process that enables them to penetrate an ovum. The sperm's cap is slowly worn away to release its enzymes. One of these, hyaluronidase, helps forge a path through the outer layer of the egg; another enzyme, acrosin, breaks down the inner layer so a small slit, only large enough for a single sperm, can be made.

Conception occurs as the sperm fertilizes the egg, their chromosomes blend, and a chemical reaction occurs that reseals the membrane. This prevents other sperm from entering and creating an embryo with three or more sets of chromosomes.

The fertilized egg is now called a *zygote* and contains twenty-three chromosomes from each parent. Over the next few days, the zygote divides in half and then quickly divides twice more. At the eight-cell stage it moves to the uterus, and, if it successfully implants, produces hCG hormone for the next three months. This sustains the corpus luteum's production of progesterone and estrogen until the placenta can take over. HCG hormone can be detected in an early serum pregnancy test.

A great deal of early pregnancy loss occurs naturally within the body. In general only about 31 percent of ova exposed to fertilization will survive to a term birth. In older women this percentage decreases.

Clearly many conditions must be ideal in both partners for pregnancy to occur and proceed to term. Physiological problems that can cause female, male, or combined infertility, as well as current medical treatments, are discussed in chapters 8 through 16.

CHAPTER 8

The Female Infertility Workup

❦ I began my infertility workup with mixed feelings. It was a
frightening, uncertain time. I couldn't get pregnant and we didn't
know why. I also felt inadequate because I wasn't fertile and angry
that tests were necessary. Yet starting the workup also felt like a
positive step. I wanted to know what was wrong and try to fix it. It
gave us both a sense of control and brought us closer together.

MOST WOMEN BECOME PREGNANT within a year of having unprotected intercourse, and couples are usually advised to try to conceive for at least this long
before beginning intensive infertility testing. Earlier testing, however, may be
appropriate for women over age thirty-five, for those with known medical problems that may affect fertility, or when anxiety is affecting the couple's marriage
or either partner's self-esteem. Such factors may include irregular menstrual
cycles or painful menses (not relieved by antiprostaglandin medication), past
history of pelvic inflammatory disease (PID), pre-natal exposure to diethylstilbestrol (DES), prolonged use of an intrauterine device (IUD), or endometriosis.
(These problems are discussed in chapters 10 and 11.)

When first attempting pregnancy, a general discussion about fertility with
your gynecologist is often helpful. This physician can provide useful information about average conception time, indications of ovulation, cervical mucus
changes, and chances of pregnancy loss.

Consulting an Infertility Specialist

If pregnancy does not occur within a year, your physician should order a
semen analysis. Gynecologists may also perform the postcoital test and perhaps
hysterosalpingogram (described below). If these tests indicate a problem, or if
fertility problems continue, it is wise to consult an infertility specialist. In most
cases the patient does not need to repeat basic workup tests already performed,
since those results can be transferred to the specialist. Selecting a specialist who
is medically competent and emotionally supportive is an important step (see
chapter 4).

TABLE 8.1 FEMALE INFERTILITY WORKUP TESTS

Procedure	Purpose	Benefits, Risks, and Inconveniences	Approximate 1992 Cost
Initial Visit— Interview, physical exam, routine lab work, semen analysis for male partner	To gather medical history of both partners, detect obvious anatomical abnormalities that may be imparing fertility	May reveal causes of infertility without necessity of more costly, invasive testing	About $250 plus any lab work ordered
Basal Body Temperature (BBT) Chart	To determine length of cycles, and based on temperature elevation, probable ovulation date	Becomes tedious and stressful, affecting couple's sex life	Cost of good, reliable thermometer
Ovulation Predictor Kit	To predict time of ovulation based on LH hormone level	May yield confusing reults; some couples may test repeatedly	$20 – $25
Postcoital Test (PCT or Sims-Huhner)	To observe the quality and cellular characteristics of mid-cycle cervical mucus and the sperm's reaction to it	Couple is pressured to have intercourse two to four hours before the office visit; pelvic exam necessary to obtain mucus sample	$75
Hysterosalpingogram (HSG)	To diagnose tubal blockages, and in some cases, uterine abnormalities	Injection of dye may clear tubes; requires clamping of uterus, which may cause cramps or discomfort; small risk of infection	$400 – $500 for radiologist and hospital charges
Serum Progesterone, FSH, LH, Prolactin	To measure level of various hormones during the menstrual cycle	Simple, non-invasive blood tests that may indicate reasons for infertility	About $50 per test
Endometrial Biopsy	To examine endometrial cells for luteal phase characteristics—a good indication whether ovulation is occuring	Can cause painful cramping—many specialists use mini paracervical block	About $250 for both physician's and laboratory charges
Laparoscopy	To view the exterior surfaces of the reproductive organs and abdomen; only reliable way to diagnose some pelvic problems, e.g., endometriosis and external tubal adhesions	Requires hospitalization (usually outpatient); stresses and risks of anesthesia and surgery	About $7,500 – $8,000 for surgeon's and hospital's charges

*Costs may vary in different geographical areas. These charges are based on an average of 1992 fees of several San Francisco Bay Area hospitals, specialists, and laboratories.

Infertility tests, drugs, and surgery are expensive. Before starting your workup, discuss the projected costs of treatment and any financial concerns with your physician. Basic infertility testing may also be available through some women's health clinics and other public or private programs. They often offer reduced fees for low-income patients or those without insurance coverage. (See chapter 3 for a discussion of the economics of infertility.)

Special Considerations for Women Over Forty

Over the last decade, there has been a notable increase in first-time "older mothers." About 20 percent of U.S. women now have their first baby after the age of thirty-five. Many, in their late thirties and early forties, conceive easily and experience healthy, full-term pregnancies. Other women encounter problems with conception and/or miscarriage as they approach their forties and, in hope of a successful pregnancy, may undergo infertility testing or treatment.

Because fertility naturally declines and the risk of pregnancy loss increases as women age, a prompt workup is especially important for women over forty who have not conceived within *six* months of unprotected intercourse. A complete and thorough evaluation can be accomplished within one to two cycles. This allows time for treatment if problems are detected, and a reasonable interim for natural or medically assisted attempts at pregnancy.

In addition to the regular workup described in this chapter, several other considerations may be helpful. Careful attention to health problems that commonly affect women over forty — such as high blood pressure, heart disease, and diabetes — is important. If not already obtained, a baseline mammogram is also advised to rule out any potential problems with abnormal breast growths or cancer. The presence of hot flashes or irregular menses may indicate an early menopause. An FSH (follicle stimulating hormone) test, administered early in the menstrual cycle, can be a significant indicator of "ovarian age" and therefore probability for successful pregnancy — either naturally or through Assisted Reproductive Technology (ART). (See chapter 14 for more discussion of the FSH test.)

Evaluation of ovulation through basal body temperature (BBT) charts or ovulation predictor kits, progesterone testing, and perhaps ultrasound tracking of developing follicles, together with the other workup tests and the male partner's semen analysis, provides more important information about the couple's fertility. Many experts believe that the workup should be devoted solely to diagnosis, regardless of the patient's age, and that treatment should be initiated only after testing is completed.

After this short and intensive testing period, the specialist and couple can analyze the data and formulate a three- to six-month plan. Depending on the workup results, the FSH level, and the couple's preferences, recommendations may be made for specific medical treatments, surgery, or natural attempts at pregnancy.

There is a tendency, especially among older infertile couples, to panic and rush toward in vitro fertilization (IVF) or another Assisted Reproductive Technology (ART). If the workup tests do not reveal any physical problems and the FSH level is within normal limits, many specialists advise couples — -even those in their early forties — to allow at least another six months for a natural conception. In many cases, the chances of a pregnancy occurring naturally, or perhaps through intrauterine insemination, are probably the same or better than ART success rates for women forty years and older. (The exception may be donor egg IVF. This complex psychological issue, which merits lengthy and careful thought in any case, is discussed in chapter 14.)

Emotional Stress of Testing

❦ The emotional stress of medical procedures has immobilized me for periods of time. My career and educational goals were often interrupted during years of tests that were expensive and time-consuming; that required specific timing and sometimes had to be repeated; that were often painful, inconclusive, and embarrassing; and that sometimes required surgery. On many occasions, I would put myself and my husband through emotions I didn't realize I was capable of — as a result of tests.

Once a couple decides to have a baby, it is a devastating and bitter disappointment when menstruation occurs each month. After years of careful contraception, it is maddening to find conception difficult or even unattainable. Anxiety, marital stress, anger, and loss of self-esteem are all common reactions. It is critical to address these emotions, as well as your medical problems, during this time. By entering the workup process with an informed and positive attitude, couples can optimize their chances of success, feel some degree of control over their treatment, and enhance their love and respect for each other.

The Initial Infertility Visit

❦ I went to that first visit feeling vulnerable and scared. I was relieved that before the physical exam we met with our specialist in his private office. He and his staff were friendly, and I felt good about seeking answers and help for my problem. But I also felt angry that I had to go through this at all.

It is recommended that both partners attend the first visit to meet the specialist, discuss their medical histories and personal concerns, and help plan the course of their workup.

The initial visit begins in the specialist's private office. The doctor will take a medical history, including the age of each partner, lifestyle habits, any medical problems, past contraception methods, marital history, present relationship, previous pregnancies by past or present partner and the outcome, past surgeries, past and present drug and medication use, and the duration of infertility.

Next, the woman is taken to an examining room and asked to undress. She is given either a large paper gown or two coverings for her breasts and pelvic area. The physician performs a physical examination, checking the thyroid gland, breasts, pelvis, heart, lungs, and abdomen. This examination will determine whether she is in good health and without obvious gynecological abnormalities.

If not performed in the past year, a PAP smear is usually done and routine blood tests and urinalysis may be ordered. If excessive body hair or other indications of hormonal imbalance are noted, appropriate blood tests may be ordered. Screening for infectious or sexually transmitted diseases may also be done.

Some specialists also introduce the BBT chart at this time. The couple may be asked to record daily basal temperature for a few cycles. To optimize chances for pregnancy, intercourse is usually recommended every other day for several days before and after the time of ovulation.

Unless the initial examination reveals a specific problem, the workup usually begins with the simple, noninvasive, and least costly tests: semen analysis, postcoital test, and blood tests. Pregnancy occasionally occurs during the testing period. Otherwise, the workup progresses to more complex, invasive, and expensive tests: endometrial biopsy, hysterosalpingogram, laparoscopy, and perhaps surgery.

If time allows, many couples continue going to tests and appointments together to ask questions, discuss test results, and plan the next step of the workup.

Semen Analysis

The semen analysis, a simple procedure, should always be done at the beginning of the workup. In the past many women endured needless tests when, in fact, the problem was caused by male infertility. This test may be ordered by an internist or gynecologist before the infertility specialist is consulted.

If the semen analysis is abnormal, another test is usually ordered before any conclusions are drawn. If a subsequent test reveals a low count or other abnormality, the couple is referred to a urologist who specializes in male reproductive problems. (For a complete discussion of this test and of male infertility, see chapters 15 and 16). If the semen analysis is normal, testing should begin with the female partner.

The Basal Body Temperature (BBT) Chart

🐛 Those damn charts! Nothing in my story has stayed more constant than my hatred for them. But I took my temperature religiously. Maybe, just maybe, if I was a good girl, I would get pregnant.

Chances for pregnancy are greatly increased by timing intercourse around ovulation. The BBT chart is a graph the patient uses to plot daily basal temperature during the menstrual cycle. It is an indirect measure of ovulation based on progesterone secretion. The woman's temperature must be taken daily upon awakening and prior to any activity. A standard oral thermometer may be used, although BBT thermometers with minute gradations are also sold.

A textbook-perfect graph will show a low baseline temperature during and after menstruation. Prior to ovulation there will be a drop in temperature, followed by a sharp rise after an ovum is released. The rise, caused by the production and release of progesterone, indicates an egg is ready for fertilization, providing other factors are also favorable. If pregnancy occurs, the basal temperature will remain elevated. Otherwise, decreased progesterone secretions trigger menstruation and the temperature falls to basal level again.

ARE BBT CHARTS OR OVULATION PREDICTOR KITS NECESSARY?

For many infertile couples the BBT chart is a source of stress and anxiety. Sex becomes scheduled, with a resulting loss of spontaneity, and disappointment increases each month that menstruation occurs. Too often couples live by the chart and find themselves only making love around their "fertile time," a pattern that can undermine even the most stable relationship.

There is much controversy among specialists about the accuracy of BBT charts. Many women do not experience sharply defined drops or rises in their cycles. In rare cases the ovaries will secrete progesterone without ovulating. Conversely, a small percentage of women will have flat temperature charts although endometrial biopsies indicate ovulation has occurred. The charts can be useful, however, to time such procedures as endometrial biopsies and postcoital tests.

Some specialists recommend using ovulation predictor kits, a more accurate, though expensive, indicator of impending ovulation. The kits detect the presence of leutenizing hormone (LH) in the urine. Intercourse is recommended both the night of, and twenty-four hours after, the LH surge is detected. Many couples, though, find predictor kits as anxiety-provoking as BBT charts. Some women report variations or gradations of color on the test sticks which lead to confusion and uncertainty about whether the surge has occurred. They often retest for several days afterward. Frantic that they will miss their fertile time, many couples feel pressured to make love almost daily while they are using the kits.

Other physicians utilize frequent sonograms for several days prior to expected ovulation, followed by an hCG shot to stimulate release of the egg(s).

The Basal Body Temperature (BBT) Chart. Note that in the first graph there was no chance for conception because intercourse did not occur at the time of ovulation. During the next cycle the timing was better and pregnancy followed.

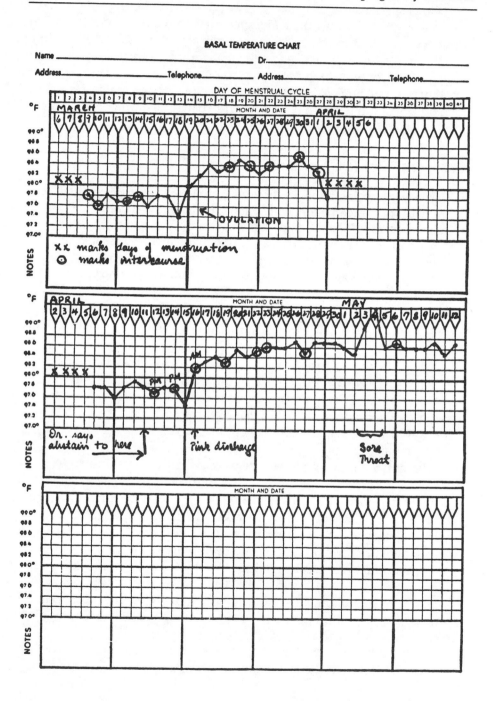

Both methods can be expensive — $40 per cycle or more for the predictor kits and $75 to $200 for the sonogram (depending whether it is performed in the physician's office or the hospital).

Other specialists believe that, after a cycle or two, charts, predictor kits, or sonograms are not worth the additional stress they usually create. Utilizing these tools for two or three months is probably long enough to determine whether ovulation is occurring and the regularity of menstrual cycles. Rather than charting for months, these experts recommend sexual intimacy through-out the cycle, and preferably every other day before and after midcycle. If neces-sary, other workup tests can be performed to diagnose hormonal or ovulation problems and determine whether fertility drug therapy is advisable.

Postcoital Test (PCT or Sims-Hühner)

❦ My gynecologist told me to come in on Day 12 of my menstrual cycle for a postcoital test, within about two hours of having intercourse. Of course, the doctor was very busy that morning. But we managed a very mechanical act of making love and trekked on in. He showed us the many motile sperm under the microscope, which was reassuring; but I also felt quite embarrassed during the visit.

This test allows the specialist and couple to observe the interaction between his sperm and her cervical mucus, both of which play a critical role in fertility.

Prior to ovulation, a thick, opaque cervical mucus blocks sperm from enter-ing the cervix. As ovulation approaches, increased estrogen levels in the blood cause the mucus to change character and become thin and stringy, with a con-sistency like raw egg whites. The mucus can be pulled and stretched between the fingers (called the Spinnbarkeit phenomenon). (See chapter 9 for discussion of cervical mucus problems.)

The postcoital test involves a pelvic examination within two to twelve hours after intercourse to obtain a sample of this mucus. Beside observing the quality of the mucus, the number and movement of the sperm are also noted. There should not be a discrepancy between the postcoital test and the semen analysis. If the male's sperm count and motility are normal, numerous wiggling sperm should be present in healthy mid-cycle mucus.

An abnormal PCT may reveal thick, cloudy, or scanty mucus and/or few or no moving sperm. The pH and acidity level of the mucus, which may affect receptivity to sperm, can also be measured. An improper chemical balance or sperm antibodies within the mucus may be among the factors responsible for an abnormal test.

It is important to note, however, that specialists disagree about the reliabil-ity and importance of the PCT. Many women have become pregnant during cycles that yielded "poor" or "abnormal" PCT results. Yet most specialists use the PCT and factor the results with the couple's other fertility test data.

Though painless, the test is likely to involve some inconvenience as it cannot easily be scheduled in advance. Some patients find it embarrassing as well. Specialists also have differing opinions about when to perform this test. Because pH and acidity factors can change within several hours, some advise couples to have intercourse two to four hours before the office visit. Other physicians prefer to wait up to twelve hours after intercourse to observe how the sperm react to the changing chemical environment of the mucus and to alleviate some of the pressure on the couple. If the suggested timing is difficult for you, or if repeated postcoital tests are necessary, discuss your concerns with your specialist.

Serum Progesterone Test and the Endometrial Biopsy

❦ My specialist smiled and said, "Your progesterone level is sky high!" This made me feel good. I tried to concentrate on this part of my fertility, which was healthy and normal.

❦ I think everyone has a different threshold for pain. Before my endometrial biopsy, I was told to take an over-the-counter pain reliever. It didn't help and I wish I was offered a stronger one. For me, the physical discomfort intensified my fear and emotional stress. I advise women to inquire about the pain or discomfort of the workup tests and ask for what they need to get through them.

These two tests investigate whether ovulation is occurring and if the uterine (endometrial) lining is being adequately prepared to nourish a fertilized egg. A simple blood test, taken between Days 21 and 24 of the cycle, measures the level of progesterone hormone. An elevated level would suggest that ovulation has occurred.

Different types of endometrial tissue form during the cycle depending on the amounts of estrogen and progesterone in the blood. Progesterone-stimulated tissue, usually present after ovulation, is necessary to sustain pregnancy. Later in the workup an endometrial biopsy may be performed to check whether the endometrial tissue has properly responded to the elevated progesterone level.

The biopsy is usually done close to menstruation, preferably one to three days before a period is expected. Couples who worry about affecting an early pregnancy may prefer to use contraception during this cycle, or to request an early blood-sensitive pregnancy test before the biopsy is performed.

A newer instrument, a small plastic catheter called a pipelle, is now being used by many specialists for the biopsy. Many patients think that it greatly reduces pain or discomfort. Others still find this test uncomfortable and their specialists administer some type of pain medication or anesthetic before the biopsy is performed. The patient is prepared for a pelvic examination. After explaining the procedure, the specialist inserts the pipelle through the cervical canal and retrieves a bit of uterine lining.

The tissue is examined microscopically. It should resemble postovulatory cells in character and hormonal content. The results of the serum progesterone and endometrial biopsy can indicate whether a problem exists within the uterus, or whether the ovaries are not producing the hormones necessary to establish a favorable endometrium.

A fertilized ovum may be unable to implant properly in a poorly developed endometrial lining, and early spontaneous abortion can occur without the woman ever being aware of a pregnancy. A progesterone deficiency or luteal phase defect can frequently be improved with hormones (see chapter 9).

Hysterosalpingogram (HSG)

> ❦ I was very anxious as I awaited my HSG, terrified that it would reveal blocked tubes. Since I'd had an IUD and probably some mild pelvic infections, I suspected that the tubes were the source of my infertility. The procedure was painful but quick. To my joy, my body told me that my tubes were open as I felt the dye pass through them. Simultaneously I saw it all on the screen as my gynecologist and the radiologist also watched. The results were so positive that I didn't mind the physical pain. Even as it occurred, I imagined I would perceive the pain of childbirth.

This X-ray study, which has replaced the outmoded Rubins' tubal insufflation test, is used to diagnose tubal blockage or uterine abnormalities. Many specialists like to attend the hysterosalpingogram test to supervise the procedure and observe the results.

The patient lies on the examining table with her legs elevated in stirrups. To control the motion of the uterus, the physician or radiologist places a clamp on the cervix, which often produces unpleasant or painful cramping. Many specialists will order use of a local anesthetic to alleviate this discomfort.

A radiopaque dye is then injected through the opening of the cervix into the uterus. As the dye moves through the pelvic organs, an X-ray machine photographs the revealed outline. If the Fallopian tubes are open, the dye spills out the ends into the pelvic cavity and is absorbed by the body. There can be a therapeutic benefit to the procedure, as the flushing of the tubes can improve their functioning. Some women become pregnant within three to six months following the test, despite long periods of prior infertility.

On the other hand, the procedure may cause tubal spasm(s) and block the flow of the dye, thereby giving a false test result. Additionally, the introduction of the dye (a foreign substance) into the sterile body cavity creates a slight risk of infection. A preventive treatment of oral antibiotics is often prescribed before the procedure and continued for several days afterward.

An HSG will not reveal adhesions on the exterior of the tubes or microscopic damage to the tubal lining resulting from a previous infection. (See chapter 11 for further discussion of these problems.)

Hormonal Blood Tests

There are many hormones involved in the functioning of the menstrual cycle. If the endometrial biopsy, postcoital tests, and HSG do not reveal a cause for continued infertility, the specialist may suggest hormonal testing as the next step. Serum (blood) tests can check the levels of estrogen, FSH, LH, prolactin, and other specific hormones in the bloodstream during various phases of the menstrual cycle.

In rare cases the test results indicate the need for further investigation of the patient's pituitary, thyroid, or adrenal glands. Referral may be made to an endocrinologist, or the specialist may recommend further blood work or, in rare cases, a magnetic resonance imaging (MRI). (See chapter 9 for further discussion.)

Hysteroscopy and Laparoscopy

❦ As part of the work-up, our specialist suggested a hysteroscopy. It revealed a number of fibroids within my uterus that might affect pregnancy. We had no idea that this might be a problem. We agreed to treat this before proceeding any further.

❦ I was afraid of the laparoscopy both because it was surgery and because of what it might reveal. I both wanted a reason for why I was infertile and dreaded knowing it. I did, however, have a great deal of confidence in my specialist. Before we went to the hospital, my husband and I took a long walk on the beach. Then we checked into the same-day surgery unit. The nurses were friendly and supportive, and the anesthesiologist spoke with me beforehand. As I went into surgery, I felt a great sense of relief. At last I would know something, and this awful uncertainty would be over.

Some specialists may recommend a hysteroscopy during the later stages of the workup or before an IVF cycle. It may be performed at the time of laparoscopy, or scheduled independently on another visit. During this procedure, a slender, lighted scope is inserted through the cervix and the uterus is slightly inflated with carbon dioxide gas or a liquid solution. The surgeon can directly view the uterine interior and check for such abnormalities as fibroids, adhesions, or polyps, which may affect fertility. Removal of smaller uterine growths and scar tissue may be possible through the hysteroscope.

Laparoscopy, which permits the surgeon to view the exterior surfaces of the reproductive organs and abdomen, is usually performed at the end of the workup. It can be a useful diagnostic tool when other tests have not revealed a cause for continued infertility. Like all surgical procedures, laparoscopy poses a small risk of adverse reactions to anesthesia or abdominal damage from the procedure itself. It is also expensive (surgeon and hospital bills totaled about $8,000 in 1992) and is usually performed under general anesthesia.

Currently, laparoscopy is commonly used for both diagnosis and surgical treatment of many pelvic problems, including endometriosis and tubal disease. Any surgery, be it "minor" or "major," can raise intense feelings. See chapter 5 for a detailed discussion of the physical and emotional dynamics of laparoscopy and major surgery.

Coping with the Stress of the Infertility Workup

❦ When my HSG revealed open tubes, we decided to spend a day rejoicing. I'd put off having the HSG for months, not wanting to know if the results were disappointing. We took a ride along the coast and had a marvelous dinner at a restaurant that had been highly recommended.

In addition to those offered in other chapters, the following suggestions may be helpful during your workup:

☐ Educate yourself about the workup tests. Learn all you can about your tests and any problems that are diagnosed. Acquiring knowledge and information often restores a sense of direction and control. Ask your physician for references. The National Office of RESOLVE (see *Resources*) and many of its local chapters also offer literature about the workup tests and various medical problems.

☐ Work together with your specialist. Take an active role in planning the course of treatment, and call your doctor when you have questions, concerns, or need more information. If you are sensitive to pain or discomfort, ask about the use of analgesia or local anesthesia.

☐ Be prepared for unfavorable test results. Some of your tests may reveal a problem. This is shocking, frightening, and disappointing news. Allow yourself time to feel and absorb these emotions. One woman gave herself twenty-four hours to "hit bottom and lick her wounds" before facing any more. Negative test results may also reveal a reason for your infertility, perhaps a problem that can be treated. In this sense they open the door for action.

☐ Celebrate positive test results. A positive test result indicates one area where your body is healthy and functioning properly. Take pride in this sign of your body's strength and well-being. Share your happiness with your mate, perhaps with a romantic dinner or special outing. If a test result is unexpectedly positive, celebrate in a big way; let your imagination run wild!

CHAPTER 9

Hormonal Problems and Their Treatment

❦ I had always thought of ovulation as such a simple task. But when I started charting those temperature graphs, I realized how irregularly I ovulated. It saddened me to think my body was having such a difficult time releasing an egg, and I dreaded taking drugs to help it happen.

THE COORDINATED SECRETION OF HORMONES that culminates in the maturation and release of a fertile egg is staggeringly complex, requiring an intricate sequence of interactions between the hypothalamus, pituitary, and ovaries. This miraculous process is described more fully in "Human Reproduction."

Between 2 and 3 percent of all women of reproductive age suffer from secondary amenorrhea (an absence of three or more consecutive menstrual cycles after puberty). Many other women ovulate irregularly. In all, between 20 and 30 percent of female infertility patients experience ovulatory problems.

Other women suffer from inadequate hormone production during different phases of the menstrual cycle. Such hormonal imbalances can contribute to such conditions as polycystic ovarian disease, hyperprolactinism, secondary amenorrhea, luteal phase defect, cervical mucus problems, or post-birth control pill syndrome. This chapter examines some of the causes of hormonal problems and current treatment options, including ovulation inducing drugs.

Factors that Can Disrupt Ovulation

There are a number of reasons why some women ovulate irregularly or suffer from secondary amenorrhea. Some have detectable problems involving the ovaries, hypothalamus, and pituitary that disrupt or halt the ovulation process. In any case, a thorough fertility workup, that includes a reasonable investigation of physical and hormonal factors, should be undertaken to diagnose any organic problems. After the workup, the couple and specialist can evaluate the benefits, disadvantages, side effects, and success rates of appropriate treatment options.

POLYCYSTIC OVARIAN DISEASE

Polycystic ovarian disease (PCO), also called Stein-Leventhal syndrome, is caused by hormonal imbalances that disrupt the ovulation process. Named for the multiple cysts that often form on the ovaries in response to these imbalances, PCO occurs in between 1 and 4 percent of all women, and about 50 percent of those who suffer from secondary amenorrhea. PCO is diagnosed by physical examination, blood tests, and ultrasound imaging of the ovaries.

Causes. PCO is a cyclical, self-perpetuating condition. Although women and men normally have correspondingly appropriate amounts of both female and male hormones in their systems, for unknown reasons women with PCO have elevated androgen (male hormone) levels. These levels are toxic to the developing follicles within the ovary. Their growth is arrested and pea-sized cysts are formed on the surface of the ovary. These cysts, many times smaller than those ovarian cysts that require surgical removal, produce some estrogen, which slows follicle stimulating hormone (FSH) production. Although leutinizing hormone (LH) levels are elevated in response to the estrogen production, ovulation does not occur because the ovarian follicles have atrophied. This results in an absence of progesterone hormone. Androgen levels remain elevated and the cycle repeats itself.

Symptoms. Women with PCO may have a history of very irregular or nonexistent menstrual cycles. Excessive hair growth on the face, breasts, and abdomen occurs in about 70 percent of patients. Other complaints may include infertility, obesity, and enlarged or multi-cystic ovaries. Elevated androgen levels may also be detected by a blood test.

Treatment. At one time, PCO was treated by surgically removing a wedge of the ovary. While this procedure is no longer recommended, some surgeons are now utilizing laser surgery to puncture as many follicle cysts as possible. This reduces androgen levels and hopefully restores hormonal balance. The long-term benefits and risks of ovarian scarring from this method are being studied.

If a pregnancy is desired, clomiphene is usually prescribed to induce ovulation. If this is ineffective, some specialists may recommend ovulation induction with hMG, FSH, or GnRH with an ovulation pump. If elevated prolactin levels are also present, treatment with bromocriptine may also be suggested. (See sections below for a discussion of these drug treatments.)

Hyperprolactinism

Prolactin, a hormone present in both men and women, is manufactured by the pituitary gland. Its production, however, is probably controlled by the hypothalamus through complex hormonal interactions. Prolactin prepares a woman's breasts for lactation during pregnancy, drops after delivery, and fluctuates while she nurses. Because many, but not all, women stop ovulating and menstruating while breastfeeding, lactation has acquired the reputation of a natural (though actually unreliable) contraceptive.

Causes. Tranquilizers, reserpine and aldomet (high blood pressure medications), tiny benign pituitary tumors (microadenomas), hypothyroidism, or unidentified factors can cause excessive secretion of this hormone (hyperprolactinism), which occurs in about 15 percent of women with ovulatory problems. This imbalance can either block ovulation, or impair the process, which may result in luteal phase defect.

Symptoms. About 30 percent of patients with hyperprolactinism have milk in their breasts, a condition called galactorrhea. (Breast milk is not always spontaneously released; in some cases, it may be detected by massaging the breasts and gently squeezing the nipples.) Other symptoms may include decreased vaginal secretions, irregular ovulation, and amenorrhea. Not all women with these problems, however, have elevated prolactin levels; conversely, women with hyperprolactinism may not experience any of the above-mentioned symptoms.

Diagnosis. Although prolactin was recognized more than a century ago, a simple blood test for measuring its presence was not developed until the mid 1970s. Specialists now consider between 0 and 20 ng/milliliter (ng=one billionth of a gram) in the normal range. Higher levels are considered abnormal and can exceed 100 ng/milliliter when pituitary tumors are present.

PITUITARY TUMOR TESTING

❦ My blood test revealed a high prolactin level. I had to have a scan of my pituitary gland done to ensure there wasn't a tumor there causing the imbalance.

Pituitary tumor? The very phrase wreaked such terror in me that I nearly fainted at the suggestion. I closed my eyes and tried to feel if something was there.

Prolactin-secreting pituitary adenomas, *which in all reported cases have been benign*, occur in 5 percent of women with secondary amenorrhea. Although this can be a frightening prospect, it is important to remember that the pituitary gland is not part of the brain but is located below it; *pituitary adenomas will not impair or affect brain function.*

When a blood serum test reveals hyperprolactinism, your specialist may recommend a CAT (computerized axial tomography) scan or an MRI (magnetic resonance imaging) to check for adenomas. Usually performed on an outpatient basis in the hospital, a CAT scan is an X-ray technique that produces a computerized picture of the brain and its adjacent structures with remarkable accuracy. The scan uses less radiation than a regular head X-ray and produces photographs of minute, carefully defined areas of the pituitary gland, which can reveal adenomas or cysts. The patient must lie still on an X-ray table for thirty to forty-five minutes, a difficult task if one feels anxious or nervous. The machine is kept in a cool room, so ask for a blanket if you feel uncomfortable. During the scan your head may be encompassed by the machine and this can cause sensory deprivation. Some patients are positioned with their heads rest-

ing below their shoulders in a recessed, padded area. This can also be disorienting. Let the technician know which position is most comfortable for you. Visualizing relaxing, peaceful scenes can relieve boredom and fear.

An MRI is a procedure that utilizes a magnetic field, rather than radiation,
to create an image of the internal organs and structures of the body. The patient
lies in a capsule-like enclosure. For several intervals of about fifteen minutes
each, the capsule is inserted in the imaging chamber for the test. The technician
will explain the procedure in advance. Most patients are offered earphones to
listen to relaxing music during the procedure. In some cases, a sedative may be
offered to patients who are uncomfortable in close quarters.

Although CAT scan or MRI films are taken by a technician, only a radiologist may interpret the tests and convey those findings to your specialist. Waiting to hear the results is often the most difficult part of the experience.

Treatment. Because pituitary adenomas are benign and rarely measure
more than 1/3 inch in diameter, surgery is rarely recommended; instead adenomas are usually treated with the drug bromocriptine. It is thought that this drug
shrinks the tumor while the medication is taken, but it is not known whether
the tumor will grow again after the drug is stopped. (Bromocriptine is described
more fully below.)

Emotional Support. A suspected pituitary tumor is a frightening prospect to many women. It is important to remember, however, that all prolactin-
secreting pituitary adenomas are benign and bromocriptine treatment offers
encouraging success rates. For reassurance and emotional support, many
RESOLVE chapters (see Resources) can refer you to other women and men who
have been tested and treated for pituitary adenomas.

Absence of Gonadotropin-Releasing Hormone (GnRH)

Originating from the hypothalamus, GnRH triggers the release of FSH and
LH from the pituitary gland. The hypothalamus may cease to secrete GnRH in
response to stress or for other unknown reasons, and this may in turn halt the
pituitary gland's hormonal activity.

At first, GnRH was administered to patients in continuous doses of either
too great or too little quantity. It has since been discovered that the brain
releases GnRH in a pulsing manner. The ovulation pump, a device that mimics
the brain's method of release, and treatment with injections of hMG (Pergonal)
are options for this condition (see discussion below).

Luteal Phase Defects

❦ Diagnosing my luteal phase problem required numerous
endometrial biopsies. I also lost several early pregnancies. I felt like I
was on an emotional roller coaster of hope, disappointment, and
grief.

The luteal phase of a woman's cycle normally encompasses the ten to fourteen days between ovulation and her next menstrual period. When this half of the cycle lasts nine days or less, or inadequate levels of progesterone hormone are secreted during this phase, the patient is thought to have a luteal phase defect (LPD). This complaint, which occurs in about 5 percent of infertility patients, is a poorly understood set of hormonal fluctuations that prevent the body from achieving or sustaining pregnancy. Women with this problem may also suffer multiple miscarriages.

Luteal phase problems may be caused by a low output of progesterone hormone, which results in an inadequate maturation of the endometrial lining. The embryo then has difficulty implanting and surviving its early gestation. It is also thought that a high prolactin level or use of clomiphene may contribute to luteal phase problems.

Diagnosis. A luteal phase defect is usually diagnosed by a low blood serum progesterone test (taken seven days after ovulation), along with an endometrial biopsy (performed a few days before the expected menstrual period) that indicates a development lag in the maturation of the endometrium of two or more days. Known to occur sporadically in many women, luteal phase defect should be documented in at least two successive menstrual cycles before a diagnosis is made.

Treatment. Luteal phase problems are usually treated with clomiphene, clomiphene and human chorionic gonadotropin (hCG), or natural progesterone suppositories. Forms of synthetic progesterone, such as birth control pills, are not recommended because they may cause birth defects. Some specialists recommend intramuscular injections of progesterone to support early pregnancy in women with a history of miscarriage. However, there is controversy among experts about whether this is effective.

Infertility specialists also differ on whether to use clomiphene to treat luteal phase defect problems. Paradoxically this drug sometimes causes luteal phase problems in women with normal ovulatory cycles by affecting progesterone secretion. Although pregnancy rates of 40 to 50 percent have been reported with hormonal treatment, the best treatment for luteal phase defect problems remains elusive.

Emotional Impact. Luteal phase problems exact a heavy emotional toll. Frequent endometrial biopsies may be required, and there are often false pregnancy hopes or miscarriages. If you suffer from this problem, be sure to seek emotional support as well as competent medical care.

Cervical Mucus Problems

The cervix contains more than a hundred tiny glands that secrete mucus throughout the menstrual cycle. This mucus, which changes character and consistency as estrogen levels shift, plays a critical role in fertility.

During most of the cycle, the cervical mucus is quite acidic, thick, and cloudy and creates a barrier that prevents bacteria, sperm, and other foreign substances from entering the uterus. When sperm encounter this type of mucus, they usually die within a few hours.

In response to the increase in estrogen levels as the body prepares to release an egg, the tiny cervical opening (os) dilates slightly, and the glands increase mucus production about thirty-fold. The mucus, composed of about 98 percent water with traces of salts and proteins, becomes thin and clear. The pH of the mucus becomes slightly alkaline, a "sperm-friendly" solution that serves as a buffer to the vagina's normally acidic environment.

Under the microscope this ideal mucus has a lacy, fernlike appearance. The mucus forms long narrow filaments with large open spaces between them. Over the course of several hours or days, the sperm swim through these spaces, enter the uterus, and move through the Fallopian tubes in search of an ovum. For up to three days, the mucus acts as a reservoir for continuous release of sperm into the uterus. After ovulation occurs, progesterone levels increase. In response, the cervical mucus becomes thick and opaque and again forms a barrier.

It is important to note, however, that each woman's body varies in the amount and consistency of mid-cycle mucus. Some women easily detect mucus in the vagina or on toilet tissue. Some can actually pull and stretch it between their fingers. Other women may feel "dry" in the vagina when, in fact, perfect mid-cycle mucus is present near the cervix. Some women also get pregnant with scanty or thick mucus.

Inadequate or scant mid-cycle mucus, however, may impair fertility in some cases. It is estimated that 10 to 15 percent of female infertility patients have a cervical mucus problem, although it is difficult to determine whether this is the *sole* factor in the couple's infertility. In many cases the cause of mucus problems is not known, although hormonal abnormalities are often a contributing factor.

The Hühner (or postcoital) test, performed during the female infertility workup, checks the quality and quantity of mid-cycle mucus and the sperm's reaction to it. "Poor" mid-cycle cervical mucus is usually thick and cellular and may contain white or red blood cells.

Treatment. There are, unfortunately, few effective treatments for cervical mucus problems. Some infertility specialists prescribe estrogen pills for seven to ten days prior to ovulation to stimulate mucus production. Possible side effects to estrogen treatment include water retention or bloating, nausea, or breast tenderness.

Intrauterine insemination (IUI), a procedure where the semen is placed directly into the uterus to bypass the mucus completely, may also be recommended. IUI offers up to a 25 percent success rate.

Premature Ovarian Failure

🐝 I was diagnosed with premature ovarian failure in my mid-thirties. It was unexpected and a terrible shock. The doctor mentioned the option of egg donor in vitro fertilization. I found myself excited about the chance for a pregnancy, yet grieving at the same time for the loss of my own eggs and genetic children.

Premature ovarian failure (POF) is a condition in which the ovaries "shut down" and cease to manufacture hormones before menopause has naturally occurred. This problem occurs in about 10 percent of women with ovulation problems associated with infertility. POF can be caused by a number of factors. There may be decreased numbers of oocytes (germ cells), destruction of these cells after birth, or an acceleration of the natural disintegration process. Sometimes exposure to radiation or chemotherapy can affect the functioning of the ovaries. An autoimmune response, some types of chromosomal abnormalities, and perhaps even a genetic tendency may also be underlying causes. In many cases, the cause is unknown.

POF is an irreversible condition. Some specialists recommend treatment with estrogen to prevent osteoporosis and atrophy of the genital tract. Although it is unlikely in most cases, pregnancy may occur in 5 percent of women with POF after estrogen treatment.

Until a few years ago, women with POF had little hope for pregnancy and often experienced the deep grief of permanent infertility. Egg donor in vitro fertilization, a recent advance in Assisted Reproductive Technology (ART), now offers a treatment option to women with POF. This procedure involves stimulating the development of eggs and retrieving them from a donor, fertilizing them with the mate's sperm, and then transferring these embryos to the patient's uterus for gestation. This complex physical, emotional, and ethical process is discussed in chapter 14.

Post-Birth Control Pill Syndrome

🐝 I took the Pill for four years. After I stopped, it was a long nine months before my periods resumed. I was afraid I wouldn't ovulate again without drug treatment.

Birth control pills prevent ovulation by suppressing the activity of the pituitary and hypothalamus glands. After the Pill is stopped, it may take from three to twelve months before the body resumes normal ovulatory cycles.

Most specialists prefer to let the body resume its cycles naturally. For about 5 percent of women who stop taking the Pill, however, a year or more will pass without a resumption of ovulation. These are usually women who experienced irregular periods before taking the Pill and may have a predisposition to ovulatory problems. In these cases, fertility drug treatment may be considered.

TABLE 9.1 "FERTILITY" (OVULATION-INDUCING) DRUGS

Drug	Function	Contraindications
Clomiphene (Brand names Clomid, Serophene)	Induces ovulation by chemically stimulating the pituitary gland to produce hormones that trigger the ovulation process	May not be appropriate for patients with large fibroid tumors, ovarian cysts or liver problems
Bromocriptine (Brand name Parlodel)	Reduces pituitary's production of prolactin hormone while it is taken	May not be appropriate for patients with pituitary tumors larger than 1 cm
Human Menopausal Gonadotropin or hMG (Brand name Pergonal), Follicle Stimulating Hormone (FSH) (Brand name Metrodine)	Stimulates ovary to develop follicles. In addition, an injection of Human Chorionic Gonadotropin required to trigger ovulation	May not be appropriate in cases of pituitary tumor or ovarian cysts
Gonadotropin Releasing Hormone (GnRH)	Triggers normal pituitary hormonal activity so ovulation can occur	Effective only in women with hypothalamic amenorrhea

NOTE: This table should be read across pp. 132 and 133. Costs based on an average of several San Francisco Bay Area pharmacies and fertility clinic charges.

Ovulation Inducing Drugs

Five different drugs have been developed to help women who ovulate either infrequently or not at all. Most experts believe that they do not improve fertility in women who ovulate regularly, and should not be prescribed in these cases. (Ovulation induction with one of these drugs, however, may be recommended for women undergoing an ART or intrauterine insemination [IUI] cycle. See *Chapters 14* and *16*.)

Before beginning treatment with any ovulation inducing drug, each infertile woman and her mate must be individually and thoroughly evaluated to rule out any other problem that may be affecting fertility.

These drugs—clomiphene, bromocriptine, human menopausal gonadotropin (hMG), follicle stimulating hormone (FSH), and gonadotropin-releasing hormone (GnRH)—are appropriate only in specific situations (see Table 9.1). Although the FDA has tested, and in some cases approved, the use of these medications for fertility problems, it is important to note that the long-term effects of these drugs on the patient, as well as her or his unborn children, are not known. It is wise as a patient, consumer, and a potential parent to educate your-

Dosage	Side Effects	1992 Cost/Cycle
Usually 50 mg/day for 5 days; dosage may be increased to 250 mg/day for 5 – 8 days if necessary	Vary in frequency and intensity with each patient; may include nausea, vomiting, visual problems, headache, insomnia, hot flashes, breast tenderness, heightened emotional sensitivity, painful ovulation, decreased menstrual flow, up to 10% chance of twins	$30 – $40
2.5 mg 2 or 3 times/day	May include nausea, nasal stuffiness, dizziness, low blood pressure, headache	$75 – $112
Controlled doses of 10 – 24 ampules given by injection for 9 – 12 days	20 – 40% possibility of multiple births; small risk of hyperstimulation syndrome; involves a great deal of emotional stress	About $50 – $70 per ampule or $450 for a kit of 10 ampules, plus $300 – $500 for ultrasounds, blood work, and office visits
An ovulation pump administers minute, pulsating injections every 90 minutes	No known physical side effects; patient must carry pump and attached IV tubing for one or two weeks or until ovulation occurs	$1,500 – $2,000 per cycle for pump rental, hormone, tubing, and monitoring

self about the history, side effects, and success rates of any recommended drug. Discuss any questions and concerns with your specialist and others who have taken the drug. Other sources of information about fertility drugs include medical articles, RESOLVE publications (see Resources), and literature from pharmaceutical companies. (Chapter 4 includes suggestions for doing your own medical research.)

CLOMIPHENE (BRAND NAMES CLOMID, SEROPHENE)

❦ Clomiphene greatly affected my moods and ability to cope. I felt these changes a day after I began the pills until about thirty-six hours after I stopped. I began to dread "clomiphene days," but was afraid that if I stopped taking it I wouldn't ovulate. Luckily I had no problem with ovarian cysts.

❦ I conceived my son after one cycle of clomiphene. I just couldn't ovulate without it. I was lucky it worked so quickly and I felt no ill effects.

Clomiphene, the most commonly prescribed fertility drug, is used primarily by women who ovulate either irregularly or not at all. Hundreds of thousands of patients have taken clomiphene over the past twenty-five years. It has been found to work best in women who ovulate occasionally, but *does not* improve fertility in those with regular menstrual cycles. Clomiphene may also be prescribed to improve progesterone production after ovulation, a common cause of luteal phase defect, and in cases of polycystic ovarian disease. Some men also take clomiphene to try to improve low sperm counts (see chapter 15).

An antiestrogen, clomiphene induces ovulation by blocking the estrogen receptors in the ovary and tricking the pituitary into producing more FSH. These hormones stimulate the ovary to ripen several follicles, which increases estrogen levels. When clomiphene is stopped, the hypothalamus detects the estrogen and prompts the pituitary to release a surge of LH, which stimulates ovulation

Is Clomiphene a "Safe" Drug? In recent years, concerns have been raised by women's health groups, and in a number of magazine and newspaper articles, about the safety and long-term effects of clomiphene use for women and those children conceived during treatment cycles or in the months after the medication is stopped.

Clomiphene has been prescribed for more than two decades to large numbers of women. Although it is an estrogen compound, chemically related to diesthylbestrol (DES), there have been no scientific findings to date that clomiphene use for ovulation induction produces detrimental, long-term effects in women or their offspring. In appropriate cases, clomiphene is prescribed in low dosages before conception occurs and should be stopped as soon as pregnancy is confirmed. DES, on the other hand, was administered for months *during* pregnancy and thereby caused damage to the developing reproductive systems of some exposed fetuses.

Although experts disagree about how long traces of the drug remain in the body, most feel that, in low dosages taken before conception occurs, clomiphene does not have any lasting, harmful effects on patients or developing fetuses. To the extent that it is not inherently dangerous or life-threatening, clomiphene is considered a "safe" drug by the medical profession. As with any medication, patients considering clomiphene treatment must weigh the possible risks of using the drug against the possible benefits.

Contraindications. Clomiphene should not be prescribed if large fibroid tumors are present, as it can cause them to grow. (Treatment in cases of small fibroids should be carefully discussed with your specialist.) This drug is also not appropriate for patients with ovarian cysts or liver problems.

Periodic Pelvic Examinations. Normally clomiphene causes some ovarian enlargement, which is usually not harmful or dangerous. Ideally a follicular cyst about an inch in diameter develops, forms a corpus luteum, and dissolves if pregnancy does not occur. Although the risk of forming other types of cysts is very low if successful ovulation takes place, a woman taking clomiphene should have periodic pelvic examinations to ensure that her ovaries are not enlarging abnormally. Your specialist will advise you on how often to schedule appointments.

Dosage. Clomiphene is administered orally, usually in doses of 50 milligrams daily for five days, beginning with the second to fifth day of the menstrual cycle. The dosage may be increased, from 100 milligrams to as much as 250 milligrams per day, for five to eight days if the patient does not respond.

Side Effects. Clomiphene increases estrogen in the body to higher levels than in a normal ovulatory cycle, which causes some side effects in many, but not all, women who take it. Some of these same problems also occur with birth control pills, another type of hormonal therapy. The intensity and frequency of side effects vary with each patient.

Reported side effects include nausea, vomiting, vision problems, headache, insomnia, hot flashes, mood swings, irritability, and breast tenderness, and in rarer instances, ovarian cysts. Because clomiphene can also cause dizziness or vision problems, be cautious while driving or performing chores requiring alertness. Immediately report any side effect to your specialist.

Because it is an antiestrogen, clomiphene may also diminish the quality and quantity of cervical mucus. If this happens, IUI treatment may be recommended (see chapter 16). Other specialists prescribe synthetic estrogen (Estrace or Premarin) from Day 8 through Day 16 of the cycle. It can be difficult to balance the clomiphene and estrogen, and dosages may need to be adjusted.

Emotional Effects of Clomiphene. Many women complain of intense mood swings and heightened emotional sensitivity while taking clomiphene. Besides causing personal frustration, these reactions may contribute to marital stress. In addition, some physicians discount their patients' complaints about the emotional effects of clomiphene, which may cause friction between doctor and patient.

Success Rate. About 70 percent of patients ovulate and about 40 percent become pregnant within a year of clomiphene treatment. Most pregnancies occur within the first three months of treatment, and there is a 5 to 10 percent chance of conceiving twins with clomiphene use.

Cost. Clomiphene is the least expensive fertility drug. A one-cycle supply of five 50 milligram tablets may range from $30 to $35 or more. As with any prescription medication, it may be worthwhile to shop around before ordering.

BROMOCRIPTINE (BRAND NAME PARLODEL)

❦ I conceived my daughter after taking bromocriptine for nine cycles. Luckily I felt no side effects from it. We stopped the drug immediately after a positive early pregnancy test. Still, my baby was exposed to the drug for several weeks and I do worry about that.

❦ The initial effects were literally staggering. For two days I couldn't stand up without having the room spin. I was ready to

give up when, on the the third morning, I got out of bed and, to
my surprise, life was back to normal.

Bromocriptine, a drug first marketed in 1978, controls hyperprolactinism
by suppressing hypothalamic activity and shrinking pituitary adenomas. *This
drug does not cure hyperprolactinism*, but it will reduce prolactin levels *while it is
taken*. Previous symptoms often recur when the drug is stopped.

Before recommending treatment with this drug, your specialist may recommend a CAT scan or MRI test to insure that pituitary tumors (adenomas) are
not causing the imbalance (see section above). Although this medication can be
used by patients with adenomas smaller than one centimeter, patients with
larger tumors may not respond as well to the drug.

Dosage. Bromocriptine is introduced slowly, usually beginning with a
fraction of a dose per day, gradually increasing daily dosage as side effects subside. This approach usually prevents sudden drops in blood pressure as well.
Eventually, a dosage of 2.5 milligrams of the drug is taken two or three times
daily with meals to alleviate nausea. The drug is also available in vaginal sup-
pository form. Its use should be discontinued when a pregnancy is confirmed.

Side Effects. Initially many patients taking bromocriptine experience
nausea, nasal congestion, dizziness (especially in the morning), low blood pressure, or headache. These symptoms usually abate with time, often after the
first few doses. While your body adjusts to the drug, it is wise to avoid sudden
changes in posture and to use caution when driving or engaging in activities
requiring alertness.

This drug has been used extensively in Europe, Japan, and the United
States since the mid 1970s. Its use has not been associated with a greater incidence of birth defects or miscarriage than occurs in the general population.

Success Rates. About 90 percent of women will ovulate with bromocriptine as long as it is taken. Pregnancy rates range between 65 and 85 percent.

Cost. Each tablet costs about $1.20. They must be taken continuously, two
to three times daily — an expense of about $75 to $112 per month.

HUMAN MENOPAUSAL GONADOTROPIN (hMG)
(BRAND NAME PERGONAL)

❦ I'm now trying hMG for the fourth and last time. I've been lucky
not to have any physical discomfort or side effects. Still, so much
rides on each attempt — physically, financially, and emotionally.

Yet this experience has also brought my husband and me
closer. He has been trained to give me some of the shots at home.
He's also come for the ultrasound tests; together we've seen the
developing follicles on the screen. It's been hard not to consider
each follicle as a "mini-pregnancy" even though they haven't
been fertilized yet! At first we even gave each one a nickname,
but we soon stopped that. It was so painful when I didn't get

pregnant. We both feel, though, that it has been a wonder to witness the growth of an egg. The ultrasound has given us a window into a miracle.

A very expensive and laboriously prepared medication, hMG is composed of purified FSH and LH hormone. Developed in the early 1960s, it is a natural hormone made from the urine of postmenopausal women. When the ovary detects hMG in the blood, it assumes that FSH has been released by the pituitary. In response, the ovary develops numerous follicles, even though the pituitary and hypothalamus have remained dormant. Ovulation, however, cannot occur without an injection of human chorionic gonadotropin (hCG), which simulates the presence of the LH surge.

This drug is most often prescribed to women with low estrogen levels who do not respond to clomiphene. It may also be used in cases of polycystic ovarian disease or luteal phase defects, or during ovulation induction for one of the Assisted Reproductive Technology (ART) procedures. In some cases hMG may be taken in conjunction with clomiphene. It is also sometimes prescribed for men with low sperm counts. The use of hMG can result in multiple fetuses and, in rare cases, hyperstimulation of the ovaries. For this reason, *only specialists experienced with the use of hMG should carefully monitor and supervise patients using this drug.*

Contraindications. Before hMG is prescribed, the possibility of pituitary tumor should be investigated. In addition, it should not be used if thyroid or adrenal problems or ovarian cysts are present.

Procedure. Treatment can begin at any time if the patient is not ovulating. In some cases, and particularly during ovulation induction for an ART procedure, the patient may take a preliminary series of GnRH agonist shots to shut down her present cycle (see chapter 11). Pharmacies sell hMG by individual units (ampules), or in kits that contain up to ten glass vials of both powdered hMG and distilled water. The powder and sterile water are mixed, and this solution is injected intramuscularly in controlled doses for nine to twelve days. Some specialists will train the patient or her husband to administer the shots, a way to involve both partners and reduce some of the necessary office visits.

During treatment the patient is carefully monitored for estrogen levels, ovarian enlargement, and cervical mucus changes. Frequent pelvic examinations, trans-vaginal ultrasound, and blood tests are performed to monitor the number and quality of developing follicles and to adjust the dosage of hMG. If more than four follicles develop (for procedures other than ART), most specialists advise discontinuing treatment until these ova disintegrate, and then resuming a new treatment cycle a few weeks later.

When an ultrasound reveals that the eggs are mature, an injection of 10,000 IU of hCG is given. Ovulation usually occurs twenty-four to thirty-six hours later.

Side Effects. Use of hMG has always carried a high rate of multiple births. Although ultrasound techniques have reduced this likelihood, there is a 20 percent occurrence of twins, 5 percent incidence of triplets, and about a 1 percent chance of quadruplets resulting from hMG treatment. Most physicians will not proceed with a cycle if more than five follicles develop, unless an ART cycle is being attempted. There may also be the risks of miscarriage or premature delivery associated with multiple births.

Many women complain of abdominal tenderness or bloatiness while taking hMG. Usually these symptoms are a nuisance, but not inherently dangerous. In about 1 to 3 percent of hMG cycles, however, excessive estrogen levels lead to hyperstimulation syndrome, characterized by ovarian enlargement, abdominal swelling, fluid retention, and weight gain. (Women with polycystic ovarian disease may be more likely to develop this problem, and some specialists prefer to prescribe FSH, discussed below, to these women rather than hMG.) Severe cases of hyperstimulation require immediate hospitalization and continued observation for one to three weeks until the swelling subsides.

Emotional Factors. A course of hMG, for either natural or ART attempts at pregnancy, requires intense, almost daily involvement in office visits, injections, examinations, and monitoring tests for nine to twelve days. Because the patient and her partner can watch the maturation of the follicles, many are extremely frustrated and disappointed if ovulation or pregnancy does not occur. In fact, some experts estimate that up to 30 percent of hMG cycles are canceled because of inadequate or excessive follicular development or early, spontaneous ovulation, That hMG is offered to women who do not respond to other fertility drugs, and is thus often a final course of medical treatment, intensifies the couple's emotional stress.

Cost. Treatment with hMG is expensive. Depending on the pharmacy and potency, ampules cost between $50 and $60 each and up to several dozen may be used each month. Costs for office visits, ultrasounds, and blood work must also be added, which may bring per cycle costs to $2,000 or more. Medical insurance coverage for hMG treatment varies between companies and group or individual policies.

Success Rates. More than 75 percent of women ovulate with hMG treatment. Between 20 and 60 percent of these patients will get pregnant, depending on the nature of their hormonal problems and whether other infertility factors are present in either partner. The miscarriage rate may be slightly higher than that of the general population.

FOLLICLE STIMULATING HORMONE (FSH) (BRAND NAME METRODIN)

This drug is sometimes prescribed alone, or in addition to hMG, for ovulation induction. Unlike hMG, FSH does not containing leutinizing hormone (LH). Combining the two drugs increases the FSH/LH ratio and may help follicle development in those women who do not respond to hMG alone. Some, but not all experts, think that FSH may be especially helpful for women with polycystic ovarian disease.

Side effects, contraindications, emotional issues, costs, and success rates of FSH are similar to those of hMG.

GONADOTROPIN-RELEASING HORMONE (GnRH) AND THE OVULATION PUMP

❦ After obtaining as much information as we could handle, we added the also necessary leap of faith. Since I do not ovulate on my own, the benefit of treatment that stimulates ovulation is clear; ovulation, however, is not enough. Months of clomiphene did not result in conception a second time. After a pause of several years, we decided an ovulation pump — a small, programmed machine that injects measured intravenous doses of GnRH — was more likely to result in conception, with fewer negative side effects. Worn on a belt for the first half of a menstrual cycle, with an unobtrusive IV line threaded down my sleeve, the pump caused me no problems. I knew it was a temporary encumbrance, and experienced no skin infection or pain at the site where a needle entered my arm. A soft, barely perceptible sound at each timed hormone infusion was the secret I literally carried with me.

❦ I consider the pump a mixed blessing. It has given me the gift to discover my body can function normally with a little help. However, inserting the needles has often been physically painful. I've also had to make a big adjustment to physically carrying the pump and tubing around for a week or two. Still, I prefer the pump and GnRH treatment in both a physical and emotional sense to hMG.

A natural hormone, GnRH can be used by women with polycystic ovarian disease or those who do not respond to clomiphene, but it does not seem to help women with a luteal phase defect. A device has been developed to administer this hormone to anovulatory women. A battery-run pump about three inches by four inches, often used by diabetics to deliver measured doses of insulin, administers a minute, pulsating injection of GnRH every ninety minutes around the clock. These small intermittent doses mimic hypothalamic stimulation of the pituitary. The body then takes over and releases the other hormones necessary for a normal cycle, although an hCG injection is often given to support ovulation.

This treatment is performed on an outpatient basis and can be started at any time. The GnRH hormone is placed in a bag inside the pump. One end of a generous length of plastic tubing is attached to the pump; the other end contains a needle, which is inserted in an arm vein and securely bandaged. The site of the needle is changed every four or five days. Long-sleeved clothing can be worn over the tubing, and the pump can be carried in a pocket or worn at the waist. The pump is needed only until ovulation has occurred.

No side effects or increased risk of multiple births from use of GnRH have been reported. Some patients, however, have had problems at the site of the needle insertion with skin irritations or infections. Because of this factor and the inconvenience of wearing the apparatus, some physicians and patients prefer ovulation induction with hMG.

Success Rates. Most patients ovulate in one to two weeks and pregnancy rates vary among clinics. Call those you are considering and ask for their success rates.

Cost. In 1992, the per-cycle cost for pump and tubing rental, GnRH drug, and monitoring charges was between $1,500 and $2,000.

Coping with Fertility Drugs

Many women and men find it difficult to separate a fertility drug's effects from the overall physical and emotional stress of infertility. If you do experience adverse reactions to any drug, notify your specialist immediately and discuss whether to continue usage or modify dosage. Also share your physical and emotional reactions with your mate. Some of the coping suggestions offered in Part One may be helpful during this time. In addition, seeking information and support from others who have experience with these medications, and periodically reassessing your goals — through a support group or with an infertility counselor — may also ease some of the stress.

CHAPTER 10

Pelvic Abnormalities and Surgical Treatment

❦ The hysterosalpingogram and laparoscopy showed my ovaries swollen with cysts and the Fallopian tubes tangled around them. My specialist reviewed the surgery with us beforehand. He said he would do his best to save both ovaries and tubes, but he was very worried about the right side. "We're dealing with threads here," he said. I closed my eyes and tried to control my fear of losing part of my body.

SEVERAL TYPES OF PELVIC ABNORMALITIES account for about 60 percent of female infertility problems. These include blockage or scarring of the Fallopian tubes, adhesions or endometriosis which may affect any of the reproductive organs, uterine growths or masses (fibroids), and pelvic problems found in some women who were exposed prenatally to the drug, diethylstilbestrol (DES).

This chapter examines the causes, diagnosis, and current surgical treatments for some of these factors. Endometriosis, a common pelvic problem that can affect female fertility, is discussed in chapter 11.

The Fallopian Tubes

The Fallopian tubes (oviducts) were first described by an Italian anatomist, Gabriello Fallopio, in the 1500s. Connected to the uterus and lying just above the ovaries, they play a crucial role in fertility. Their job is to retrieve an ovum as it is released from the ovary, move the sperm toward it, and transport the fertilized egg (embryo) back to the uterus for implantation. They also secrete essential chemicals vital to proper ovum and sperm interaction. Rarely, an embryo will implant in the tube and begin an ectopic pregnancy. In most cases, however, the embryo is successfully transported to the uterus.

The oviduct's external appearance has been described as a smooth muscular tube about four inches in length, that gradually widens to a trumpet-shaped opening containing delicate, gracefully waving tentacle-like ends resembling a sea anemone in appearance and movement. The *infundibulum* is the trumpet-like end that nestles close to the ovary. The rounded distal opening, where the ovum enters, has a diameter of between 1/4 and 1/2 inch. Fringelike projections called *fimbria* grasp the ovum as it is released from the ovary and fertilization usually occurs in this part of the tube. Fimbria can be destroyed by inflammation and do not regenerate themselves.

The infundibulum tapers into the *ampulla* section, a slightly narrower passage that runs about half the length of the tube. This in turn narrows into the *isthmus*, only about 1/8 inch in diameter, which opens into the uterine cavity at the proximal end. Sperm are deposited in the vagina during intercourse, pass through the cervix, are transported by both their own locomotion and uterine contractions up the uterus, and enter the tube at the isthmus.

Normally, numerous hairlike projections called *cilia* line the interior mucus membrane of a Fallopian tube. Interspersed among the cilia are *secretory cells*, which release a fluid that fills the tube. The ovum floats and the sperm swim in this medium. The cilia also facilitate transportation by beating in only one direction and by inducing contractions of the muscular walls of the tube.

The Fallopian tubes are especially fragile and vulnerable to infections and to diseases such as endometriosis. In response to these conditions the tubes become inflamed, summon millions of white blood cells to destroy the invading cells and form scar tissue (adhesions) during the healing process. Adhesions vary in appearance and composition, from tough, webby, or fibrous bands to filmy bits or layers of tissue. Even filmy adhesions can impair the delicate functioning of the tubes. If the infection continues unchecked, the tubes will continue to scar and eventually will close. Rather than allow an infection to spread to the abdomen (a life-threatening condition), the tubes often seal off their ends, sacrificing fertility to ensure the body's survival.

Acute and Chronic Salpingitis (Pelvic Inflammatory Disease)

Pelvic inflammatory disease (PID) is a term commonly used to describe an infection or disease of the pelvic organs. Although pelvic infections often enter through the cervix and can affect the uterus and ovaries, it is usually the Fallopian tubes that suffer fertility impairment. The most fragile and delicate part of the reproductive system, they are also the most seriously affected by infection.

The medical term for PID of the Fallopian tubes is *salpingitis*, and the disease may be present in either acute or chronic form. Acute salpingitis is the active stage of inflammation, usually caused by infection from either a sexually transmitted disease or use of an intrauterine device (IUD). It is often a silent and symptomless process; many women are unaware that they have an infection and do not seek treatment. Infertility specialists rarely see a case of acute salpingitis; instead they see its aftermath. Perhaps years after the original infection, a woman attempts unsuccessfully to conceive. During an infertility workup her specialist discovers chronic salpingitis in the form of tubal blockages, scarring, adhesions, "clubbed" (sealed) ends, or chronically inflamed tissue.

CAUSES OF SALPINGITIS

An epidemic of sexually transmitted diseases, coupled with the use of intrauterine contraceptive devices by many women, has made salpingitis a major health problem in the 1990s. Not surprisingly, the fertility of teenagers and older women alike has been affected. Salpingitis alone now accounts for more than 30 percent of female infertility problems.

Sexually Transmitted Diseases (STDs). According to the Centers for Disease Control, about 12 million Americans contract some type of STD every year and about 25 percent of these cases occur among teenagers. In addition to the well-known venereal diseases syphilis and gonorrhea, more than twenty new varieties of STDs have been identified. These microbes may be bacterial or viral and are passed by genital, oral, or anal sexual contact. If a woman or her mate has had multiple sexual partners, she has a good chance of contracting one of these diseases during her lifetime. For those who are at risk, periodic testing for sexually transmitted diseases is advisable to prevent future fertility problems. The most common STDs are chlamydia and gonorrhea.

Chlamydia is a cross between a bacterial and a viral disease. It is often symptomless and is difficult to diagnose, although some women experience mild to severe abdominal pain or discomfort, a high- or low-grade fever, painful intercourse or menses, spotting between periods, vaginal discharge, or fatigue. Infected men sometimes complain of painful urination or pain after intercourse. Although both sexes can contract chlamydia, it seems to affect fertility most often in women. Men usually act as carriers, although their fertility can also be impaired. Chlamydia can live in the pelvic region for many years and will slowly scar the reproductive organs if left unchecked. To prevent reinfection, both partners are treated with antibiotics such as tetracycline or erythromycin for ten to fourteen days.

Gonorrhea is a bacterial disease that is usually spread through sexual contact. Symptoms in women may include cervical discharge, painful urination, abdominal pain, fever, and vomiting. Some women, however, have no symptoms in the early stages of the infection. Men may have a discharge from the penis or painful urination, although some experience no obvious symptoms. If left unchecked, gonorrhea can result in PID and other complications. Treatment is usually attempted with penicillin; some physicians use tetracycline if the patient is allergic or sensitive to the penicillin drugs.

Intrauterine Devices (IUDs). Although these were once thought to be safe and convenient contraceptives, most physicians now regard IUDs as potentially dangerous devices that have contributed to fertility problems in many women. It has also been suggested that the threads attached to IUDs, which pass through the cervix and into the vagina, often serve as "ladders" to the uterus for infectious bacteria and viruses. Thousands of women, or an estimated 1 percent of all IUD users, subsequently developed salpingitis.

Several different types of IUDs have been prescribed over the years. The Dalkon Shield has received the most publicity as an IUD that has caused injury or fertility impairment in many women. Following lengthy litigation that resulted in a court-awarded settlement, a claims resolution process has been created for women who were injured by Dalkon Shield use. More than 200,000 claims have been filed to date. For those who submitted claims before April, 1986, there may also be funding available for infertility treatment. For further information, contact the Dalkon Shield Trust (see Resources).

It is now believed that *most* IUD devices can cause reproductive problems, and that IUD users roughly double their chances of developing salpingitis compared with women who do not use these contraceptives. Their use is rarely recommended.

DIAGNOSIS OF CHRONIC SALPINGITIS

Once ovulation and cervical mucus factors have been checked, the infertility specialist usually studies the condition of the Fallopian tubes. A pelvic examination may sometimes, but not always, reveal tubal or uterine tenderness, decreased organ mobility, or a palpable mass suggesting salpingitis.

Several workup tests can be performed to check whether the tubes are open (patent) and free of blockages or adhesions. Hysterosalpingogram (HSG), laparoscopy, and perhaps hysteroscopy can often determine whether the tubes are open and if adhesions, fibroids, or endometriosis are present. (See chapter 8 for further discussion of these tests.)

The presence of chronic salpingitis is often not discovered until laparoscopy, usually the last procedure of the standard female workup. During laparoscopy, pelvic problems can be assessed and, depending on their location and severity, may also be treated surgically at that time.

Surgical Treatment for Pelvic Abnormalities

❦ The surgery removed my right ovary and repaired my left tube from an ectopic pregnancy. Moderate endometriosis was also found. As I came out of the anesthetic and heard this, I thought, "How will I get pregnant now?"

The Evolution of Microsurgery. The technique of surgery by microscope, or microsurgery, was first used about sixty-five years ago. It was initially adapted for gynecological procedures in the late 1960s, and is now widely utilized in fertility surgery, most commonly on Fallopian tubes and ovaries damaged by inflammation, infection, previous sterilization (tubal ligation), or endometriosis. (See chapter 11 for additional discussion of surgery for endometriosis.)

Previously such surgery was performed without a microscope (macrosurgery) and was not very successful in terms of subsequent pregnancies. The advent of microsurgery provided greater magnification of the affected area, more delicate and precise cutting and suturing, and gentler handling of the tissues. The needles and suturing material used are significantly smaller than those used in macrosurgery. In addition, equipment and techniques are being constantly improved and refined in this surgical specialty.

In the past five years, there have been rapid and exciting advances in surgical technique — particularly in the area of laparoscopic surgery, which also provides magnification of the operating field. Most procedures, which once required major surgery with a two- to five-inch pelvic incision (laparotomy), are now performed on an out patient basis through the laparoscope. Usually only a tiny incision through the navel is required, and perhaps several other small incisions to insert other surgical instruments. Often these corrective surgeries are done at the time of diagnostic laparoscopy; in a few cases, they may be rescheduled soon afterward.

Many specialists now recommend laparoscopic surgery for up to 90 percent of their patients who require pelvic surgery. Procedures that, just a few years ago, involved up to a five-day in-patient hospital stay and three to six weeks of convalescence are now done on an outpatient basis. Patients are able to return home the same day and resume normal activities within a week. For women and men alike (laparascopic surgery is being increasingly utilized in male reproductive treatment), these technological strides have significantly reduced the duration, trauma, disability, and expense of surgery as well as loss of wages and time from work.

Indications for Laparoscopic Surgery. Once the Fallopian tube or its lining is irrevocably damaged, it cannot be replaced, restored, or regenerated. Attempts at tubal transplants have not been successful to date. There are, however, many cases where tubal blockages, adhesions, ligations, or cysts of the reproductive organs can be bypassed or removed with surgery in an attempt to restore fertility.

Following an infection, blockages, adhesions, or scarring of the tubes can occur in a number of locations — at the proximal end near the uterine junction, throughout the middle section of the tube, or at the distal opening near the ovary. Blockages near the fimbria, which can result in clubbed ends, commonly occur and may be especially critical to fertility. Fimbria or cilia scarred by infection cannot be restored or replaced. Damage to these delicate structures can seriously impair fertility or increase the chances of tubal pregnancy.

Depending on the location and extent of the tubal, ovarian, or uterine impairment, laparoscopic surgery, major surgery (laparotomy), or an Assisted Reproductive Technology (ART) such as in vitro fertilization (IVF) may be recommended. Each patient must be individually evaluated to decide which treatment is appropriate. This is a prudent approach as pregnancy rates are highest with the initial laparoscopic or major surgery and decline with subsequent attempts. (See chapter 11 for further discussion of surgical treatment for endometriosis.) In some cases, pregnancy rates after microsurgery are so low that IVF may indeed be a more viable option.

Surgery, whether it is a "minor" laparoscopic procedure or a "major" laparotomy, can be an intense, traumatic experience for many patients. Chapter 5 presents a thorough discussion of the physical, emotional, and psychological dynamics of pelvic surgery and anesthesia.

Who Should Perform Laparoscopic or Major Surgery? An infertility specialist should perform these surgeries because the techniques require intensive training and experience to master. The surgeon must carefully control bleeding, precisely cut and suture diseased areas, and handle this delicate tissue gently to minimize new adhesion formation. These techniques are costly to learn, and continuing education is necessary to keep up with technological advances. A specialist should ideally handle one to two cases per week to keep in practice.

To optimize chances for subsequent pregnancy, a range of surgical techniques must be appropriately utilized, and good clinical judgment exercised, by a trained and experienced physician. As one specialist remarked, "Booking a flight on a supersonic jet is futile if your pilot can't fly the plane!" Some sources of referral for infertility specialists are your gynecologist, women's health clinics, or RESOLVE (see Resources).

Laparoscopic Surgery

🐾 Having had a number of surgeries, I can tell you that videolaseroscopy provided validation for, and understanding of, the pain I had been having. It is one thing for a physician to tell you what he or she did, but it is another thing indeed to actually *see* what the source of the problem actually is. Seeing what was wrong and what was done has emotionally and physically helped me deal with my problem. It is also a useful tool and record for the physican and any future doctors you might consult.

As previously stated, many specialists are performing up to 90 percent of pelvic surgery procedures, on an out-patient basis, through the laparoscope. Both electrosurgery, which utilizes an electrical current, and laser techniques are often combined with other tools, such as the Argon Beam Coagulator, to make incisions or remove or vaporize adhesions, cysts, ectopic pregnancies, and fibroids.

Laser. Laser, an acronym for Light Amplification by Stimulated Emission of Radiation, was first adapted to pelvic surgery in 1969 and is now widely used. Electrical energy is applied to either a gaseous or crystal source to produce powerful, concentrated, sometimes-visible wavelengths of light. Each type of wavelength laser interacts with tissue in slightly different ways, enabling extremely precise and carefully controlled cutting, evaporation, and coagulation. Blood vessels are sealed during this process, which some experts believe minimizes the risk of subsequent scar tissue formation. In many instances, it is safer to use laser, rather than electrosurgery, near delicate or critical organs and structures such as the Fallopian tubes, blood vessels, and bowel.

Currently, several types of lasers are available: the CO2, KTP 532, Argon, and neodymium Yag (Nd.Yag). The CO2 is currently the most widely used because it is the easiest to control and the least penetrating of all the varieties. With this laser, the directed beam absorbs the water in the targeted tissue and releases steam that instantaneously vaporizes the surrounding tissue within one millimeter. Use of the KTP 532, a fiberoptic laser, and the Nd.Yag is considered riskier near critical organs, although the former may be extremely effective in coagulating bleeding surfaces. The Argon laser has limited applications at this time. In the near future, adjustable wavelength lasers may be available, which offer all these properties in one instrument.

Despite its amazing capabilities and attendant media attention, the laser is not a magic cure-all. It is simply a precise way to cut or destroy abnormal tissue. By setting and focusing the energy level of the laser, the surgeon can make a fine incision that also coagulates the tissue. Although the speed of laser surgery may reduce operating time and thereby diminish some of the risks of anesthesia, experts disagree about whether sole use of the laser results in less subsequent adhesion formation. Because it does not seem to offer better pregnancy rates than electrosurgery, many specialists regard the laser as an invaluable tool when used in tandem with other techniques.

Argon Beam Coagulator (ABC). One of the latest developments in advanced surgical technique, the ABC was approved for surgical use in late 1991 and has enabled fertility specialists to safely perform even more complex procedures, such as uterine fibroid surgery, through the laparoscope. The ABC directs an electrical current to the tissue through a stream of inert argon gas. Unlike the CO2 laser, the ABC is a smokeless technique that effectively stops tissue bleeding.

TYPES OF LAPAROSCOPIC SURGERY

Several intriguing variations of laparoscopic surgery, which have greatly expanded its application, have recently been developed.

Videolaserlaparoscopy is being increasingly utilized by surgeons. Beside the small incision through the navel required for laparoscopy, several additional incisions between one-quarter to one-half inch are made below the navel or in the lower abdominal wall for this procedure. A tiny videocamera is attached to the laparoscope that provides the surgeon with an excellent, high-resolution view of the operating field. The specialist can also stand up straight during the entire procedure, and experiences much less fatigue than during a regular laparoscopy, where he or she must lean over for an hour or more to look through the instrument. The camera also videotapes the surgery, providing an invaluable record for diagnosis, recommendation for treatment, and consultation with other experts.

Pelviscopy enables surgeons to perform more complex procedures that formerly required major surgery. Through a half-inch incision made through the abdominal wall, adhesions, some ovarian cysts, most ectopic pregnancies, and many smaller uterine fibroids can be removed with and through the laparoscopic instruments. Some of the procedures now performed through laparoscopy and/or pelviscopy include:

□ salpingoneostomy: the closed (clubbed) distal end is opened; in some cases, the ends may be cut and folded back, although some surgeons prefer to use major surgery for this procedure;

□ adhesiolysis: the cutting of adhesions from the reproductive organs or bowel;

□ laparoscopic linear salpingostomy: the removal of an ectopic pregnancy; in about 5 to 20 percent of cases, some fetal tissue may remain necessitating treatment with medication, or possibly another laparoscopy or major surgery, for complete removal of the pregnancy tissue;

□ treatment of some types of ovarian cysts and endometrial impants (further discussed in chapter 11).

Hysteroscopy. In some cases, a hysteroscope may also be utilized during laparoscopic surgery to treat such uterine problems as small fibroids (up to five centimeters), adhesions, and some anatomical irregularities.

Tubal Catheterization and Balloon Tuboplasty. This fairly new, non-surgical technique is often appropriate for proximal tube blockages. A series of catheters containing slender guidewires or tiny balloons, similar to those sometimes used to clear blocked arteries, is carefully directed by X-ray, vaginally guided ultrasound, or through a hysteroscope into the uterus. The catheter is then carefully inserted through the proximal opening of the tube to the blockage. In many cases, gentle pressure will clear the blockage and restore full tubal function. Catheter and balloon tuboplasty has been most effective for women with dislodgeable blockages near the uterine junction. Success rates of up to 40 percent have been reported.

When Is Major Surgery Recommended?

In 5 to 20 percent of patients, a laparotomy requiring an abdominal incision and, in some cases, inpatient hospitalization, may still be recommended. Such cases include:

□ removal of large uterine tumors (fibroids) and repair of congenital uterine abnormalities;

□ proximal tubal blockages that do not respond to other techniques;

□ some types of ovarian cysts, extensive adhesions or presence of endometriosis;

□ the possibility of malignancy;

□ reversal of tubal ligation (reanastomosis). About 1.5 percent of American women who have had tubal ligations, or 15,000 to 20,000 per year, opt for a reversal. In some cases, these decisions are prompted by remarriage; others tragically lose a child and wish to become pregnant again. Most specialists recommend major surgery for this procedure;

some are performing this surgery, with smaller incisions and delicate technique, on an outpatient basis.

In this event, the patient, her mate, and their specialist can decide whether major surgery will be done immediately after laparoscopy or at a later date. Some women and physicians prefer to discuss the findings of the laparoscopy and then schedule major surgery at a later time. Others may want surgery to proceed immediately after the laparoscopy without the patient regaining consciousness. (See chapter 5 for further discussion of anesthesia and major surgery.)

Risks and Disadvantages of Microsurgery

Because it is so precise and meticulous, microsurgery often requires several hours or longer to complete. Patients are subject to the attendant risks of regional or general anesthesia. The procedures themselves carry a small risk of hemorrhage or perforation of the bowel.

If major surgery is required, patients can expect a two- to five-day hospital stay and a convalescence of at least two to four weeks. Any type of surgery is expensive, as specialized equipment and highly trained personnel are needed. In 1992, an outpatient laparoscopic surgery ran about $8,000. Major surgery, with a three-day hospital stay, can range from $10,000 to $13,000. (Estimates include surgeon, anesthesiologist, and related hospital charges, such as operating room and recovery room time, semi-private room, and medications, and vary widely between patients. Coverage for infertility surgery also varies among insurance carriers and individual policies. See chapter 3 for further discussion.)

Women who have a history of tubal problems and corrective surgery also have a risk five to ten times greater of ectopic pregnancy (5 to 10 percent) than those in the general population (about 1 percent). Depending on the overall condition of the tube, there is also a risk of ectopic pregnancy if the fimbria are damaged or absent. (See chapter 13 for a discussion of the emotional impact of pregnancy loss.)

Success Rates

Pregnancy rates for tubal surgery depend on the location of the blockage or adhesions, the length of remaining tube, the skill of the surgeon, and other fertility factors of the partners, such as age and sperm count or motility. If the fimbria remains intact and a sufficient length of tube is saved, pregnancy rates ranging from 10 to 70 percent are reported.

Successful reversal of a tubal ligation depends on the original site of sterilization, as well as the length of remaining tube, skill of the surgeon, and fertility factors of the partners. Pregnancy rates of 30 to 90 percent have been cited.

Adhesion Formation Following Surgery

After surgery the body sometimes forms scar tissue (adhesions), of varying texture and consistency, during the healing process. In most cases this does not create a problem. It is, however, an unfortunate occurrence in terms of fertility surgery. Subsequent adhesion formation may contribute to continued fertility problems.

In an attempt to inhibit scarring, some specialists prescribe antibiotics and other drugs that are administered intravenously immediately after surgery. Other surgeons place special solutions or substances in the abdominal cavity during surgery to discourage adhesion formation. And newer "barrier" methods, which separate tissue surfaces, are currently undergoing clinical trials to test their effectiveness. Still there is a 50 to 70 percent chance that adhesions will form, which may impair tubal function. This scarring usually occurs within the first few weeks after surgery, and there is no way to know beforehand which patients will be affected. To date, no single approach other than good surgical technique has been proven effective in preventing adhesion formation.

Some specialists will perform a laparoscopy sometime after surgery for a second look. At this time adhesion formation is fresh and can often be broken up through the laparoscope. If pregnancy does not occur after six to twelve months, other specialists recommend a second laparoscopy to check whether scarring has again impaired tubal patency and function. Although "second-look" laparoscopies are effective in reducing adhesions, they do not seem to increase subsequent pregnancy rates. Experts feel that they may be helpful to some, but not all, patients.

Second and Subsequent Laparoscopies or Microsurgeries

The chances for pregnancy are 5 to 25 percent (or about halved) with the second surgical procedure and steadily decrease with subsequent attempts. Assisted Reproductive Technology (ART) currently offers a 10 to 35 percent chance for pregnancy, depending on the procedure, ages, and fertility factors of the partners (see chapter 14). The couple and their specialist may consider ART, adoption, or child-free living a better option after one unsuccessful microsurgery attempt.

DES

❦ As a DES daughter, I am resigned to feeling a bit schizophrenic about infertility treatments. I have been harmed by exposure in utero to an unsafe, ineffective yet very popular reproductive therapy of our parents' generation. My harm includes infertility and loss of a premature baby following infertility treatment. Yet I have also benefitted from current treatments that ultimately allowed me to have a healthy baby. I am resigned especially to reaching decisions about medical intervention when there are no clear answers — indeed there is disagreement — among the experts. The experience of DES exposure reminds us that much is unknown about effectiveness and long-term safety of treatments and that many reproductive therapies are experiments that will not prove successful.

Diethylstilbestrol (DES) is a synthetic form of estrogen, which over the years, has been used as a lactation inhibitor and additive to poultry and livestock feeds. Between 1941 and the early 1970s, DES was prescribed to at least two million pregnant American women (in an estimated 10 percent of all pregnancies during this time) to prevent miscarriage. Its use during pregnancy continued for nearly two decades even though studies performed in 1953 found DES ineffective in preventing miscarriage. "DES daughters and sons" are those offspring whose mothers took diethylstilbestrol during pregnancy.

DID MY MOTHER TAKE DES?

There is a wide range of known and suspected side effects associated with DES exposure, although experts often disagree about diagnosis and treatment. It is helpful for DES offspring to discover the dosage and length of time they were exposed pre-natally. When both patient and physician have this information, early detection and careful monitoring of health-related problems is possible.

Unfortunately there are many women and men who are unaware of their prenatal exposure to DES because their mothers are not sure whether they took the drug during pregnancy. DES Action USA, a nationwide consumer advocacy group, urges anyone born between 1941 and 1972 to "ask your mother." They can provide information and suggestions for tracing medical records. (In many states, patients have a legal right to information contained in their medical records.) DES Action USA has many chapters and is an excellent resource for emotional support, information, and medical referrals (see Resources).

EFFECTS ON HEALTH, FERTILITY, AND PREGNANCY

Many DES children are now in their childbearing years and their experience is providing important data about the drug's effects on fertility. Researchers have discovered a spectrum of suspected and known DES side effects. Correlations to menstrual irregularities, decreased fertility, ectopic pregnancy, and early miscarriage are suspected. In some offspring known side effects include anatomical abnormalities of the reproductive organs that may cause pregnancy complications in DES daughters and decreased fertility in both DES-exposed men and women.

As a result of their prenatal exposure, some DES daughters have structural or cellular abnormalities of the vagina, cervix, Fallopian tubes, or uterus. For example, the uterus may be T shaped or unusually small or the Fallopian tubes may be abnormally shaped or smaller in diameter than those of nonexposed women. Some DES daughters have problems with cervical mucus production, ovulation, conception or embryo implantation, miscarriage, premature deliveries, and tubal pregnancies. There has been less research and study of DES sons, though some experts suspect that some of these men may have problems with undescended testicles or benign cysts of the reproductive tract resulting from their in utero exposure to the drug.

It is important for DES daughters or sons concerned about health, fertility, or pregnancy issues to find specialists or obstetricians familiar with this drug and its long-term effects. A DES daughter should have a special examination periodically (as recommended by her physician) for careful scrutiny, a complex Pap smear of the cervix and vagina, and perhaps a special test of the cervical cells.

Because DES daughters have an increased risk for tubal pregnancy, weakened cervical muscles, and pre-term uterine contractions, early confirmation and close, continuous monitoring of pregnancy is also important. Many medical centers recognize these tendencies, carefully monitor DES-exposed pregnant women, and often refer them to premature labor prevention programs. It is important to remember, however, that an estimated 80 percent of DES daughters will have at least one successful pregnancy.

Continued research on the long-term health and fertility effects of DES exposure is needed. At the time of this writing, however, the funding of a number of DES research projects is in jeopardy. Some programs are being funded on a year-to-year basis; other grants may be discontinued permanently. For more information and ways to help, contact DES Action, USA (see Resources).

CHAPTER 11
Endometriosis

❦ I developed ovarian cysts that contained endometriosis. My tubes were also stuck to the ovaries with scar tissue and couldn't move freely to pick up the eggs at ovulation. It's been hard dealing with both infertility and endometriosis — which can be a serious problem itself — at the same time.

I've been lucky that I haven't had any physical pain during my cycle and little menstrual discomfort, but having endometriosis — and losing parts of my ovaries with each surgery — has affected my self-image and feelings about my body. It has impaired my fertility and I've had to make decisions about surgery, medications, and whether to try to get pregnant sooner than I had planned.

I'm determined, though, to live a happy and fulfilled life. I continue to educate myself about endometriosis and the latest developments in treatment, make informed decisions, eat well and exercise regularly, and find support among other women with this problem.

❦ I've had problems with the symptoms of endometriosis for more than ten years and, for the past five, have undergone surgery and drug treatments with Lupron, Synarel, and Danocrine. During this time, I've had pain throughout the month and "periods from hell" — bad cramping and heavy bleeding for up to a week. Some days I've had to stay in bed.

When endometriosis is this severe, it permeates every part of your life. It is emotionally draining and creeps into your work and affects your relationships with family, friends, and lovers.

I reached a turning point a few years ago. I accepted that this would be a health issue throughout my reproductive years, and looked until I found a physician with education, training, and interest in endometriosis. I read about this subject, ask lots of questions before deciding on any treatment, and belong to an Endometriosis Association support group.

THIS DISEASE IS NAMED AFTER THE endometrial cells that normally compose the lining of the uterus and are expelled each month during menstruation. Endometriosis is caused by the growth of these cells outside the uterus — most typically on or within the ovaries and tubes (collectively termed the adnexa),

Endometriosis.

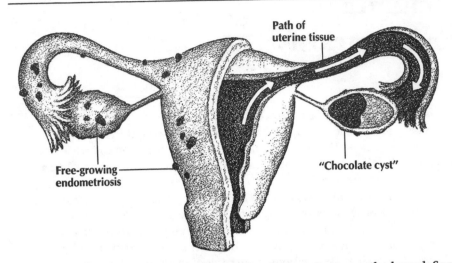

Path of
uterine tissue

Free-growing
endometriosis

"Chocolate cyst"

the exterior of the uterus, within the abdominal cavity, or on the bowel. Some experts, in fact, suggest that there may be a much greater incidence of endometrial implants on the peritoneum (abdominal lining) than previously thought. In very rare cases, endometriosis has also been found in the lungs, heart, arms, and legs, and in the scars of previous Caesarean sections.

Endometriosis was identified by physicians more than eighty years ago, and knowledge about this disease has progressed with research and the advancement of gynecological surgery. The more experts discover about endometriosis, however, the less they seem to understand this enigmatic condition. Women who have the severest manifestations, such as large cysts or massive scar tissue in the pelvis, may have minimal pain or discomfort. Conversely, women with mild endometriosis may experience intense pain with menses and intercourse.

Like the tissue lining the uterus, endometrial implants grow with the fluctuations of estrogen and progesterone hormones during the menstrual cycle. The body sometimes builds cysts (endometriomas or "chocolate cysts") around the foreign cells, and hormonal stimulation may also cause these cysts to grow. Endometriosis may also grow on the reproductive organs and bleed painfully during menstruation. The inflammatory response to these implants, along with hormones (prostaglandins) released by the implants, may contribute to the pain some women with endometriosis experience throughout their cycle and/or during menstruation. (Some women with endometriosis, however, experience little or no pain.)

In 1979, the American Fertility Society devised a classification system to categorize different stages of endometriosis, provide a prognosis for the chances of conception, and report pregnancy rates following treatment. Stages 1 and 2 refer to minimal and mild signs of endometriosis, usually without ovarian or tubal disease; Stage 3 describes moderate disease; and Stage 4 encompasses severe findings of implants, cysts, and/or adhesions. Experts note that there is no correlation to the degree of pain or other symptoms experienced by women in any of these stages, to the recurrence rates subsequent to treatment, or to pregnancy rates for women with a limited degree of endometriosis.

How Does Endometriosis Affect Fertility?

The link between infertility and endometriosis has puzzled physicians for decades, and is probably associated with multiple factors unique to each woman. Between 30 and 40 percent of women who have endometriosis encounter fertility problems, and about 20 percent of infertile women are diagnosed with this problem — often at the time of diagnostic laparoscopy.

Endometriosis rarely causes Fallopian tube blockage, although scar tissue can restrict tubal motility. While there seems to be an association between endometriosis and infertility, there is no direct scientific evidence that minimal or mild endometriosis decreases fertility.

What Causes Endometriosis?

Although it is not known what causes endometriosis, the most common theory suggests that blood and endometrial cells back up through the uterus and tubes (retrograde bleeding), and implant or attach to other reproductive organs. The tissue responds to the usual hormonal fluctuations of the menstrual cycle, triggering repeated inflammatory responses at the site of the disease, that over time result in scar tissue or adhesion formation. The Fallopian tubes, ovaries, and uterus may be affected, and in rarer cases, the abdominal wall, bowel, and ureter.

Although many experts think retrograde menstrual bleeding occurs in most women, only some will develop endometriosis. And of this group, some, but not all, experience fertility problems. It has been suggested that the tendency to develop endometriosis may be hereditary, but this theory has not been scientifically substantiated.

Medical research has also associated chemical substances called prostaglandins with endometriosis. These hormones are normally released by the uterine lining (endometrium) before the menstrual period, causing uterine contractions like menstrual cramps or labor pains. Women with endometriosis may have higher levels of prostaglandins in their pelvic fluids or tissues than other women, and some researchers suspect these chemicals may interfere with the motility (rhythmic contractions) of the Fallopian tubes. This may impair the tubes' ability to move the sperm up toward the ovum or the fertilized embryo back down to the uterus. Higher levels of prostaglandins may also lower the level of progesterone produced by the corpus luteum, which is formed after the ovum is released from the ovary, and thus affect the luteal phase of the menstrual cycle.

Several other theories of possible causes of endometriosis have been suggested. Some experts think endometriosis may sometimes spread to other parts of the body through the blood or lymph system. This theory may explain the extremely rare incidence of the disease in areas outside the abdominal cavity, such as the heart, lungs, or arms. Another theory posits that endometrial cells may migrate during female fetal development to other areas of the abdomen, and after puberty, develop into endometriosis at these sites.

Other, often controversial, literature has been published, by several medical specialists and The Endometriosis Association (see below), suggesting a possible link between an allergic reaction to candida albicans, a yeast that is naturally found in the body, and the development of endometriosis. These experts think that if the candida yeast grows unchecked, normal immune system function may be suppressed or impaired in some women, fostering the growth of endometriosis. Other fertility experts are skeptical of their reasoning, citing a lack of documented scientific data to substantiate this theory.

Which Women Develop Endometriosis?

Endometriosis is diagnosed in about 20 percent of infertile women. It is also found in 15 to 25 percent of all female surgical patients and in 2 to 4 percent of teenage girls who undergo abdominal surgery. The disease process probably begins in the early teen years, shortly after the onset of menstruation. Interruption of the menstrual cycle by pregnancy, breastfeeding, or oral contraceptives often temporarily arrests its progression, although some women develop endometriosis after birthing or nursing one or more children. If the disease continues to develop, it usually reaches its maximum severity in a woman's thirties and early forties. For most women, the onset of menopause and cessation of menstruation halts the disease process and its related symptoms.

The Endometriosis Association has compiled a Data Registry based on more than 3,000 women's case histories. Ninety-three percent of the respondents were Caucasian, averaged thirty-one years of age, and reported a median income level of $35,000 per year. Sixty percent of these women experienced their first symptoms of endometriosis before the age of twenty-five, and received their initial diagnosis up to ten years later. Of those surveyed, the following symptoms were noted: 96 percent had pain throughout their cycles and/or during menstruation; 80 percent had some problem with fatigue, and 44 percent experienced fertility problems.

Endometriosis seems to affect women of every race, socio-economic class, and income level. Although women who have experienced many years of menstrual cycles uninterrupted by pregnancy or lactation may have a greater chance of developing this disease, medical experts still do not know why some women develop endometriosis and others do not. As with many diseases, there is probably a complex set of components that affect the patient's experience, including heredity, hormonal function, reproductive history, immunologic status, uterine anatomical factors, and reactions to medical and surgical treatment.

Symptoms

Some women experience noticeable and quite uncomfortable symptoms with endometriosis. Others report little or no pain or discomfort, and are often surprised when endometriosis is diagnosed by laparoscopy.

Depending on the location of the implants, symptoms may include pain throughout the cycle or with menstruation, painful intercourse (particularly with deep penetration), lower abdominal cramps, heavy and/or irregular vaginal bleeding, rectal pain with defecation, urinary discomfort, and infertility. The degree of pain does not necessarily correlate to the severity of the disease. An inability to get pregnant may occur in 30 to 40 percent of women with endometriosis. In fact, the desire to become pregnant may bring a woman to the infertility workup that reveals the disease.

The Emotional Dynamics of Endometriosis

❦ Receiving a diagnosis of any disease is a painful and frightening experience, and endometriosis is an especially distressing diagnosis to receive. You are told that little is known about the disease, that it may recur in about 50 percent of women after treatment, and that it may affect fertility, although experts aren't always sure why. You have to absorb all of that, worry about whether you'll ever be able to get pregnant if you haven't had children or want to have more, and wonder whether it will come back and when. All your instincts say, "Do something, fight it." But there doesn't seem to be anything you can do to prevent or cure endometriosis — not even surgeries, drugs, or a healthy lifestyle. And a lot of the literature suggests that "competitive" or "aggressive" women are the ones who get it. So then you wonder whether you brought it on yourself!

❦ I am thirty-three years old, single, and part of a vastly populated generation that is caught somewhere between "Friday Night Bars," video dating services, and spending time alone. We all have some sort of grieving process for the loss of our fertility. And my realization of it coincided with an event in a friend's life.

Two years ago, during my initial stage of anger and "Why me?", a good friend became pregnant. A friend without endometriosis. She and her husband were overjoyed. The pregnancy was unexpected. They had been married for thirteen years and a few months earlier decided to "consider" starting a family. Nature and failure of birth control produced the baldest and most charming little fellow named Casey. During her pregnancy I had a shower and invited what we call our "women's group." Everyone was overjoyed and came bearing cuddly baby gifts. I was never jealous of my friends and their families — but after our party celebrating Karen's life, I cried. Why couldn't my closest friends share in my pain with a similar energy that they used to celebrate Karen's joy?

We all lose our fertility at some point in our lives. And to steal an image from poet Donald Justice: "We must learn to close softly the doors to rooms we will not be coming back to." Women with endometriosis may have to learn to close some doors early — and single women with endometriosis may have to learn to close these doors alone.

Rebecca Mormann

A diagnosis of endometriosis often foreshadows a chronic, painful, and frustrating experience. Some women must face the consequences of this disease throughout their reproductive years: physical discomfort, emotional stress, frequent medical visits, fertility problems, and perhaps surgery or drug treatments. In many cases, women must cope with both an illness and a fertility problem at the same time. Single women confront a sometimes frightening and painful problem without a partner's love and support, and often fear the loss of their fertility before they feel ready to bear a child.

Many women with endometriosis feel a loss of control over their childbearing choices. They are often advised to become pregnant as soon as possible and to complete their childbearing quickly, before the disease progresses or further jeopardizes their fertility. They may feel pressured to have a child (or more children) before they feel ready, yet fear they may not get the chance if they hesitate. Yet if they do try to become pregnant and do not conceive after a few months, women may also worry that the disease will worsen and further impair their fertility.

Many women with this disease, regardless of their marital status or sexual orientation, also encounter stereotypes unique to endometriosis. In the past, the medical literature has often suggested that endometriosis is a "career woman's" or "schoolteacher's" disease developed by "driven, ambitious, over-anxious, and/or perfectionist" women. These stereotypes, often confusing and frightening, may foster feelings of guilt or self-blame about having endometriosis. With continued research and education, such characterizations are being recognized as unfair and scientifically unsubstantiated profiles of women struggling with an often painful and traumatic disease.

Suggestions for coping emotionally with endometriosis include educating yourself about the disease, finding emotionally supportive health professionals knowledgable about diagnosis and treatment, and seeking reassurance and understanding from other women who have endometriosis. The Endometriosis Association, founded and directed by Mary Lou Ballweg, is an excellent resource for medical literature, video- and audiotapes, on-going research, referrals, newsletters, workshops, conferences, and an international network of chapters and support groups (see Resources). For suggestions for additional readings about endometriosis, see the Bibliography.

Diagnosis and Treatment

❦ We were surprised when my specialist found minimal amounts of endometriosis during a laparoscopy. It didn't affect my ovaries or tubes and I didn't have any pain or unusual bleeding, yet I had been unable to become pregnant after years of trying.

❦ Max had tears in his eyes. I asked him what the doctor had found. He only smiled and said he loved me very much. The doctor would be in soon to talk to me. Not such good news, I thought.

It was one of the worst cases of endometriosis my surgeon had ever seen. My ovaries were grossly enlarged — nearly five times normal size. The Fallopian tubes were blocked and wrapped around my swollen ovaries. Endometriosis was in my large bowel as well. I had no chance of conceiving a child at present. With drug and surgical treatment, I might have a chance. My doctor thought I'd had endometriosis for probably fifteen years, judging from its severity.

A medical history that includes irregular, painful, or heavy periods and a pelvic examination may suggest endometriosis. Occasionally nodules can be felt by physical examination at the back of the uterus. Although a hysterosalpingogram is an important diagnostic test to check the condition of the Fallopian tubes, it is not a reliable test for the presence of endometriosis.

Almost all specialists feel it is necessary to perform a laparoscopy to diagnose endometriosis. This procedure is often used to examine the intra-abdominal area of patients who have pain or undetermined problems. During laparoscopy, the surgeon may find implants or cysts ranging in color from clear, yellow or white, to darker growths (often called "powder burns"), which may be blue, red, brown, or black in appearance. Many experts now think the implants are initially clear in color and darken as the disease progresses. Endometriosis may be found on or within the reproductive organs or in the abdominal lining (peritoneum).

Once endometriosis is diagnosed, the patient and physician must decide on short- or long-term treatment goals that may include relieving painful symptoms, arresting the progession of the disease, and restoring or preserving fertility. Although there is no known cure for endometriosis, it can be treated with surgery to remove the implants, adhesions, and/or cysts, or with drug therapy to shrink the growths. After treatment, it is hoped that the reproductive organ function will be improved and, if desired, pregnancy can occur.

SURGERY

❦ I've had both videolaseroscopy and major surgery (laparotomy) using electro-cautery to treat long-term, chronic endometriosis. The laparoscopic surgery was done on an outpatient basis, and I was back to my regular routine within a week. I also noticed a big difference between the two techniques in terms of pain. I felt lots of discomfort and burning sensations following major surgery; after the laparoscopic procedure, I felt immediate relief and little discomfort.

In many cases, corrective surgery may be performed at the time of diagnostic laparoscopy. In recent years, operative laparoscopy, using tiny videocameras, electro-cautery, lasers, and other advanced techniques, has been effectively utilized in many cases of endometriosis to destroy or vaporize implants and adhesions. (See chapter 10 for a more detailed discussion of surgery.)

In cases of severe endometriosis, the specialist may elect to remove as many implants or adhesions as possible through the laparoscope, or in rarer cases, with major surgery. Afterward, the physician, patient, and her mate can evaluate the efficacy of drug treatment alone or combined with further surgery, or perhaps the option of Assisted Reproductive Technology (ART), which may offer better pregnancy rates than second or subsequent surgeries. (See chapter 14 for discussion of ART.)

If the patient opts for further surgery, some specialists may recommend a course of drug treatment to shrink the implants or cysts before the operation (see below). During the operation, some substances may be placed in the abdomen to try to keep the organs from adhering to each other. Immediately after surgery, some physicians also administer drugs intravenously to discourage adhesion formation. Antibiotics are commonly used to prevent infection.

Pregnancy Rates after Surgery. Following surgical treatment for endometriosis, the following pregnancy rates have been reported: 45 to 75 percent in cases of Stage 1 or 2 (minimal or mild) endometriosis, if no impairment of the ovaries or Fallopian tubes is present; for Stage 3 (moderate), up to 60 percent; and 35 to 48 percent for women with Stage 4 (severe) endometriosis. Most pregnancies occur within two years of surgery. In some cases, a pre-operative course of drug treatment may be recommended to shrink implants, thus reducing both the amount of tissue requiring removal or handling during surgery, and the total operating time needed for the procedure. Some studies report improved pregnancy rates of 5 to 10 percent following drug treatment (discussed below).

Recurrence of Endometriosis/Adhesions after Surgery. If a pregnancy does not occur within twelve to eighteen months, another laparoscopy may be recommended to reassess the situation. Unfortunately the first surgery itself may cause adhesions since the body often forms scar tissue while healing.

Surgery does not cure the disease. Endometriosis can and does recur in nearly 50 percent of patients within five years of treatment. If the woman wishes to become pregnant, it is recommended that conception be attempted as soon as possible after treatment. Pregnancy rates are highest within the first two years after surgery and then decline.

DRUG THERAPY

To date, no drug treatment has proven effective in improving fertility for women with endometriosis. In many cases, pregnancy rates are just as high with "expectant management" (no treatment at all) than with drug treatment. Like surgery, drug treatment may be used to relieve severe or painful symptoms, arrest the spread of the disease, and perhaps preserve remaining fertility. Each woman must weigh the side effects of these medications against the possible benefits of treatment.

Drug treatment with one of the gonadotropin-releasing hormone (GnRH) agonists, danazol, or birth control pills may be suggested prior to, or following, surgery to further shrink implants in cases of severe endometriosis; as a treatment alternative to surgery (although many specialists routinely remove endometriosis surgically at the time of laparoscopy); and for reduction of pain, bleeding, and other symptoms for women with chronic, long-term endometriosis.

GONADOTROPIN-RELEASING HORMONE (GnRH) AGONISTS

❦ I have taken the GnRH agonists for relief of pain and bleeding from severe endometriosis. First I tried monthly injections of Lupron, which didn't suppress my cycles. I switched to the nasal spray for awhile, but that didn't work either. I found daily injections of Lupron worked. The side effects were pretty bad at first. I had lots of hot flashes and joint pain to the degree that it was hard to type at work. I was also moody and irritable. The symptoms lasted about six weeks and then subsided. Relief from the pain of endometriosis has given me my happiest days in four years. I plan to continue taking the injections for six months and then take a bone-density test.

These synthetically created chemicals imitate the actions of natural GnRH hormone in the body. Up to two hundred times more potent than natural GnRH, the agonists may be used to either stimulate hypothalamic function or shut it down completely. When dispensed through hourly pulses through an ovulation pump, a normal menstrual cycle is often restored in women who are unable to ovulate naturally (see chapter 9). If introduced in a continuous stream, hormonal activity is suppressed, and ovulation and menstruation cease. No longer stimulated by the hormonal cycle, endometrial implants shrink.

The GnRH agonists are sometimes prescribed for several reasons: for treatment of endometriosis, temporary shrinkage of uterine tumors (fibroids), and some ovulatory problems; and before initiation of an ART cycle (see chapters 9 and 14).

GnRH agonists are currently available in two forms. Nafarelin (brand name Synarel) is a nasal spray usually administered twice a day. Leuprolide (brand name Lupron) is injected once a month over a course of six months for treatment of endometriosis. (Daily injections of leuprolide are commonly used for several weeks before the initiation of an ART cycle. They may also sometimes be recommended for suppression of the cycle for endometriosis if less frequent injections are ineffective.)

Studies have shown that GnRH agonist treatment results in subsequent pregnancy rates comparable to danazol treatment with fewer side effects. The agonists may also be more helpful to women with severe pain related to endometriosis. Many women report relief of symptoms for twelve to eighteen months after the medication is stopped. Others experience a recurrence of pain two to five months after treatment is halted. Cost per cycle is about $300.

Side Effects. Women taking one of these drugs should be closely monitored for side effects, and if necessary, dosages may be adjusted. Hot flashes, similar to those experienced by menopausal women, are usually reported with GnRH agonist treatment. Less common complaints include vaginal bleeding and dryness, hair loss, pain with intercourse, decreased sex drive, headache, insomnia, depression, and weight loss or gain. There may also be up to a 6 percent loss of bone density while the drugs are taken. Most women regain some of the loss, but a permanent loss of 1 to 3 percent may occur. Some specialists recommend a bone scan following treatment. At this writing, only one six-month course of GnRH agonist treatment is recommended until more studies are available on its long-term effects.

DANAZOL

❦ For seven months I consumed four capsules of danazol daily. My horrendous periods stopped the first month of therapy. That was the good part. The worst part was that I gained thirty pounds and grew hair on my face.

❦ I have taken danazol for five months. I have not gained any weight or experienced any other negative effects. In part I attribute my feeling of good health to the absence of menstrual periods which, since the age of eleven, have always been painful and nauseating. Secondly, the pressure to get pregnant is gone. Our sex life has improved because we again make love when the mood strikes us, rather than when a schedule tells us.

Danazol (brand name, Danocrine), derived from a derivative of a male hormone, acts directly on the ovaries and reduces their hormonal output to continuous, flat levels. Without normal estrogen production, FSH and LH production from the hypothalamus is suppressed, preventing ovulation and menstruation while the drug is taken. Although drug therapy does not remove existing scar tissue or ovarian cysts, it can arrest the disease temporarily so pregnancy can be attempted.

Initial daily dosage is 800 milligrams (mg), taken two to four times daily to suppress hormonal activity. After two months, the dosage is often reduced to

600 mg, and then cut again to 400 mg two months later. Subsequent pregnancy rates of 30 to 50 percent, depending on the severity of the endometriosis, have been cited. Cost is between $100 and $200 per month, depending on dosage.

Side Effects. Although individual reactions to danazol vary tremendously, mild symptoms are experienced by about 80 percent of women taking the drug and some women report severe reactions. Side effects can include weight gain, hair growth on the face and chest, fluid retention, fatigue, acne, vaginal dryness, and deepening of the voice. Abnormal hair growth and voice changes may remain even after the drug is stopped. Some women also experience vaginal spotting and bleeding caused by changes in the uterine lining. If symptoms become severe, most physicians and their patients agree to stop danazol treatment. It is hoped that the lower dosages now being prescribed will reduce the occurrence of these problems. Danazol should not be prescribed to patients with high blood pressure or heart or liver problems.

BIRTH CONTROL PILLS

Oral contraceptives are most commonly prescribed to treat this disease, although their effectiveness in treating endometriosis has not been proven. They stop ovulation, although withdrawal bleeding occurs when the monthly cycle of pills is completed. They are considerably less expensive than danazol or the GnRH agonists, and their side effects are usually milder. The use of birth control pills carries a small risk of blood clotting problems, and are not recommended for women with high blood pressure, gall bladder, liver, or heart problems, epilepsy, migraine, or a history of cancer. Cost is $15 to $20 per month.

Side Effects. Side effects of the pill include weight gain, breast tenderness, depression, and vaginal bleeding.

EFFECTIVENESS OF DRUG THERAPY
FOR OVARIAN ENDOMETRIOSIS

In ovarian endometriosis, scar tissue often binds the ovary to the side wall of the pelvis or to the Fallopian tube and partially covers it. Even if the patient is ovulating, that envelope of scar tissue can block the ovum from entering the tube.

Endometrial implants, from two to two hundred millimeters (up to eight inches), may also be present in large cysts within the ovary. Drug therapy is usually not effective for cysts more than several millimeters in diameter. The cyst will continue to grow and may leak endometriotic tissue elsewhere in the pelvis, or cause discomfort and pain during the menstrual cycle. Surgery is usually more successful than drug therapy in treating ovarian endometriosis.

CHAPTER 12

Immunological and Unexplained Infertility

❦ After many tests our specialist found we had a sperm antibody problem. He wasn't sure if this was causing our long-term infertility or not, but it was the only problem ever diagnosed. He suggested we might use a condom for six months and then try to get pregnant again, or we could consider intrauterine insemination. It's frustrating that so little is known about sperm antibodies, and it's difficult to find other infertile couples with this problem.

❦ We've tried to get pregnant for six years without success. Both of us have been tested and no physical problem was ever found. Some people who hear this are quick to say, "Well then, your infertility must be psychological." That's so unfair and so painful to hear. No one wants a baby more than we do.

Immunological Infertility (Sperm Antibodies)

THE PRESENCE OF SPERM ANTIBODIES (immunological infertility), which can occur in both men and women, may contribute to or cause fertility impairment in 5 to 10 percent of infertile couples. Immunological infertility has, however, generated a great deal of controversy in the medical community. Experts disagree about the effects of sperm antibodies on fertility and about which couples should be tested or treated. Many researchers now think the presence of antibodies reduces the likelihood of pregnancy but does not prevent it.

Antibodies are protein substances (immunoglobulins) that are produced by the body's immune system and attack and destroy foreign cells. In most cases they protect us from illness. Unfortunately, antibodies sometimes consider sperm as foreign cells. In these cases they may attach themselves to the sperm and cause problems with motility or penetration of an ovum.

Sperm antibodies can appear in the blood of both men and women and may also be present in the cervical mucus, uterine lining, Fallopian tubes, seminal plasma, or on the surfaces of the sperm. To confuse matters they may appear in the blood but not in the reproductive tract and vice versa; or there may be low levels of antibodies in the blood and high amounts in the cervical mucus or semen. Antibodies present in the reproductive tract are more likely to affect fertility, and those which adhere to the surface of sperm are considered the most clinically significant. For example, those present in the cervical mucus may attach to the sperm and precipitate a quivering or shaking response that hinders their motility.

CAUSES

It is thought that some women's immune systems develop antibodies after prolonged exposure to sperm. In some cases a temporary development of immunoglobulins may also result from an infection or intrauterine insemination (IUI). (IUI may trigger antibody formation by placing a greater amount of sperm in the tubes or uterus than normally occurs after intercourse.) In either case this allergic reaction probably exists toward all sperm rather than just those of one partner.

The occurrence of sperm antibodies in men is poorly understood. It is known that sperm occasionally wander out of the reproductive tract into the blood and cause an immune reaction. In fact 50 to 75 percent of men who have had a vasectomy will have measurable sperm antibodies afterward. Yet those antibodies sometimes disappear after a vasectomy reversal or, if they remain, may not impair fertility. Any inflammation or injury of the genito-urinary tract may also result in antibody formation.

EFFECT ON FERTILITY

The degree of fertility impairment may depend on the type of antibody developed, its reaction to the sperm, and its concentration in the reproductive tract. In addition the place where the antibody attaches to the surface of the sperm seems to be critical. Although those attached to the end of the tail don't seem to hinder motility, antibodies that adhere to the main section of the tail can decrease or halt its movement through the cervical mucus. Those that attach to the head of the sperm can affect its ability to penetrate the outer covering of an ovum.

TESTING FOR IMMUNOLOGICAL INFERTILITY

When no other organic cause can be found for a couple's infertility during the workup, the specialist may recommend testing for sperm antibodies in both partners. It may also be appropriate to screen couples whose postcoital or cervical mucus penetration tests show clumping, shaking, quivering, or immobilization of sperm, those who have not achieved a pregnancy within twelve months of a vasectomy reversal, and those considering in vitro fertilization (IVF).

In the past, several laboratory tests have been used to detect sperm antibodies in either partner. Semen was mixed with blood and/or cervical mucus in a test tube and the incidence of clumping (agglutinization) or immobilization was observed. A positive result was reported if 10 percent or more of the sperm reacted to the antibodies.

A more sophisticated test called the immunobead binding test has since been developed. In this test the sperm are washed from the ejaculate and centrifuged. They are then mixed with microscopic beads that have been coated with antihuman antibodies (usually taken from a rabbit). The sperm are studied to note which antibodies have developed (referred to as IgG, IgA, and IgM), where they have attached to the sperm's surface, and the percentage of total sperm with antibodies. This important information can give the specialist a better idea of how or why the antibodies are impairing the couple's fertility, although a cure for this problem remains elusive. If 50 percent or more of the sperm react to the antibodies, or if antibodies are attaching to the heads and upper tails of a significant number of sperm, a couple may be diagnosed with immunological infertility. A positive result, however, does not necessarily indicate this is the sole, or even a contributing, cause of the couple's infertility.

TREATMENT

The indications for and effectiveness of treatment for immunological infertility also generates controversy among medical experts. Some specialists think the treatments discussed below are worth a try in a case of sperm antibodies; others are skeptical of their effectiveness.

When the antibodies occur in the female partner, the couple may be advised to use a condom each time they have intercourse for a period of six to twelve months. This treatment presumes that the female partner's immune system will relax once the sperm are removed from her reproductive tract. When sperm are later reintroduced, it is hoped that antibodies will not immediately form and pregnancy can occur. There is little evidence, however, that this treatment is effective in reducing the presence of antibodies. Although success rates of 40 to 50 percent have been reported, these studies have been criticized for poor scientific methodology and controls.

Treating an antibody problem in the male is also difficult. Cortisone, which suppresses the immune system, may be prescribed for three months (a complete cycle of spermatogenesis) or sometimes longer. Its use can produce adverse side effects such as headache, insomnia, weight gain, nervousness, mood swings, and in rare cases, ulcers, acne, and possibly long-term arthritic damage to the hip joint. Success rates of 20 to 40 percent have been reported, although methodology and controls have also been questioned in these studies. Since the spontaneous pregnancy rate is about 25 percent, many urologists don't consider cortisone treatment worth the effort.

In some cases intrauterine insemination is attempted after the ejaculate is centrifuged, the seminal fluid poured off, and donor seminal fluid or a chemical solution added. Reported pregnancy rates are about 25 percent with this method. Some couples with immunological infertility may be candidates for one of the Assisted Reproductive Technology (ART) techniques (see chapter 14).

UNEXPLAINED INFERTILITY

In about 10 percent of infertile couples, no organic cause can be found for their problem. This is called unexplained or "normal" infertility, which is a particularly inept adjective: There is certainly nothing "normal" about infertility or the stresses and heartache it brings.

Unlike those with a specific diagnosis, couples with unexplained infertility cannot focus their energy on a specific medical problem or treatment. They do not know what they are fighting or when to give up hope for a pregnancy. Their friends and relatives often suggest their problem is stress-related or even psychological in nature. Among infertile couples, they are most likely to hear the infamous advice, "Just relax" or "Take a vacation — you'll be pregnant next month."

In some happy instances, pregnancy *will* spontaneously occur. Other couples try for years without success. Although there is no specific treatment for this problem, many ART programs are now accepting some couples with unexplained infertility (see chapter 14). Other couples also consider the options of adoption or child-free living discussed in chapters 17 and 20.

CHAPTER 13

Pregnancy Loss: Medical Facts and Emotional Aftermath

❧ I got pregnant shortly after beginning infertility testing. Our thrill was short-lived as we lost the baby in the eighth week. This has been the most difficult part of our infertility.

Some memories fade, but I can remember the days preceding my miscarriage very clearly. I still remember how stunned I was when I went to the bathroom and saw blood. That shocked feeling was so overpowering I just sat there in that restroom for several minutes, then went to my sisters to seek reassurance that they had both spotted during their successful pregnancies.

The next three days were an agony. Finally one night I began bleeding heavily and passing clots. I made two trips to the emergency room with my husband only to be told to wait and expect cramps. I was not at all prepared for the intensity of the pain that was actually labor. It was 4 A.M. and I hadn't slept all night. I kept rationalizing what the pain could be. I knew an aspirin would help but thought it would be bad for the baby. I had to go to the bathroom but was afraid if I got up I would miscarry. That is what happened. I sat on the toilet and it was all over.

My husband and I have no regrets about picking up and looking at what should have been our baby. It seemed perfectly natural to us to say hello, and goodbye, and I love you.

INFERTILITY IS USUALLY associated with an inability to conceive. Some infertile couples, however, may conceive easily only to lose one or more pregnancies before term. Their fertility problem involves an inability to carry their pregnancy to a live birth. Pregnancy loss may occur through miscarriage, ectopic pregnancy, or stillbirth.

Miscarriage

❧ When I was first pregnant, my doctor estimated the due date, gave me vitamins, literature, and a schedule of appointments. I miscarried within a few weeks. No one ever mentioned to me that

20 percent of pregnancies fail. Never a word even whispered about the possibility. The miscarriage was devastating to me.

If I had been warned of the possibility, I would have had some preparation, some small bit of caution in my joy. Every woman I've spoken to who has experienced miscarriage has gone through the same plunge from euphoria into hell.

❧ For those who have been sheltered from death and have not suffered the loss of anyone close, it can be the greatest loss of your life.

For many years pregnancy loss was a taboo subject rarely discussed by couples between themselves or even with their doctors. Even today many people feel uncomfortable or embarrassed when miscarriage is mentioned.

Pregnancy loss is often regarded as a rare event that "couldn't ever happen to me." Actually, miscarriage (medically termed spontaneous abortion) is a common occurrence. *More than 50 percent of conceptions do not continue more than two weeks past fertilization.* This loss may be expelled in a heavier-than-usual period that is only a day or two late. In such cases the woman may not even realize she was pregnant.

In women up to age thirty-five, about *15 to 20 percent of confirmed pregnancies end in miscarriage*, with well over three-quarters of these losses occurring during the first trimester. The incidence of pregnancy loss rises with maternal age. A forty-year-old woman has a 25 percent chance of miscarrying a confirmed pregnancy; this risk jumps dramatically to nearly 50 percent for women forty-five years or older.

In addition, there is a 1 to 2 percent occurrence of ectopic (tubal) pregnancy. (Experts estimate that there is up to a 3 percent ectopic pregnancy risk associated with Assisted Reproduction Technology. See chapter 14 for further discussion.) And about one out of every hundred pregnancies in this country end tragically in a stillbirth.

For some women miscarriage is a sudden, unexpected shock. Others experience symptoms of impending miscarriage for several days or weeks before it actually occurs. Their breasts may lose their fullness and tenderness, and light spotting or bleeding may begin. One woman described it as "just not feeling pregnant anymore."

During a *threatened miscarriage*, vaginal staining or bleeding occurs but the cervix remains closed. Many women, in fact, experience some spotting or bleeding during their pregnancies. In many cases, this bleeding stops after a few days and the pregnancies continue successfully. If, however, cramping as well as bleeding occurs and the cervix dilates, miscarriage is usually inevitable. A *complete abortion* expels all fetal tissue from the uterus, usually over a period of several days. If the symptoms continue but the fetal tissue is not expelled from the uterus, it is termed an *incomplete abortion*. A *missed abortion* describes a similar situation where fetal tissue remains or the fetus has died in utero, but symptoms have subsided. A dilation and curettage (D&C) is often required to remove an incomplete abortion. Many missed abortions will eventually be naturally expelled.

WHAT CAUSES A MISCARRIAGE?

❦ The most startling thing about a miscarriage is the light it sheds on what no longer exists: your pregnancy. Early pregnancy, however welcome, can be rather dreamlike, the growing child a pleasant idea instead of a concrete reality. A miscarriage, in all its messy, bloody *physicality* suddenly makes the pregnancy and your feelings toward that child seem very real indeed.

Ironically, I was the most conscientious of mothers-to-be. I rested in the afternoon; I took prenatal vitamins and extra iron; I fretted over whether there were enough leafy green vegetables in my diet. I read pregnancy books, haunting the childbirth shelves at local bookstores.

And I noted, with nervous concern, the fact that my occasional light spotting indicated a possible spontaneous abortion. I tried not to agonize when my midwife and my reading told me that most first trimester miscarriages were inevitable and their causes difficult to fathom.

Perhaps she was right. I don't know, and that's the most frustrating thing of all. For all our medical advances — all the test tube babies and artificial hearts — much of the human body, our reproductive systems included, remains a mysterious labyrinth.

Melanie Lawrence

Miscarriage usually occurs when the body senses an abnormality in the fetus and rejects it to end the pregnancy. Such first trimester miscarriages are usually random events. An abnormal egg or sperm, a faulty union between them, or a chance mutation during early gestation is probably responsible, and the odds are heavily against a recurrence. Most specialists do not consider one miscarriage an indication of any physical or hormonal problem. Second trimester miscarriages, on the other hand, are unusual. These are both emotionally traumatic and physically exhausting because the woman usually goes into labor. In some instances, miscarriage can be caused by several factors. An insufficient uterine lining, caused by abnormal progesterone levels, may not properly nourish the embryo during early pregnancy and the fetus may be expelled. Infection, some kinds of disease, smoking, and environmental toxins can also cause early miscarriage. Second trimester pregnancy loss may result from weakened cervical muscles or by anatomical abnormalities or tumors of the uterus. Immunological factors, discussed below, may also cause a woman's body to reject a fetus before the twenty-fourth week of gestation.

In the past, medical experts advised women who had suffered three or more miscarriages, or a second trimester pregnancy loss, to consult an infertility specialist or obstetrician experienced in the management of difficult pregnancies and/or habitual miscarriages before attempting to conceive again. Now specialists recommend a workup after a second miscarriage or a single second-trimester pregnancy loss. Recognizing that many women who have had one miscarriage are understandably distressed about a recurrence, many physicians encourage a consultation appointment to review concerns, provide information, and discuss the possibility and appropriateness of testing. Don't hesitate to arrange such a consultation if it will alleviate some of your anxiety.

REPEATED MISCARRIAGE

❦ I sit here with cramps and the dreaded anticipation of my forthcoming period. Once again, I am reminded of my infertility. My husband and I have been trying to have a baby for two and a half years now. Or more specifically, a viable pregnancy. I have had three miscarriages. I do have some good news, I suppose. My latest blood tests reveal I have elevated anticardiolipin antibodies which is apparently the cause of the miscarriages. Treatment once pregnancy occurs is baby aspirin, and perhaps heparin and/or gamma globulin. If getting pregnant wasn't such an issue maybe I'd look forward to this. I'm nearly thirty-four and I understand that my chances of getting pregnant each month diminish as I grow older.

Many women experience one or perhaps two miscarriages, often with accompanying feelings of grief and loss, and then successfully birth one or more children. There are, however, those who suffer three, four, or more pregnancy losses without carrying a child to term. Understandably, these women and their mates experience enormous grief and anxiety, and often view pregnancy as a frightening prospect.

The risk of recurrent miscarriages in a woman who has experienced two prior pregnancy losses is about 25 to 30 percent. Although the recurrence rate for future miscarriages remains around 33 percent, the medical community describes a woman who suffers three or more consecutive miscarriages as a "habitual aborter." This is an especially painful phrase for a woman, who so yearns to carry a child, to hear.

For those coping with repeated pregnancy loss, seeking a compassionate and emotionally supportive, as well as medically competent, specialist is essential. Equally important is finding reassurance and support from other women who have experienced repeated losses. Your specialist or local RESOLVE chapter (see Resources) may be able to help you connect with others.

Diagnostic Tests and Studies. Recurrent miscarriages are sometimes caused by an abnormality in the husband or wife, rather than a chance maldevelopment caused by a faulty union of sperm and egg and include hormonal, infection, or immunological problems, uterine abnormalities or chromosomal defects in one or both of the parents.

Each woman who suffers recurrent miscarriages must be individually evaluated and treated. Depending on the patient's history and number of pregnancy losses, a variety of studies may be appropriate: blood tests to check for Rh compatibility, anemia, thyroid, progesterone, and other hormonal functions; cultures for infectious microorganisms such as mycoplasma; and hysterosalpingogram, hysteroscopy, endometrial biopsy, or laparoscopy to investigate possible uterine or hormonal problems. (See chapter 8 for a discussion of these tests.)

In some cases of repeated loss, a karyotype — a picture of chromosomal configurations obtained by culturing and staining a blood sample to highlight the pairs of chromosomes — may be recommended. An abnormal sequencing of chromosomes is found in about 5 percent of couples who suffer repeated miscarriages.

In addition, the woman and her partner may need medical advice regarding activity restriction, frequency of office visits, and additional financial costs.

Current Treatments. Treating the problem of recurrent miscarriages has long frustrated and perplexed medical experts. Although successful pregnancy rates of 60 to 80 percent are reported with some of the following procedures, between 40 and 60 percent of patients similarly enjoy a subsequent, healthy term pregnancy with no treatment at all.

However, some couples who have suffered repeated losses prefer to optimize their chances and opt for one of the following procedures:

- □ drug therapy with hormones such as progesterone or bromocriptine for luteal phase defect problems;
- □ antibiotic treatment in cases of infection;
- □ a "cerclage" procedure that literally sews a weakened cervix closed to hopefully prevent a second- or third-trimester miscarriage;
- □ surgery for uterine fibroid tumors and anatomical or other abnormalities (see chapter 10 for pelvic abnormalities and Diethylbestrol-related issues and chapter 5 for a discussion of surgery);
- □ careful supervision of the pregnancy with frequent monitoring, office visits, and if necessary, bed rest.

IMMUNOLOGICAL CAUSES OF MISCARRIAGE

❦ I had nine miscarriages before I found a doctor who diagnosed an immunological problem. When I became pregnant again, I took Prednisone daily. It took awhile for me to realize that I really was going to have a baby. After so many losses, both of us had become numb and reluctant to even hope the baby would make it. For months, I checked the toilet tissue for blood. My obstetrician decided to see me weekly, from the start, just to help me control my anxiety. Weekly I'd look forward to hearing the heartbeat of my baby. Occasionally I'd panic and then she'd see me midweek, letting me listen. Without that level of support, I would not have been able to function.

Over the past several years, there has been intensive research and debate regarding the link of immunological factors to repeated miscarriage. Experts often disagree about the actual incidence of the problem, causal theories, proposed treatments, and resulting pregnancy rates. Despite the controversy, several newly developed tests and treatments may enable many women who have suffered multiple miscarriages to birth a healthy, full-term baby.

Some experts have proposed that as many as 30 percent of women who repeatedly miscarry suffer from one of two types of immunological problems: alloimmune or autoimmune.

An *alloimmune* problem may develop when the mother's and father's tissue is too similar or compatible in chemical composition. Normally, in the first few weeks following implantation, the father's cells within the embryo send chemical signals to the mother's body. Sensing these messages, she produces blocking antibodies that coat the embryonic cells. Although technically a "foreign" body, the developing fetus is protected from the mother's immune system and is allowed to flourish and grow.

Many researchers now theorize that if the parents' tissues are too similar, the mother's body will not recognize the embryo's chemical signals, fail to produce the blocking antibodies, and eventually reject the fetus. Without fetal immunoprotection, a miscarriage is inevitable. Blood testing for HLA antigen or anti-lymphocyte antibodies, *which must be run by a reliable laboratory,* is used to suggest an alloimmune problem.

The current treatment, which is controversial among the experts, is to inject either the father's or, to introduce an even greater contrast, a donor's white blood cells into the mother's bloodstream. This would provide a concentrated exposure to a foreign cell chemistry that is perhaps 10,000 times stronger than that normally emitted by the embryo. The mother's body now recognizes the signals and produces the blocking antibodies that allow a normal pregnancy to develop. Successful term pregnancy rates of 60 to 80 percent have been reported. Without treatment, subsequent live-birth rates of 40 percent are usually cited.

An *autoimmune* problem occurs when the mother's body produces antibodies to certain chemical substances produced by the fetus — commonly fat cells. Cardiolipins, produced by the fetus' heart, are often the catalyst to an autoimmune reaction from the mother. One theory suggests that after a miscarriage, fetal cells may enter the mother's bloodstream and cause antibody formation that affects her blood-clotting mechanism. When she conceives again, clotting occurs near the placenta and another miscarriage ensues.

Diagnosis is made by an anticardiolipin antibody blood test. Again, the reliability and quality control of the laboratory is of prime importance. Treatment depends on the severity of the problem. Low doses of baby aspirin, daily dosages of Prednisone (a steroid and immune system suppressant), or heparin (an anti-clotting drug) may be prescribed. There may be side effects from steroid use, such as possible future hip bone deterioriation, which can result in arthritis.

Because of the underlying autoimmune problem, some women also experience pregnancy complications such as toxemia. Pregnancy rates up to 70 percent have been reported following treatment; control group studies of women who did not opt for treatment report pregnancy rates of 40 to 50 percent.

EMOTIONAL AFTERMATH OF PREGNANCY LOSS

❧ I miscarried this morning. There will be no baby. The world seems flat, colorless. I cry. Cry harder. It does no good. I sit on the sofa and stare out the window. A young mother pushes a stroller down the street.

We have to tell our family. I make my husband do the phoning. I'm so embarrassed, ashamed. I've let everyone down, especially my husband. Perhaps he should have married a younger woman I pack the maternity clothes to send back to my sister. She phoned this morning to tell me she's pregnant again.

Why did I miscarry? A genetic defect? Abnormal hormone level? I question and requestion the doctor. The medical reasons are unclear and somehow not really important in the bleak aftermath of miscarriage. Miscarriage, I hear again and again, is a common occurrence. But cold statistics in no way numb the pain. According to my doctor some women view a miscarriage as a pregnancy that never was; others see it as the death of a child.

I wish I was one of the lucky ones. Now everything is a constant reminder. The crib goes to the basement, eventually to Goodwill. Even diaper commercials bring a flood of tears. My sister tells me to control myself. "After all, you were only two months pregnant." She's right, of course. I must be overreacting. Still, I can't stop crying.

The doctor wants me to come back and see her if I'm not pregnant again in several months. I don't keep the appointment. I can't face all those pregnant women in the waiting room. Most of all, I can't face the fear now synonymous with a second pregnancy.

I seem to be bombarded by babies. It seems as if someone phones each week with news of another pregnancy or birth. Every day brings a new baby-related crisis, and seeing friends with children becomes impossible. Everywhere there are babies and pregnant women with toddlers in tow. Even going to the supermarket becomes an ordeal of grief.

The months slip away, but I still cry daily. My husband is understanding and supportive, but I'm sure he's getting tired of tears. It's been a year since my miscarriage — a year heavy with unfulfilled dreams and rememberings.

Some women and men think of miscarriage as nature's way of ending an abnormal pregnancy and experience little grief afterward. Others view pregnancy loss as the death of their child and a major life crisis. They may carry this pain for some time, even though successful pregnancies follow.

One or both mates often form a deep attachment to the baby as soon as pregnancy is confirmed and are unable to accept the possibility of miscarriage. They are truly *expecting* a child from the first weeks of pregnancy and the baby becomes the central focus of their life. Even though the due date is months away, they may fantasize the sex or eye color of their baby, pick out names, and buy clothing and furniture for the nursery. When the pregnancy ends, their hopes and dreams are shattered. If this is their first miscarriage, they are often unprepared for the intensity of their reactions.

> ❦ My doctor asked me how I could grieve over a "blob." I answered that I grieved for my BABY that I had lost. For four months I did nothing much but cry. I really didn't know why I was so depressed.

Many couples grieve for their baby just as they would mourn the death of a living loved one. The thought that they may have other children is little comfort now. This special, beloved baby is gone and cannot be replaced with someone else. *It is a real loss they have the right to mourn.*

Our society often denies or downplays the intensity of pregnancy loss. To many people, the fetus is a nonperson and its loss a nonevent. Those who mourn are bewildered by this attitude, finding it difficult to express their grief to others. Burying these feelings, they often experience depression or lethargy and do not recognize these reactions as grief.

Grief may begin with numbness and shock, followed by anxiety, tears, or depression. People and things related to pregnancy and babies may seem ubiquitous and evoke powerful feelings. Many women feel empty and hopeless, fearing they will never be pregnant again. Depression may last for months or longer. Some women become preoccupied with their loss and endlessly review the pregnancy, the first signs of trouble, the physical experience of the miscarriage, and their emotional reactions.

Mourning is a gradual process. At first there may be weeks or months of uncontrollable weeping and sadness, but these usually lessen with time. It is important to obtain plenty of emotional support, from those who acknowledge your loss and respect your right to mourn, during your grief. Many find it helpful to talk with others who have experienced pregnancy loss. It is a common occurrence; you will be surprised how many of your friends and relatives have also miscarried. There are also a number of local, regional, and national organizations that provide support for pregnancy loss (see Resources).

One woman, who suffered multiple miscarriages, suggests yielding completely to this critical and necessary time of grief and healing. She wept deeply and frequently, each time visualizing the pain flowing out of her body and dropping into the ocean. Many also find a memorial rite of great solace. Surrounded by those who share their feelings of loss, they can express the love, hope, and dreams they carried for their babies. Some name their child and bury the precious toys and clothing they had carefully selected before the baby was conceived. Others write poetry or an epitaph for their child.

During this time, some colleagues, friends, and relatives may be confused by the length or depth of your grief. You may wish to tell them about your feelings and ask for their understanding and patience. After a while there will be more easy days than difficult ones. Reminders may continue to recall the sadness of your loss, but the daily, incessant grief passes. (In cases of persistent, long-term grief, private counseling may be of great help.)

CONFLICT BETWEEN PARTNERS

Some couples find that the miscarriage has affected the partners differently, and communication problems quickly surface.

> ❦ My husband didn't show any emotion while I cried constantly. I misinterpreted that and thought he didn't care, that he didn't really want the baby. I was very angry with him.

A woman often openly grieves immediately after a miscarriage. Coping with physical as well as hormonal changes, she may take time off from normal activities to convalesce. The dramatic drop in her hormonal levels, coupled with the trauma of her loss and perhaps lack of emotional support, often results in intense emotions and mood swings.

For a man, an early pregnancy may seem a bit unreal. His wife is not "showing," they may not have heard the baby's heart beat, and his body is not going through any physical or hormonal changes. Although he is saddened by the loss, the pregnancy may not be as real to him. Many men are also deeply frightened by a miscarriage. They may be terrified by the bleeding and worry that their wives will be permanently harmed or even die. Ectopic pregnancies and other serious medical crises exacerbate these fears.

Concerned about his wife's physical and emotional health, he may suppress his own grief about the miscarriage and take on the role of the "strong one." He may also feel genuinely relieved that his wife has survived the ordeal. With good intentions, he may voice the same cliches as others. Many wives misinterpret this effort and this "strong silence" as apathy about their loss.

In addition to dealing with the miscarriage's effect on their lives, the man is probably also working full time. He may have to tell family and coworkers about their loss and cope with the solicitous questions and sympathy of others. This compassion is usually directed toward his wife; rarely does anyone ask how *he's* feeling or coping. This reinforces his isolation and the expectation that he remain "under control." Coming home may also be upsetting if his wife is constantly miserable.

His life, too, becomes pressured and unhappy on all fronts. It is little wonder that as their wives become stronger and their grief subsides, many men take their turn at falling apart. Their buried grief now surfaces in the form of tears, depression, or anger. It may take months, perhaps years, for both partners to complete their mourning and heal from this experience.

One or both mates may also be afraid to attempt another pregnancy. Although most physicians feel it is safe to conceive again three cycles after a miscarriage, the husband may be afraid to subject his wife to another physical and emotional loss. She may fear that the next pregnancy won't take and they will go through this despair again.

GUILT

❦ I can't even guess at how many times I tortured myself with the reminder that I had gotten pregnant before and didn't really want to be, and that must have been why I lost the baby and why I was unable to conceive again. I was being punished for taking my fertility for granted, for not being grateful enough when I had the chance, for assuming that I had a right to choose and control when I would become a mother.

❦ I have counseled women who have guilt feelings about their miscarriage caused by comments from unthinking acquaintances, such as "You really were too active," "I told you not to lift those boxes," and so forth.

It's hard to absorb the loss, hear those comments, and not feel some guilt.

"Why did it happen to me? What did I do wrong? Was it because we made love the night before?" These are all common questions after a miscarriage. Knowing why can become an obsession. Seeking to put blame somewhere may seem important, and some couples place it on themselves. Thoughtless questions and comments from others often intensify feelings of blame and guilt.

Try to remember that most miscarriages are inevitable and not anyone's fault. If feelings of guilt or anxiety persist, you may wish to consult your physician about testing for physical problems and get professional counseling about your feelings before attempting pregnancy again.

CHANGES IN BODY IMAGE

❦ I remember hating my body after my miscarriage and not wanting to appear sexually attractive to anybody. One day on the street some man made a comment about my body and I became very angry.

After a miscarriage a woman experiences a number of psychological and physical changes. Shifting hormonal levels, for example, can cause moodiness and irritability. She may also be disappointed or angry with her body, regarding it as inferior or inadequate for failing to hold the pregnancy. Some women have difficulty adjusting to a nonpregnant state and have an eerie feeling that they are still carrying a child.

The physical changes following a miscarriage last for only a few weeks. The body usually returns to its normal state, and menstrual cycles resume in about six weeks. Negative self-images, however, may last much longer. Gentleness with yourself and support from those who understand pregnancy loss, for as long as needed, is integral to healing physically and emotionally.

REMARKS OF FAMILY AND FRIENDS

❦ With all good intentions I was told by many that I shouldn't feel too bad about the miscarriage because I could always get pregnant again — as if Pinky had not been a real person to us; as if our dreams and hopes and plans had never existed.

❦ I'll never forget my neighbor's comment after we lost the baby: "Well at least you never knew him." I DID know him. He moved and kicked inside of me. I patted him and talked to him and loved him. I had hopes and dreams for him and wanted him so much. I knew him. I just didn't get to keep him.

"There will be other children. It was meant to be. Something was wrong with the child. It's all for the best." These are sentiments often expressed after a miscarriage. Although well-intentioned, such remarks may not comfort the couple at all. Instead they convey the message that there is no cause for grief or depression. "It all happened for the best" is a particularly painful cliché. The couple wanted a baby and now they don't have one. The baby didn't get a chance to live. It is hard to see how that is for the best.

Instead of well-intentioned homilies, couples who have suffered a miscarriage need validation of their feelings and permission to express them. By recognizing its importance they can face their loss squarely and openly grieve.

A frank discussion with close friends and relatives may benefit everyone. Let them know what helps and what hurts in terms of advice, conversation, social events, visits, and so forth. You may also need to establish some physical and emotional distance from those who remain insensitive. "Your Healing Rights," a chart included at the end of this chapter, may also provide some helpful suggestions.

OTHERS' PREGNANCIES

❦ Once while trying on clothes, I overheard a conversation between two women, one of whom had just delivered. They were casually discussing how many more children they planned to have. I started weeping silently and couldn't leave the dressing room until both had left.

❦ I remember a close friend having a baby around the time of my miscarriage. I called her at the hospital and wished her well, but asked her not to call me or ask me to come see the baby.

Envy and jealousy of pregnant friends and relatives are common reactions after a miscarriage. They have something you wanted so badly but lost. At the same time you may feel happiness and excitement for them. Some women also have a superstitious fear of passing their misfortune on to their pregnant friends. These ambivalent emotions can be confusing and frightening.

Try to examine your feelings and reactions. Does the idea of socializing with pregnant friends seem overwhelming? You may want to call, express your feelings, and ask for their understanding while you grieve. Some couples decide not to socialize with these acquaintances for awhile, while others choose to limit their contact to those pregnant friends sensitive to their loss.

PREGNANCY LOSS AFTER INFERTILITY

❦ **I tried for nine years to get pregnant and just lost a baby two months ago. I am scared to join a miscarriage support group, because they're all fertile people who have lost babies but have this gleam of hope. I, on the other hand, am not sure if I do have another chance.**

Infertile couples, after spending years trying to conceive, are often devastated when a pregnancy loss occurs. They often feel this was their only chance at pregnancy and they "blew it."

It is also difficult for these couples to find emotional support. Many of their infertile friends have never experienced pregnancy or miscarriage, and most couples who miscarry will be able to conceive again. For empathy and reassurance, your physician or RESOLVE (see Resources) may be able to refer you to others who have suffered a pregnancy loss after long-term infertility.

TRYING AGAIN AFTER A PREGNANCY LOSS

❦ **My fears of having another miscarriage never really disappeared, even though my next pregnancy was anxious but uncomplicated.**

Those who try to conceive after a pregnancy loss are a little wiser and sadder. These women have lost not only their babies, but also the innocent elation others feel with the first news of pregnancy. They know about miscarriage firsthand and realize it can happen again.

To increase your chances for success, be sure to give your body enough time to recover from fatigue, blood loss, and any anemia that may have resulted from the miscarriage. Most physicians advise a three-cycle wait before trying to conceive again. This also gives you some time to grieve and heal from the loss. With these precautions, you have a 70 percent chance for a successful pregnancy if no other fertility problem is present in either partner.

Most women feel anxious until they pass the point in pregnancy at which they lost their first baby — be it six, ten, or twenty weeks or birth. Expect to feel concerned and uneasy until then. You will probably have more than the usual amount of fears with this pregnancy. This is also an anxious time for your mate; take care to comfort and support each other

Although you may often feel anxious or concerned, try to enjoy your pregnancy whenever possible. Work closely with your obstetrician and call whenever you feel concerned. You may also want to talk with other couples who have experienced healthy, full-term pregnancies after a miscarriage.

COPING WITH REPEATED PREGNANCY LOSSES

❦ As I write this I am pregnant for a fifth time. My first four pregnancies ended in miscarriage. I have told only a few people. I know that I cannot bear to hear people say, "Oh, how wonderful! Congratulations!" It is impossible to convey to most of them that no, it is not wonderful, at least not at this point; that being pregnant is frightening and anxiety-producing and a situation in which daily life feels like walking on eggs.

My husband and I rarely talk about this baby. We don't really allow ourselves to think of "it" as a baby yet. I am superstitious and in a state of emotional neutrality. I am merely waiting. It is not a pregnancy celebrated and enjoyed.

Yet way deep down, there is a very secret, very private place that all the self-protective, insulating behavior does not seem to penetrate. Tiny, light-filled fantasy images scamper out for whole moments at a time before they are ruthlessly squelched and shoved back inside the dark recesses of safety. "Will she have a funny, lopsided smile like her father's? Will I nurse him here by this window?"

Hope is always there, in little glimmers, impossible to deny. Yet, like a general marshaling huge armies, I fortify against those feelings. When, and only when, I hold that baby in my arms, will I allow myself to feel that pent-up explosion of joy.

❦ When deciding whether to attempt a second pregnancy, the major dilemma for my husband and me was the near certainty that taking this deliberate step of infertility treatment would, if successful, lead again to the dangers of a premature delivery. Would high-risk care prolong that pregnancy far enough to avoid the serious health risks for a very premature newborn? Would medications to stop pre-term labor harm the unborn baby?

I conceived during my second cycle with an ovulation pump, even though a postcoital test suggested I would not. Unlike my first pregnancy, I knew I required high risk obstetric care. At twenty weeks gestation, I strapped myself to a different machine, a home uterine monitor that detects contractions. Though somewhat anxious, I was reassured to know we were more likely to catch early signs of preterm labor that, in my first pregnancy, went unnoticed until it was too late to prevent delivery. Each day, I relayed by phone to trained nurses a reading of contractions for two hours or more of monitoring. By twenty-one weeks, I was having small contractions. My doctor examined me. My cervix, already damaged by prenatal DES exposure and a cone biopsy, was effacing. I passed the next sixteen weeks on bed rest, taking oral medications aimed at slowing persistent contractions; except for three precarious weeks spent in the hospital, I was able to remain at home, using the monitor. I would never describe the time as enjoyable, but at thirty-seven weeks, all faded quickly into the joy and relief of a healthy newborn.

Unlike those who cannot conceive, women who repeatedly miscarry may begin their pregnancies easily. Then time and again, perhaps only weeks after confirmation of their pregnancy, they miscarry. This is a heartbreaking problem that brings grief and fear with each loss.

If you repeatedly miscarry, seek a medically competent and emotionally supportive specialist who is experienced with multiple miscarriage and high-risk pregnancy. Before you try to conceive again, the specialist may suggest preliminary tests or preventive treatment (see "Repeated Miscarriage" section above). Frequent office visits may be necessary to monitor the baby's development and your own health. To ensure a successful outcome some women may also require bed rest or hospitalization for part or all of their pregnancy.

It is important to have realistic expectations about your future pregnancies and seek emotional support from others with this problem. There is, however, new hope for women who repeatedly miscarry. Technological advances in the fields of autoimmune pregnancy loss and high-risk obstetrics are helping more of these women achieve and sustain successful pregnancies.

Ectopic Pregnancy

❦ First, there were the gas pains, sharper than any I'd ever experienced. Brief episodes at first, then a later, all-night episode that drove me crawling to my medical textbooks.

"Ectopic pregnancy . . . the pain is frequently of colicky variety and in one of the lower abdominal quadrants . . . It frequently disappears for some hours or days before rupture occurs, only to reappear."

My physician's face was easy to read: "I think you have an ectopic. I'm afraid the only thing we can do is surgery. When did you last have something to eat?"

Surgery now . . . today . . . no time to prepare.

In many ways, the immediate post-op period was easy. There was no more worry about an uncertain diagnosis. The pain was definite in origin, the surgery showed the remaining tube to be normal, allowing me denial of the full impact of the event. Of course there would be future pregnancies and children. But when alone in my room, I felt a bottomless emotional pain. The only baby that my husband and I ever made, that I had conceived, was gone. My right Fallopian tube, a part of my childbearing apparatus, was gone too. My body had been cut open to remove them. I felt empty.

My husband shared the loss in many ways. He spent the nights in the hospital with me, sleeping on a cot. Once we were home, he bandaged my incision daily, enabling me to shower. We exhaustively discussed and reviewed what had happened.

Talking with other women who had experienced ectopics was invaluable. I've been surprised at how much alike our reactions have been. All have described grieving periods of several months duration, feelings of lowered self-esteem and femininity, and serious concerns regarding our ability to have future children, despite medical assurance of our probable fertility.

Not so helpful were the frequent well-meaning comments from others such as, "Everything will be fine, you only need one tube"; "I think if I'd had an ectopic pregnancy, I'd be over it by now"; or "It may be a blessing in disguise; there could have been something wrong with the baby."

Ectopic pregnancy involves multifaceted loss: of the baby that would have been; perhaps of a valued body part (the Fallopian tube); and of self-esteem and femininity. Because it does not always result in sterility, the impact of reduced fertility is often not acknowledged by others. The decreased fertility was real to us, even if a successful pregnancy eventually occurs.

In about 1 percent of all pregnancies, a fertilized egg will implant somewhere outside the uterus. Usually this occurs in one of the Fallopian tubes. Such a pregnancy is termed ectopic or tubal. While it remains in the tube, an ectopic will result in a positive hCG serum pregnancy test and cause basal body temperature to remain elevated.

The fetus can grow only for a few weeks in this tiny area. As the tube stretches to accommodate the growing embryo, cramping, bleeding, or severe abdominal pain results. If the fetus is not removed, the tube will rupture. The resulting internal bleeding and attendant shock create a life-threatening condition.

Ectopic pregnancy requires immediate, competent medical care. It is critical to seek help before a rupture occurs. If the ectopic is caught early, the surgeon may be able to remove the fetus and save part or all of the affected Fallopian tube.

Although any woman can develop an ectopic pregnancy, there does seem to be a higher incidence among those who have used intrauterine devices (IUDs) or have tubal adhesions or scarring resulting from pelvic inflammatory disease or previous tubal surgery. Only 50 percent of women who have had an ectopic pregnancy will conceive again, and 10 percent of them will suffer another tubal pregnancy. This information, usually conveyed shortly after a woman's pregnancy loss, often magnifies the emotional impact of this experience.

Ectopic pregnancy evokes many of the same reactions as miscarriage. It also is a critical condition that requires emergency surgery and many women lose part or all of a Fallopian tube during the procedure. It is common to feel depressed, angry, and empty after losing both a part of your body and a pregnancy. This has been both a miscarriage and a life-threatening emergency. After an ectopic many couples are afraid to attempt pregnancy again.

Emotional support from women who have experienced tubal pregnancies can be of great comfort; expert medical advice may be of help if you are considering another try at pregnancy.

Stillbirth

❦ SONG OF SAMANTHA

God, my baby is gone, gone
    where I cannot go,
Gone where I cannot care for her
    as I did
She grew inside me, now they tell me
    she's stillborn
Still, still, still . . . they tell
    me she's dead,
Not waiting down the hall, not
    needing me any more.
Still, still, still she is
    my baby
And my tears fall like rain.
My belly is empty but I am alone.
She came but did not stay
    and my tears fall like rain.
Others have theirs, but my baby
    is gone
And my tears fall like the rain.

> —From a brochure on stillbirth,
> by Ronna Case, Chaplain,
> Eskaton American River Hospital

Stillbirth is a heartbreaking conclusion to pregnancy. Occurring about once in every hundred births, it is defined as the death of a fetus in the third trimester of pregnancy or during labor and delivery. Some women discover their baby has died in utero during their last trimester, perhaps during a routine prenatal visit. They may have an agonizing wait of several days or longer before labor begins or is induced. Other women begin normal labor fully prepared to deliver a healthy, live baby. They may learn of the baby's death during labor or upon delivery.

In cases of in utero death detected before delivery, some women and their physicians decide to use general anesthesia for the birth; others opt for a milder anesthetic or even natural childbirth. Afterward the woman's body goes through postpartum changes: Her hormonal levels alter drastically and her breasts fill with milk. While her body changes to nurture and nourish a child, her heart and mind struggle to absorb the horror of the loss of her baby.

The first and most agonizing question after stillbirth is "Why? What made this happen?" In some cases anoxia (lack of oxygen), umbilical cord dysfunction, toxemia, or diabetes may affect the growth and health of the fetus. The placenta may separate from the uterus *(abruptio placentae),* or implant between the baby and the cervix *(placenta previa).* Infection caused by premature rupture of the waters or too stressful a labor may also be contributing factors. Unfortunately, however, the cause of death cannot be determined in up to 70 percent of the stillbirths that occur.

GRIEVING AND COPING

❧ I struggle with my memories of the stillbirth. I couldn't keep all the emotions filed and bottled inside. I am thankful we had close friends outside our immediate family to talk to. But mostly it helped to talk with my wife. I found that sharing our feelings with each other brought us closer together than we had ever been. We had planned together for our child, prepared ourselves for the new addition, dealt with the pregnancy for nine months, decorated the nursery together. Yet our baby was gone.

❧ Sad, quiet day. I miss feeling the baby move so much. I keep waiting for twink twink but it isn't there. My sense of time is very strange. I can't seem to conceptualize when next week is, how many days are left in this week, how many days have gone by since the baby died. I'm constantly surprised by time — that it's only 2:30 or that it's already midnight.

I realize now that I live for the mail arriving as if I'm waiting for the healing message to come today from someone. Today there were no cards or personal messages in the mail. I was terribly disappointed.

We can pick up the baby's ashes today. I find drinking feels great. I don't want to eat. It's some kind of self-punishment thing — ignoring my body. My body feels like it's been pummeled to death.

Woke up this morning with an image of a baby with a sticker on her which says "out of print"— like a book I guess. We had a lovely goodbye party for Amelia. Too bad it wasn't a hello. Each person arrived at the party individually but when the group was formed, there was a strong feeling, a solidarity, love, whatever.

The process was almost visible but the only thing I can think to liken it to is bread rising. My friend said to me that after her baby died she felt like she had a stain on her soul.

I talked to another friend today, a psychiatrist, and said my time is still odd. I can't remember details, I forget appointments. She says that happens to people who've been traumatized. They're prepared to cry, to be upset, but they're not prepared to have part of their minds nonfunctioning. I've realized in the last week that one thing I'm grieving for is the pregnancy — I didn't get to complete it. I want to be pregnant still, to finish it.

I think one reason this is so hard on me is that it took so long to believe I was really going to have a baby and now it's taking a long time to realize that I'm *not*.

Stillbirth carries all of the aftermath of other pregnancy losses plus its own unique pain. The couple must deal with many intense emotions in quick succession, including the shocking discovery that the baby has died in utero or during delivery. This death is totally unexpected and they usually do not have time to absorb and accept the loss before it occurs.

Following the stillbirth, both parents experience deep grief at a time when difficult decisions must be made. A fetal death certificate must be completed to be signed by the physician. In most cases the couple must decide whether to view or hold their child or give their baby a name, and take his or her picture. Someone must notify relatives and friends and make funeral or burial arrangements.

Sherokee Ilse, a pregnancy loss counselor and mother who authored *Empty Arms* after her own stillbirth experience, has found the following suggestions helpful for couples dealing with the immediate aftermath of this tragedy and the ensuing period of grief:

- ☐ Decide whether you want to remain on the post-partum floor or transfer to a private room on another floor of the hospital. Some women prefer to stay in the maternity wing to grieve and have their loss acknowledged. Others find the proximity of new parents and babies too painful. In this case, ask to be transferred to another area of the hospital.
- ☐ Ask your physician and one of the floor nurses to inform those staff members who will interact with you about your loss. This may spare you from explanations to caregivers unaware of your tragedy.
- ☐ Some couples prefer to spend as much time together as possible to comfort and support each other. Most hospitals will put a cot in the room so your husband can remain with you overnight. Other women and men, when in the midst of deep grief, need solitude. If your mate is overwhelmed by the death and temporarily unable to offer consolation, call on trusted family or friends to stay with you.
- ☐ To soften another surge of grief, you may request a shot to dry up the milk that comes in a few days after the birth. If you prefer not to use

medication, bind your breasts and apply warm compresses to ease the pain until the milk dries up. This usually takes several days.

☐ Strongly consider holding and naming your baby. Though heart-wrenching, this focuses your grief and gives you a chance to say hello before you must say goodbye.

Some couples or partners who find this too overwhelming, prefer that their mother, father, or another loved one view or hold their child for them. Most hospitals take a picture of the baby and, if you wish, will keep it in a file. You may also want to obtain other permanent keepsakes — a lock of hair, handprints, and footprints. It is comforting to know you can request these keepsakes at any time. Many parents find that they become increasingly important and treasured over time.

☐ You don't have to bear your grief alone either now or in the months to come. Seek emotional support and assistance from trusted friends and relatives. There are also local, regional, and national support groups, staffed by those who have experienced stillbirth, whom you can call for solace, understanding, and support (see Resources).

After any pregnancy loss — be it miscarriage, ectopic pregnancy, or still-birth — many women and men are profoundly affected for months or years to come. Above all, be gentle with yourselves and try to understand and support each other. The following chart, reprinted with permission of The Ferre Institute, Inc., provides additional suggestions for healing.

Your Healing Rights

FORTUNATELY, all of us have a natural desire to heal and to feel better. This is a time to respect your needs and instincts, and to be gentle to yourself. Remember that you have some specific healing rights.

1. You have the right to be informed—Knowing the facts helps protect you from being misled. Know what happened, be aware of implications for the future, see your medical records, expect expertise, take notes, and ask questions.

2. You have the right to make decisions—It is your body, your baby, your partnership, and your future. It is up to you to choose whether or not you should be on a maternity ward, whether you want a private room, whether you would like visitors, and whether you would like an exception to rules so your partner can stay with you after visiting hours. In addition, you have choices to make about what you'll do with your maternity clothes and your baby items. Don't allow others to be "helpful" and make quick choices for you; instead, use others as sounding boards to help you decide which options are best for you.

(continued)

3. You have the right to protect yourself—There is no reward in punishing yourself. For now, avoid those situations that you know will be difficult. Don't wonder if you'll make it through the week. Instead, aim to make it through the next hour and then the next hour.

4. You have the right to take time—Respect your need for time; hurting and healing take time. The amount of time needed varies with each person. No one can do your healing for you. Unfortunately our society resists anything that happens slowly. Grieving and healing are hard work and can't be rushed.

5. You have the right to receive support—Be receptive to those who wish to help even though this may not be easy for you. Find appropriate support. Remember that those who care the most about you may not be the best choices for support. You shouldn't have to justify to anyone why you feel the way you do. If you feel out of control and can't seem to pull yourself together, consider seeking help from a counselor or therapist so that you can be guided through your grieving.

6. You have the right to be sad and be joyful—After your loss you have many uncomfortable feelings such as weariness, numbness, disappointment, inability to concentrate, betrayal, loneliness, helplessness, anger, guilt, and emptiness. You can't believe how sad you feel or how many tears you can cry. Don't try to ignore your feelings. You will be sad, but don't allow your sadness to control you. Others have survived their grief, and in time, you will too.

Happiness doesn't always come easily so nudge yourself to find it. Laughter and joy are healers. Do things that you enjoy doing; pamper yourself a little. Push yourself if you feel you are becoming lethargic or reclusive. Celebrating bits of joy doesn't dishonor your loss. Finding joys is one of your choices; focus on joys that help you to heal.

7. You have the right to remember your baby—Your memories are an important part of your life. Healing doesn't mean forgetting or making the memories insignificant. Healing means refocusing. If it is possible, you may see, touch, name, and photograph the baby. You may wish to save a lock of hair, take a footprint, or have a memorial service. You may want to request an autopsy and see the report. Later it may be comforting to do something tangible like planting a tree, selecting a special piece of jewelry with the birthstone, or donating to a charity. On the anniversary you may want to share a special time with your partner.

Reprinted with permission from "Miscarriage: Surviving Pregnancy Loss," published by The Ferre Institute, Inc., New York; principal author Jody Earle.

CHAPTER 14

Brave New ART: Creating Families Through Assisted Reproductive Technology

❦ Susan had used an IUD contraceptive for about fifteen years. She never had any pain, bleeding, or other symptoms, and had annual check-ups. During those years she worked diligently on her teaching career, wasn't involved in a permanent relationship, and didn't want children. She and Matt found each other in their late thirties. Happy and in love, they planned a lifetime together and at least one child.

The IUD was removed and three months passed without a pregnancy. An old fear surfaced that Susan recalled from adolescence. She sensed she was infertile. Secretly she marked tiny dots on the calendar with each period, and then as she became more frantic, little x's every time she and Matt made love. Matt noticed her preoccupation, and after eight months, they agreed to consult a specialist. At the initial interview, Susan lied and said they'd been charting for a year. She couldn't face another cycle without help.

They progressed through the workup quickly. The tests revealed a varicocele and slightly low sperm count for Matt and a blocked right tube in Susan. Matt underwent surgery. Soon after, they began clomiphene, ultrasounds, hCG shots, and intrauterine inseminations. It was a nightmare for Susan. Since childhood, she had been afraid of needles, hospitals, and medical procedures. She was, however, more terrified of never having a child.

With the approach of her thirty-ninth birthday and the failure of the ninth IUI attempt, Susan and Matt assessed the situation. Their home was filled with tension, frustration, and unhappiness. Only two weeks of the month were bearable; then her period came and they were devastated again.

Their physician told them that in vitro fertilization was an option. Susan and Matt looked at each other. The only thing they knew about high-tech procedures was that their insurance didn't pay for them. Yet they longed for a baby and nothing else had worked.

In 1978, THE DRAMATIC CONCEPTION and birth of the world's first "test-tube" baby ushered in a new, swiftly evolving, and often turbulent era of infertility technology. Since that miracle, in vitro fertilization (IVF) has been enthusiastically discussed and widely publicized. To date, more than 40,000 children worldwide have been born through IVF, 10,000 or more in the United States.

IVF is a highly technical, complex process that usually involves ovulation induction with fertility drugs (natural cycle IVF is offered by some programs), ultrasound-guided aspiration of a number of eggs from the mother, and laboratory evaluation and fertilization of those ova with the father's sperm in a plastic dish. *(In vitro* literally means "in glass," but plastic dishes are now commonly used.) The fertilized eggs (embryos) are then incubated and transferred, through the cervical opening, into the mother's uterus with the hope of a successful pregnancy and birth. The two- to three-week treatment protocol and subsequent ten-day wait until the pregnancy test is often described by IVF couples as a careening roller coaster ride of hope, impatience, exhilaration, disappointment — and at times — despair.

Over the past fifteen years, there has been a rapid proliferation of knowledge and a refinement of IVF technique. A new "generation" of technological advancement is occurring in this field every two or three years! Accordingly, numbers of successful pregnancies are being reported by programs established both in the United States and abroad.

In addition, several high-tech variations of IVF have been developed for appropriate patients — a veritable alphabet soup of acronyms collectively termed, together with IVF, Assisted Reproductive Technology (ART):

GIFT (gamete intrafallopian transfer) is a process in which one or more eggs are aspirated from the ovary and then, together with her mate's sperm, injected into the patient's Fallopian tube(s), usually by laparoscopy, for natural fertilization and implantation.

ZIFT (zygote intrafallopian transfer) or TET (tubal embryo transfer) combines GIFT and IVF techniques by transferring embryos fertilized and incubated in the laboratory into the Fallopian tube(s) rather than the uterus.

FET (frozen embryo transfer), as its name suggests, involves the transfer of previously fertilized embryos into either the Fallopian tubes or uterus during a hormonally enhanced menstrual cycle.

Egg donor IVF and the surrogate gestational mother options, among the most controversial of ART permutations, involve a third party. Egg donor IVF uses ova donated by another (often younger) woman, fertilizes them with the sperm of the recipient's mate, and transfers the embryos into her tubes or uterus for gestation. In the gestational surrogate mother option, eggs are retrieved from the genetic mother, fertilized with her mate's sperm, and the embryos are transferred to another woman's uterus for gestation and birth.

Unquestionably these advances are intriguing medical options, renewing hope for many infertile couples who do not respond to other less invasive or expensive procedures. In fact, this is often the last resort for many couples who have already endured years of unsuccessful medical treatments and surgeries that often offer higher success rates than ART. Cautious and thorough consideration of all aspects of these options is critical.

Although success rates are slowly rising with improved clinical and laboratory technique, ART procedures are still in an early stage of development. Consequently, live, full-term birth rates vary markedly between clinics and are often discouragingly low — although some approach natural conception rates for some patient age groups. These are also expensive options, not always covered by insurance; many couples borrow money or deplete their savings to finance this effort.

There is also a great deal of myth, misunderstanding, and controversy surrounding these advances. The unsolicited advice offered to infertile couples now has a new twist: "Don't worry. You can always have a test-tube baby!" Such statements mistakenly presume that ART is an easy, inexpensive, highly successful, or stress-free experience. At the same time, other segments of society vehemently argue that ART options are inequitable, unethical, or exploitive to patients or involved third parties, and therefore inappropriate avenues for infertility resolution.

Nevertheless thousands of couples, some clinging to mere shreds of hope, will seriously consider this final medical effort. ART is an extremely stressful and expensive undertaking, and, depending on the partners' ages and individual fertility factors, *only about 10 to 35 percent of ART attempts culminate in a live, full-term baby.* For many, if not most, patients, these high-tech efforts will be yet another painful and costly disappointment.

If you are considering the ART option, a thoughtful and practical evaluation of its benefits, risks, and challenges is a wise investment. It is helpful to obtain advice and counsel from professionals knowledgable about ART and other couples who have undergone the procedures, and to gather reliable and accurate information about all aspects of this option. Interested couples and single women who approach the high-tech arena as cautious and informed consumers, and who carefully research the decision-making and clinic selection process, medical indications and procedures, risks, costs, success rates, emotional and psychological dynamics, and ethical ramifications of these new frontiers, enter the process aware of its challenges and realistic about their chances for success.

Indications for ART

❧ Isabella, born in Argentina, had two children during her first marriage and underwent a tubal ligation after the birth of her second son. Several years after her divorce, she moved to the United States. She married Phillip in her mid-thirties and they decided to have one child together. Isabella underwent microsurgery to reverse the ligation

After two years passed without a pregnancy, she opted for IVF. Two attempts failed with the same program. She and Phillip have decided on one more try. Her employers are supportive of her efforts, agreeing to a "flex-time" schedule on the days she must commute two hours each way to a new IVF program. Her medical insurance policy will cover part of the expense.

IVF or other ART procedures may be an appropriate treatment for a number of infertility problems:

☐ Tubal blockages, adhesions, or ligations. Depending on the location and extent of tubal damage, laparoscopic or microsurgery may yield a higher success rate than IVF. If a pregnancy does not occur within twelve to eighteen months of surgery, IVF may be preferable to subsequent surgery. Many specialists feel that IVF is not as physically traumatic, is less expensive, and offers better success rates than repeated surgery. Other patients with severe tubal problems may be referred directly to IVF.

☐ Endometriosis that does not respond to surgical or medical treatment. Again, IVF may be more successful and less invasive than repeated surgical attempts. For women older than thirty-five with endometriosis, some specialists advise primary treatment with an ART option rather than a year or more of medical or surgical treatment.

☐ Cervical mucus problems that have not responded to intrauterine insemination (IUI) treatment.

☐ Infertility traced to sperm antibodies.

☐ Some types of male infertility, such as low sperm count or poor motility, and cases where fertility drug treatment (for the male) has not resulted in pregnancy.

☐ Long-standing unexplained infertility, in which no physical problem can be found in either partner.

In most cases, the ART option should be recommended ONLY after other less invasive procedures or treatments have not succeeded over a reasonable length of time. In all cases, both partners should be thoroughly evaluated and tested before an ART procedure is attempted.

Making the Decision

❦ Christine, a thirty-four-year-old nurse, was diagnosed with endometriosis six years ago. Since then, laser and electro-cautery surgery has been performed twice through the laparoscope. Clomiphene treatment and six unsuccessful intrauterine inseminations followed each surgery. Then she and her husband, Joe, took a three-year break. During that time, the couple investigated both adoption and child-free living.

The years of infertility have taken a considerable toll on their relationship. Marital counseling helped them heal some of the wounds and clarify their goals. Both want a biological child and have decided to resume treatment. They have limited financial resources and no insurance coverage for ART. Their families have offered to help with the expense.

The physical, emotional, ethical, and financial demands of ART, as well as its success rates, must be carefully weighed before a couple or single woman decide on this option. Most prospective candidates have already experienced several years of infertility stress and treatment; many women have undergone surgery. This experience will again stress individual self-esteem and an already taxed relationship.

Age must also be considered. Fertility naturally declines, and miscarriage rates increase, as women reach their thirties and forties. This affects ART success rates. Women older than thirty-five should also consider the higher incidence of birth defects such as Down's syndrome for this age group, and decide whether they are comfortable with such prenatal testing as amniocentesis.

When deliberating any important choice, it often helps to take a few days to individually consider key issues and questions. After this private reflection, the couple can share their goals and thoughts as they search for common ground and direction. Some questions and issues relevant to the ART option include:

- ☐ Have we pursued other less invasive and costly fertility treatments for a reasonable length of time before considering ART?
- ☐ Why do I prefer the ART option to other possible resolutions such as adoption, child-free living, or donor insemination?
- ☐ Am I familiar with the procedures, success rates, and requirements of the ART process?
- ☐ Am I willing to undertake the considerable physical and emotional stress of this experience?
- ☐ Do I have any religious or ethical reservations about any aspect of this process?
- ☐ What are my feelings about cryopreservation (freezing) of embryos? About donation of unused embryos to another infertile couple or to medical research?
- ☐ What about the possibility of a multiple pregnancy? How do I feel about pregnancy reduction (abortion of one or more fetuses) if a multiple pregnancy occurs?
- ☐ Am I between thirty-five and forty years of age or older? How will my age affect the ART process and my chances for success?
- ☐ Can we afford the expense of several attempts? Have we researched our insurance coverage for this option?
- ☐ Can I handle the disappointment of one or more unsuccessful attempts?

☐ How many times would I try ART before pursuing other options?
☐ How will I select an ART program? What attributes and features are important to me?
☐ Are we getting enough emotional support?
☐ Where do we stand as a couple on this decision? Does one partner prefer this option more than the other? Should we seek private or marital counseling while in the process?

As feelings and opinions gel, the process of joint decision-making begins with often tentative, sometimes emotional or impassioned conversations Although many feelings may surface, this is the time to honestly communicate hopes, fears, doubts, and preferences. ART is a time-consuming as well as difficult physical and emotional experience. This option is not appropriate for everyone, and *no one should feel obligated or pressured to try any of the ART options.* There are other alternatives for every infertile couple, such as adoption or child-free living.

Repeated discussions over a period of time are often necessary before a couple reaches an agreement. Participation in an infertility support group can help clarify their goals during this process. Couples may, however, find themselves "stuck" and unable to reach a mutually agreeable decision. In these cases, a consultation with an infertility therapist may be useful.

As with any fertility treatment, it is important to enter ART as a couple that is clear about what this choice means to each partner, is committed to the decision and the relationship, and is able to encourage and support each other throughout the process. (See chapter 2 for further discussion of decision-making as a couple during infertility.)

Selecting an ART Program

❦ Cindy and Hal, both thirty-five, have been trying to get pregnant for ten years. A workup done seven years ago showed a low sperm motility factor for Hal. All Cindy's test results were normal. They underwent six unsuccessful ART attempts with one program.

Flat broke and emotionally bereft, they took a break from medical treatment. During this time they adopted their son Toby through an independent adoption. Although parenting Toby has brought them great joy, the pain of their infertility remains. They still want to birth at least one child.

After Toby's second birthday, Cindy and Hal again discussed medical treatment. Since their insurance covered part of the expense, they agreed to another ART attempt. This time they are more involved patient-consumers, carefully researching a number of programs before choosing one. Besides investigating the success rates for male-factor problems at each program, they also want to learn about each ART option and which ones may be appropriate for them.

Selecting a program among the myriad now available can be a daunting prospect. In some metropolitan areas, there may be a half dozen or more local ART clinics in operation. Couples residing in less populated or rural areas must also consider the cost of travel as well as the attributes of distant programs.

Your specialist may be able to advise you about various ART programs and their quality. Referrals from other ART patients and RESOLVE's National Office may also be helpful (see Resources). And it is beneficial, as a medical consumer with considerable emotional and financial resources at stake, to do some investigation and research of your own.

The American Fertility Society (AFS) and its affiliated specialty group, the Society of Assisted Reproductive Technology (SART), are also excellent sources for referrals and information. In an annual edition of *Fertility and Sterility*, the AFS publishes the "IVF Registry," a compilation of the success rates of 180 participating programs across the country. (Some ART clinics have yet to achieve a live, full-term birth, and not all programs report their statistics to the AFS registry.) Each year, the AFS also produces an annual edition of "clinic specific" statistics with further data about individual programs in the United States, Canada, and abroad (see Resources for ordering information).

Once you identify several prospects, call or write for detailed information about their medical staff, guidelines, candidacy requirements, costs, and success rates. As you narrow the field of possible programs, consider the following factors:

The ART Team. Ask for the qualifications and experience of each member of the medical team. The AFS recommends staff expertise in reproductive endocrinology, male reproduction (urologist or andrologist), laparoscopic surgery, ultrasound technique, embryology, tissue culturing, and cryopreservation. The expertise of the laboratory personnel and quality of the facilities are crucial to the success of an ART attempt. Is the lab staff available, if needed, at all times? Are they experienced with embryo cryopreservation? For male-factor couples, experience with sperm micromanipulation may also be critical.

Waiting Lists. How long is the wait for the initial interview? Are psychological evaluations or pre-program counseling recommended or required? After acceptance, how long is the wait to begin a treatment cycle?

Cost. At the present time, the federal government does not grant funding for either ART research or services. Each ART program is thus self-supporting, and patients are required to pay for full costs themselves, through insurance coverage, or a combination of both. Depending on the program and type of procedure, the 1992 cost for ART ran between $8,000 and $10,000 or more per attempt (charges are much less for either natural cycle IVF or frozen embryo transfer). If applicable, also add cost of travel, up to two weeks of accommodations, and perhaps wages lost from work to the expenses

Many programs require that the entire cost be paid before each attempt; others offer a payment plan. Ask for an expense breakdown, itemizing each step of the medical and laboratory process and whether advanced monies are refundable if the cycle is cancelled for any reason.

Medical insurance coverage for ART varies tremendously. Some carriers will cover all of the cost. Others will pay for only part of the expense — perhaps ovulation induction medications, laboratory charges, or specific medical procedures. A few states have mandated insurance coverage for some infertility procedures, including ART. (See chapter 3 for a discussion of the economics of infertility.)

Availability of Counseling and Support Groups. Is there a counselor or psychologist on the program staff? Are fees for such services additional or included in the cost? Are patients referred out for counseling? Are these therapists professionally and/or personally experienced with infertility and ART issues?

Success Rates. Success rates are of paramount concern to any interested couple. Unfortunately, these figures can be misleading. An excellent clinic may have a lower over-all success rate for a particular factor if they accept women older than forty. Another may report a high pregnancy rate (40 percent or more), but not adjust the figures for subsequent pregnancy losses. Some clinics have yet to report a live, full-term birth.

Ask how long the medical team has been working together and how they compute their success rates. How do they factor in multiple pregnancies, transient "biochemical" pregnancies, ectopic pregnancies and miscarriages, and patients who drop out from different stages of the protocol? Do they report to the IVF Registry? What are their live, full-term birth rates for *your age group with your fertility factor(s)*? (See pages 208–210 for further discussion of success rates.)

You may then compare this information, and other issues important to you, with the candidacy requirements of the programs. Before making a decision, some couples prefer to visit the clinics to meet the physicians. For many, the "right" program combines medical and technological excellence with that intangible chemistry of team esprit, warmth, concern, and emotional support.

Requirements for ART Candidates

❦ This obstacle on our uphill struggle took us by surprise. Matt and I simply couldn't choose a program. We had to be *accepted* into one — pass their test for which we couldn't study or prepare the right answers. All we could do was apply and wait for their judgment. Again we felt out of control and physically inadequate.

Each ART program has its own screening procedures and criteria for acceptance. All will require your previous medical records, infertility workup test results, and surgery reports. In most cases, the clinic will assume that the patient has tried other methods of medical treatment before attempting ART. Most programs also require that applicants meet most or all of the following requirements:

☐ Ability to ovulate. The woman must be capable of ovulation, have at least part of one functioning ovary, and respond to the fertility drugs that will stimulate the formation of one or more eggs. (Egg donor IVF, discussed below, is an option for women who do not respond to ovulation induction.)

☐ Age. Most programs will accept women up to age forty, and many are extending their age limits to forty-four or older. Because there is some decline in fertility in the mid-thirties and early forties, some programs give priority to women older than thirty-five. (See the egg donor IVF section below for another option for women older than forty.)

☐ Rubella immunity. Before ART is attempted, it is wise to test for rubella immunity and be vaccinated if necessary. If the mother is not immune and contracts rubella during early pregnancy, birth defects could result.

☐ Male partner fertility. Presumably a complete semen analysis of the male partner was performed during the workup. In addition, the Sperm Penetration Assay (SPA) is often done before an IVF attempt to check the sperm's ability to penetrate an ovum. (See below and chapter 15 for further discussion of this test.) ART is sometimes appropriate for male-factor infertility. If this is not feasible, some programs will perform ART using donor sperm (see chapter 16).

☐ Counseling. Many clinics require pre-program interviews, psychological evaluations, and/or counseling to assess the couple's ability to cope with the emotional and physical stress of the IVF experience. The process is usually described in detail, and the couple is informed of potential health risks and chances of success. In addition, they are urged to plan for alternative resolutions if ART should not be successful. Not all programs have ongoing counseling and psychological services available during the process. If you undertake ART, you may wish to secure emotional support from a counselor or support group.

The Medical Process of In Vitro Fertilization

❧ Everything happened so quickly. We went in for the initial interview. The doctor greeted us and then examined me. He said that his team had studied our records of the past year and thought I was definitely an IVF candidate. They had a cancellation and we could begin now. NOW? Matt and I were dazed. We both had to get blood tests immediately, and Matt had to give another semen sample for the first series of tests.

I started to shake and cry in the lab. I held out my arm, closed my eyes, and said, "Please just do it fast." In the parking lot, Matt gently removed both our bandages, pressed our forearms together, and said, "Blood brothers, Susan. We'll do this together."

Most programs will run several preliminary tests and procedures to gauge the couple's probability of success and to determine which ART option is most appropriate for their fertility factor(s).

TABLE 14.1   THE IN VITRO FERTILIZATION MEDICAL PROCESS

The IVF process is both stressful and costly (1987 fees range from $4,000-8,000 per attempt, depending on the program and procedures used). At each step, many patients either drop out voluntarily or fail to respond to treatment and are unable to continue. Only 10-20 percent of those who begin are blessed with a live infant nine months later. The complete procedure follows these steps:

To begin treatment cycle	shut down current cycle with GnRh shots and administer ovulation induction drugs for 9 to 12 days; monitor follicular development through blood tests and ultrasound.
If eggs develop,	retrieve ova through ultrasound guided vaginal aspiration.
If retrieval successful,	evaluate ova in laboratory for maturity.
If ova are fertilizable,	collect semen from male partner.
If semen is collected,	culture and incubate ova and sperm.
If fertilization and normal cell division occur,	transfer fertilized eggs into patient's uterus.
	Perform pregnancy test after 10-14 day wait.
If negative (80-90 percent)	couple must decide whether to try again.
If positive (10-20 percent)	natural progesterone may be given during early pregnancy.
If miscarriage does not occur,	live term infant is born nine months later.

FSH blood test. Researchers have noted a correlation between the level of follicle stimulating hormone (FSH) in a woman's blood and her "ovarian age"— a factor that does not necessarily coincide with her chronological age. The ovarian age of a forty-two year old woman, for example, may actually be "younger" than that of a thirty-six year old.

The level of FSH is measured on the third day of the menstrual cycle. A "high" FSH reading (above 15 milliInternational Units per milliliter— mIU/ml) often indicates the presence of fewer, older follicles that are not releasing adequate amounts of estrogen. To compensate, the hypothalamus generates large amounts of FSH to stimulate estrogen production in the ovary and initiate a cycle. Women with high, early cycle FSH readings are usually, but not always, older (forty and up) and are often unsuccessful with IVF — either in the ovulation induction or the transfer stages. A high FSH reading often translates into a 5 percent chance for ART success.

Physicians, however, often advise several FSH tests before drawing a conclusion. Clomiphene, for example, can temporarily elevate FSH levels and it may take a month or two for the body to stabilize after the drug is stopped.

Pelvic Ultrasound, Hysterogram, or Hysteroscopy. Many specialists perform a pelvic ultrasound to rule out cysts or other abnormalities and obtain a baseline reading of the uterine lining thickness before a treatment cycle is attempted. Others advise a hysterogram or hysteroscopy to visualize and assess the condition of the uterine cavity.

Sperm Penetration Assay (SPA). Before initiating a stressful and costly ART treatment cycle, many experts prefer to run a SPA (hamster egg test) to confirm that the male partner's sperm can indeed fertilize his partner's eggs. Although the semen analysis run during the workup may be normal, there is sometimes a hidden male-factor problem that is revealed by the SPA (see chapter 15 for a detailed discussion of this test).

A positive SPA result is reassuring, but a negative one doesn't necessarily mean that the ART attempt will fail. Care must be taken that the test is run properly with at least twenty to thirty hamster ova, and with a control group of donor sperm, before any conclusions are drawn. A negative result is a concern and, in such cases, some specialists advise patients to consider the alternative of simultaneous fertilization of retrieved oocytes with both the mate's and donor sperm. This is a complex psychological and emotional decision and, like egg donor IVF, one which should be given lengthy consideration beforehand. (See "Egg Donor IVF" in this chapter and chapter 16 for discussion of donor gamete issues.) In some male-factor cases, however, micromanipulation techniques or adjustments with nutrients and follicular fluid may be performed in the lab. With such care, pregnancy rates for these couples may be improved.

Screens for mycoplasma, AIDS, hepatitis, herpes, gonorrhea, chlamydia, and other viruses or infections. Blood samples are screened for a number of bacterial or viral agents that may cause health problems or perhaps increased risk of miscarriage. Many clinics prescribe a routine course of antibiotics for several days before the procedure as a safeguard against present infections, or any that may occur during treatment.

Sperm Survival Test. In addition to the SPA, some programs utilize this test to determine the longevity, motility, and forward progression of the sperm. After twenty-four hours, 70 percent of at least 20 million sperm should be alive and moving. In cases where fewer survive, the lab may compensate during the ART process with various energy supplements and multiple inseminations of the follicles every few hours.

Selecting the Appropriate ART Technique

❦ The medical team sat around the conference table with well-studied sheaves of records and screening test results before them. They carefully considered one case at a time, listening intently as each colleague debated the best option for the couple.

They all agreed on IVF for Susan and Matt. Although only one Fallopian tube was closed, they worried that a previous pelvic inflammatory disease infection had subtly damaged the patent one. They didn't want to increase the risk of a tubal (ectopic) pregnancy with GIFT or ZIFT, although given her age, those success rates were higher. They would also discuss Matt's low sperm count with the lab team.

IVF would also be the best choice for Isabella and Phillip. Although an HSG showed the tubes open after her microsurgery, they were concerned about their patency and the risk of an ectopic pregnancy.

The team thought GIFT was the best option for Christine and Joe. Her tubes were open and Joe's sperm count and SPA test looked good.

Hal's motility problem concerned everyone, as did Cindy's prior unsuccessful IVF attempts. Donor egg IVF or use of donor sperm had been suggested to the couple, but they were adamant about using their own gametes. Since Cindy's tubes looked normal and healthy, the team recommended ZIFT and possible micromanipulation of sperm.

The four couples would enter the ovulation induction stage at the same time.

Every ART specialist has acquired different training and clinical experience in these procedures, and some carry a bias toward one type of technique over another. For example, a number of programs prefer to use IVF with all patients regardless of the fertility factors. Others will utilize GIFT or ZIFT if there is no history of tubal problems.

Although medical expertise is critical in the choice of treatment, couples can still be involved in the decision-making. Together with your specialist, discuss why one method is recommended rather than another, and the differences between their advantages, risks, costs, and success rates.

Natural Cycle IVF

Some programs offer the option of "natural cycle" IVF, which is attempted during a normal menstrual cycle without the use of ovulation induction drugs. A shot of hCG and progesterone and estrogen hormones, however, are usually prescribed to better time ovulation and retrieval, and to prepare the uterus for the embryo transfer.

Many specialists do not advocate or recommend this option. They feel the chances for pregnancy are enhanced when a number of eggs are retrieved, fertilized, and transferred. Other experts argue that it is worth at least one try. It is less expensive than standard IVF (running about $2,500), may afford reasonable success rates to younger women, and offers the advantages of an endometrium not affected by massive doses of drugs and a dramatically decreased risk of multiple pregnancies. As with any ART procedure, a skilled laboratory staff is essential.

Standard IVF Protocol

Most IVF cycles will involve nine steps, occurring over four weeks.

STEP 1. Halting the Current Menstrual Cycle with Gonadotropin-Releasing Hormone (GnRH) Agonists

❦ We entered a strange and exciting new world. We were given explicit instructions that we followed to the letter. Matt was trained, with the help of Dr. X's nurse, a video, and an orange, to give me shots. We started with daily injections and it wasn't too bad. The needles were small and I didn't have any side effects. When I got scared, I closed my eyes and imagined my body as a mesh, opening up to receive this medication and prepare myself for the baby. It took fourteen days for my period to start.

Many, but not all, IVF programs begin the protocol with daily injections or inhalation of a GnRH agonist, such as Lupron or Synarel, that stop hormonal production and shut down the patient's current cycle. Menstruation occurs in seven to fourteen days. To suppress a natural surge of LH hormone and possibly spontaneous ovulation, treatment with a GnRH agonist may be continued until the retrieval. (See chapters 9 and 11 for a discussion of the GnRH agonists and the ovulation induction drugs and their side effects.)

STEP 2. Ovulation Induction with Fertility Drugs

❦ My first sonogram showed a couple of cysts. Dr. X monitored them for two days and told me we might have to cancel the cycle. I was devastated — we had already spent fourteen days on Lupron shots. But he finally decided to go ahead. We bought a kit with about ten days worth of Pergonal in it. Matt had to break off the top of the glass vials and mix the drugs together. Dr. X started me on three amps a day. Matt gave me the shots in the evening. These were intramuscular shots and those needles were BIG. Again I overcame the fear and imagined this baby and what good parents we would be.

❦ Susan has always been afraid of needles, so the challenge was definitely increased when we moved on to Pergonal. I'm generally pretty clumsy and usually think I can't do anything mechanical, but I wanted to be involved in this for Susan. The Pergonal is not ready-made, and requires breaking glass vials, mixing the powder and fluid, and drawing it up into the syringe before giving the shot. I was always afraid of either shattering the glass and cutting myself, or worse, accidentally getting bits of glass into the solution. For a guy who almost flunked chemistry, it was a pretty heady experience. After the solution was prepared, I would give Susan just a little notice and then give her the shot, while I talked about relaxing, opening up, and imagining the baby we were trying to have.

Maybe not all men would be as worried about their ability to give the shots, but I'm sure that the involvement and the sense that "we" were making this baby would be a feeling that many would share.

The IVF cycle is initiated after menstruation begins. Superovulation (stimulating the development of a number of oocytes) is attempted with injections, once or twice daily, of Metrodin (FSH), Pergonal (hMG) or a combination of both, for eight to twelve days. Some programs vary this "recipe" by combining either FSH or hMG with clomiphene. In these cases, a GnRH agonist is usually not used because that drug does not combine well with clomiphene.

Specialists feel that the primary advantage of using fertility drugs is to stimulate the development of a number of eggs that can be taken from the ovaries, fertilized outside the body, and transferred. This increases the chances that one of those eggs will successfully implant and develop. Unfortunately, large doses of such medication are often used, unless natural cycle IVF is attempted (see section above). These drugs may produce unpleasant physical and emotional side effects in some women, and their long-term effects on the body are not known — important factors to weigh when considering the use of ovulation induction medications.

STEP 3. **Monitoring Follicular Development**

❦ I began daily blood tests and sonograms. Matt couldn't take any more time off, so I went alone to the lab every morning at 7:30 — bleary-eyed but still scared. I quickly realized that the same four of us were there every day. We talked to each other as we waited to be called. I grew to care for them all, but I especially loved Isabella. She was beautiful and so kind to me. She left her home every morning at 5 A.M. to get to the lab in time. We shared a lot. I told her how afraid I was of needles. She told me this was her last try; she couldn't take anymore.

Everyday we all met and asked anxiously, "How are you doing? Is everything okay?" We'd speak about how nerve-wracking this was, how much we wanted these babies, what we had been through already. But there was also an etiquette. You never asked how many follicles were developing or anything too personal. Every morning Isabella held my hand and told me I would do fine. She waited while they took my blood and then we walked together to the clinic for the sonograms. And the nurses were wonderful — they gave us so much support.

We all traded phone numbers. And every night we each called Dr. X's number and listened to the tape for our instructions. One night I heard: Susan, two amps in the morning, two in the evening; Isabella, four amps; Christine, three amps; Cindy, three amps. Sometimes I took two shots and the others only one. I worried about this and wondered what was wrong with me.

Day after day this went on. And one by one the women advanced to the hCG shot. Their names dropped off the tape. Isabella had also moved on. I continued to take the Pergonal and had to buy a second kit. I was beside myself; it felt like everybody was graduating but me. I was forever computing where the other women were in the program. Finally, after the twelfth day, Dr. X said we had three, possibly four follicles. I was ready for the next stage. That evening Matt gave me the hCG shot.

Over a six- to twelve-day period, several methods are used to monitor the development of follicles, the fluid-filled sacs within the ovary that contain the eggs. After hMG and/or FSH is administered, frequent (often daily) blood tests are required to assess estrogen and LH levels. Cervical mucus, retrieved by pelvic examination, may also be tested to determine whether ovulation is imminent.

Ultrasound, the bouncing of high-frequency sound waves from the ovary, is also done frequently to track the growth of the follicle(s). In this painless ten-minute procedure, the woman lies on a table, is prepped for a pelvic exam, and a slender instrument is inserted into her vagina. Her reproductive organs become visible on a screen and a picture is taken of the developing follicles. The specialist evaluates this information daily. Are there too many follicles developing or too few? Are they growing normally? The medications are constantly adjusted according to the number of developing follicles and their rate of maturation.

As they increase in size, the follicles secrete increasing amounts of estrogen. They usually each contain an ova, although the team may find an empty sac during aspiration. When blood tests and sonograms show peak estrogen levels and follicles approximately fifteen to twenty millimeters in diameter, an hCG shot is given to enhance development. Ovum retrieval, by ultrasound-guided aspiration, is usually scheduled within thirty-six hours of this injection. Spontaneous ovulation occasionally occurs; in such cases the treatment cycle is cancelled.

STEP 4. Assessing Endometrial Morphology

Some specialists also test the serum progesterone levels and measure, through ultrasound, the growth of the uterine lining during this stage. Research has indicated that if the ovulatory phase and the endometrial development are not in synchronization, the chances of an ART success are doubtful. Some experts feel that in this case it is important NOT to proceed. They recommend retrieving the eggs, fertilizing them, and freezing the embryos for implantation in a subsequent, natural cycle when the endometrium is more receptive.

STEP 5. Retrieving the Eggs

❦ Two days later we drove to the hospital for the aspiration, furiously computing. How many follicles actually have eggs in them? Of those, how many will fertilize, how many implant? We finally figured we had a 50 percent chance of one aspirating, fertilizing, and implanting. God knows how we got that number.

I was both excited and scared. While they put the IV in my arm, I looked around and saw Isabella walking toward me! I realized that she had come in today for her transfer. She held my hand and said, "Isn't this exciting?"

I broke the rules and asked her how many eggs she had. She said sixteen and then she left for her procedure. I was devastated. Sixteen! I asked Matt why we were even there. I had three, four at the most. The nurse took my hand and said, "Susan, it doesn't matter. They only transfer four. You've got what you've got. It's going to be all right."

The sedation took and I was really groggy. They aspirated all four. I had secretly worried that the pressure would be too much, and Matt wouldn't be able to give a sample. Afterward he came into the recovery area, smiled at me and whispered, "They put me in a room with a video and a couple of Playboys. I produced enormous, unbelievable, copious amounts of semen, Susan." I began to cry.

The ART team attempts an ultrasound-guided aspiration of the follicles through the vagina. This outpatient procedure is usually performed with intravenous sedation, carefully monitored and adjusted by the anesthesiologist. A needle attached to a catheter is guided, by ultrasound, through the vaginal wall (about $1/16$ inch in thickness) to the ovary. The follicle sac is punctured and the egg and its fluid aspirated. The process is repeated for each egg. Many women can feel each puncture, and some find the procedure quite uncomfortable or painful. If the patient is extremely anxious or uncomfortable, stronger sedation, or perhaps regional or general anesthesia may be used.

Most patients develop between four to ten eggs; some produce many more. In most cases, the attempt to withdraw at least four eggs is successful; the surgical team is rarely unable to retrieve at least one egg.

In most cases, the patient's mate will provide a semen sample within five hours of the aspiration. He is asked to abstain from ejaculation for a least forty-eight hours prior to the collection. For many men, this is an anxiety-producing situation. Some programs will store a previously collected, frozen semen sample. Often this "insurance" is enough to alleviate the anxiety. If not, the frozen sample is available for the fertilization, although success rates using fresh sperm are often higher.

After the woman has sufficiently recovered from the aspiration and any anesthesia administered, she and her mate leave the clinic to eagerly wait for the completion of the fertilization and incubation process, and for the call to return for embryo transfer.

STEP 6. The Critical Role of the Laboratory: Ovum and Sperm Preparation, Fertilization, and Incubation

❦ The success of an IVF attempt hinges on the quality of the lab. I know of programs where they turn out the lab lights at 5:00 and go home, in effect saying, "Vaya con Dios, Eggs!"

I tell every patient that lab personnel must be available whenever needed, and those gametes and embryos should be carefully tended. Don't accept anything less.

❦ I love to meet with ART patients, explain exactly what happens in the lab, discuss methods we can use to overcome certain problems, and show them pictures of each stage of embryo development. I want to help them in any way I can through this difficult experience. Most really appreciate this effort and are fascinated with the biological process. Some have been in other ART programs and never knew what went on in the lab. There was this void between aspiration and transfer where they just waited and worried.

The critical role of laboratory staff and procedure in the ART process cannot be overemphasized. Many experts believe that if fertilization does not occur within the first twenty-four hours after insemination, the chances for pregnancy are almost nil. Meticulous laboratory technique and careful evaluation, monitoring, and handling of the couple's eggs, sperm, and developing embryos, according to their unique fertility factors, can enhance the chances for a successful IVF cycle.

Many embryologists and lab personnel also welcome and enjoy interaction with patients (or those considering ART), and encourage phone calls or meetings to explain lab procedure and answer questions.

Ovum Preparation. After retrieval, each egg is evaluated for maturity, washed, and cultured in a plastic dish. A chemically balanced, sterile medium, similar in composition to human Fallopian tube fluid, is then added. Some labs will check, over the next four to six hours, for the development of the polar body. The emergence of this cell, which mirrors the genetic information of the main cell body, indicates normal maturation progress. Efforts may also be made to synchronize the development rate of all oocytes aspirated. The eggs are incubated, at body temperature, for about seven hours.

Sperm Preparation. The semen sample is washed to separate the sperm from the seminal plasma. It is centrifuged until the heavier sperm cells form a pellet beneath the fluid. This liquid is replaced and the stronger, more motile sperm swim up into this new medium. In some cases of low sperm motility, processing with a "percol" solution may be used instead. During sperm preparation, the membrane over the head of the sperm will undergo a process called capacitation, enabling them to fertilize an egg.

A sample is drawn and evaluated before fertilization is attempted. The embryologist notes the quantity of sperm and their motility, as well as the quality of the culture medium. Nutrients may be added or the chemical composition of the fluid adjusted.

Fertilization. About seven hours after aspiration, if the gametes are mature and ready, the embryologist adds between 50,000 and 500,000 sperm to each dish. They are then incubated for about seventeen hours, under precise conditions of humidity, temperature, and gaseous air content, which replicate those within the body. After several hours, there should be a noticeable breakdown of the cumulus layer. If sufficient numbers of sperm are not binding to the zona, more may be added. If none have bound after four hours, a few programs may try micromanipulation techniques. (These techniques are still experimental, offer very low success rates, and are utilized in only a few clinics. See chapter 15 for further discussion.)

The pro-nuclei stage usually occurs about twelve hours later, followed by the first cell division fifteen to eighteen hours after insemination. The fertilized eggs are now called zygotes. During natural reproduction, a zygote immediately divides and continues to do so for four to five days as it travels down the Fallopian tube. When it reaches the uterus, it contains either thirty-two or sixty-four cells and is called a preembryo.

During the IVF process, the zygote is allowed to divide for about two days, to the two- to eight-cell stage. Although an IVF zygote is significantly less developed when it reaches the uterus than its natural counterpart, pregnancy rates are highest when transfer is within two days of retrieval.

STEP 7. **Embryo Transfer**

❦ The day after the retrieval, the embryologist called and said all four of our eggs had fertilized and divided. We were on top of the world! She told us to come in early the next morning, which was my thirty-ninth birthday. When we woke up, Matt said, "Happy birthday. Let's go get a baby!"

I was so excited. When we got there they took Matt into the lab to look at the embryos. I was given a sedative and rolled to a darkened room where Dr. X was waiting with the catheter. I was very drowsy and relaxed. He gently dropped the embryos in and told me to rest. They put the bed in a head-down position and I lay there for three hours and slept. Later, I dressed slowly, moving as little as possible. They took me out to the car in a wheelchair. Matt reclined the seat, drove home, and gently helped me up the stairs and to our bedroom.

> Dr. X advised three days of bed rest, but I stayed there for four. Matt left drinks and sandwiches by the bed each morning. I read and rested and thought about the baby. I started progesterone shots right after the aspiration and continued them every day. Now we had ten days to go before the pregnancy test.
>
> I did as little as possible and stayed very quiet. I wanted to call Isabella, but didn't dare. I didn't want to hear that she was pregnant. No one called me, either.

The embryo transfer is done at the clinic as an outpatient procedure. No anesthesia is required, although some patients are offered a sedative. The patient is prepped for a pelvic exam, a speculum is inserted in her vagina, and her cervix is cleaned. The embryos are immersed in a protein-enriched drop of culture fluid and placed in a slender catheter attached to a syringe. The catheter is threaded through the cervix and into the uterus, where the embryos are injected.

Specialists often have different guidelines about how many embryos to transfer Some programs will transfer no more than four embryos in an ART cycle regardless of the couple's preferences. Depending on the patient's age, the maturation and quality of the embryos, the number of previous ART attempts, and the couple's feelings about abortion in the case of multiple pregnancy (selective termination or pregnancy reduction), other specialists may transfer up to six embryos to the uterus (IVF) or tubes (ZIFT). (See discussion of the ZIFT procedure below.) Additional, unused embryos may be frozen in liquid nitrogen and saved for a future natural cycle attempt. (See the discussion of cryopreservation below.)

After embryo transfer, most women remain in bed for three to six hours. One to two days of rest is commonly advised, followed by a week or two of limited activities. After leaving the clinic, the couple must wait an endless ten days before a pregnancy test can be done.

STEP 8. **Progesterone Support**

During normal fertilization, the corpus luteum (the follicle sac remaining in the ovary after ovulation) secretes increasing amounts of progesterone hormone to sustain the pregnancy until the placenta can take over. Some ART teams fear that the aspiration process affects the corpus luteum and its subsequent progesterone production. It is also thought that the use of high doses of fertility drugs affect the endometrial lining and the chemical balance within the body.

Many experts believe the chances for successful pregnancy are increased by hormonal support either after aspiration or embryo transfer. They prescribe natural progesterone, through suppositories or daily injections, for the first eight to ten weeks of pregnancy or until menstruation occurs. Some programs also offer the options of weekly injections of synthetic progesterone (no correlation with increased risk of birth defects has been found to date) or hCG boosters. Other programs discontinue progesterone supplementation after a positive pregnancy test.

STEP 9. **Pregnancy Test**

❧ Ten days later I went in for the pregnancy test. I was very frightened. This was it. Matt and I had used all our savings and already I was wondering how we'd find more money if it didn't work.

They took the blood and said they would give the results to my gynecologist. The test came back with a number, not a positive or negative result. My gynecologist said, "I wish that hCG number were higher."

I asked, "Am I pregnant or not?"

She said, "I don't know. We'll run it again in two days." Totally confused, I called Dr. X's office. They were ecstatic and thought I was pregnant. We ran it again in two days. Same thing. My gynecologist said, "Wish that number was higher."

Dr. X's nurses were screaming, "This is wonderful, this is fantastic."

My emotions were seesawing up and down. I took another hCG test two days later and yet another three days after that. Finally, my gynecologist and Dr. X agreed that I was pregnant.

I remained cautious, not quite believing. Several weeks later, Dr. X had me come in for a sonogram. He pointed to the screen, smiled and said, "We have one viable pregnancy."

"Do you mean I'm going to have a baby?" I asked.

Again he pointed at the screen and said, "Susan, look. Look! One baby!"

Then I caved in. Crying, I slowly lifted myself from the table and hugged him.

A pregnancy test is usually done ten to twelve days after an IVF transfer — earlier than a serum hCG test would be ordered in a normal pregnancy. Consequently, many obstetricians unfamiliar with the IVF process may not understand early test results.

An IVF specialist will look at the hCG level on the first test and, based on that number (usually above 25 mIU/ml [milliInternational Units per milliliter]), predict the probability of a viable pregnancy. In these cases, a sonogram to confirm a uterine pregnancy and heartbeat is performed five weeks after transfer. Some programs continue progesterone injections until the eighth to tenth week of gestation; others discontinue this medication when pregnancy is confirmed. The patient is then referred to an obstetrician for pre-natal care and delivery.

If the hCG level is in the borderline region, another pregnancy test will be ordered in two or three days. The level of hCG hormone should double in that time. If the number remains low, the patient will be given a negative result, asked to stop the progesterone injections, and expect a period in a few days.

Most programs advise a one- to three-cycle rest period between attempts. There is usually no restriction on the number of times a couple can attempt ART, but because of the expense and emotional stress, most couples try one to three times. After three or four — and certainly a maximum of six — unsuccessful attempts, many experts feel that standard IVF probably will not work. In such cases, egg donor IVF may be an option for the couple, as well as adoption and child-free living.

Success Rates

❧ On the day she took the pregnancy test, Cindy recognized those now-familiar feelings of excitement, hope, fear, and dread. This was it — try number seven and probably her last. She couldn't think about or concentrate on anything else, and as she had six times before, gave up the idea of going to work. Instead she went hiking on a favorite trail near her home, not far from a pay phone. Several times, she walked to the phone and called the clinic. On the third try, Dr. X came on the line. Cindy took a deep breath and said hello.

"I'm really sorry, Cindy, but the test was negative."

Tears rolled down her cheeks. With great effort, Cindy muffled a sob and thanked Dr. X for his help and said she couldn't talk anymore right now. He asked her to set up a talk appointment when she was ready. Cindy hung up the phone and cried for a long time. Then she called Hal.

Christine and Isabella received similar calls that day from Dr. X. For several weeks, all three women were sad and tearful. Their mates were similarly frustrated, sad, and concerned about their wives. All three couples, in their own way and time, grieved yet another loss in their infertility struggle.

❧ I feel horrible when I have to call the three out of four ART patients who don't get pregnant. We all feel the loss. In a sense, my patients WERE pregnant — they had viable embryos inside of them. Some are angry and upset with me. Others are confused. They say, "But everything was going so well. What went wrong?"

Most, like Isabella, Christine, and Cindy, just express their sadness and thank me for taking care of them. I urged them, as I do all my patients, to come back to review their experience and future plans, and if necessary, to bring closure to their treatment.

There is a great deal of confusion about interpreting the success rates of ART programs. Some clinics report pregnancy rates as high as 40 percent, while others claim a 10 to 15 percent success rate.

Why is there such a discrepancy? Some programs may not accept candidates older than a certain age or with multiple fertility factors. Patients may also drop out of the program at each stage: Some women do not respond to the fertility drugs and ovulation does not occur, or one or more eggs may not be aspirated during the retrieval. Success rates may vary between IVF and other procedures such as GIFT, ZIFT, and egg donor IVF. Statistics can also be skewed by including only women who successfully complete the transfer stage of a procedure. When pregnancy does occur, percentages can also be misleading. Some programs may report all pregnancies achieved in a sample of patients as successes, and not adjust the figures for transient hCG rises or subsequent miscarriages and ectopic pregnancies.

When considering an ART program, *determine how many live, full-term births have resulted in relation to the number of patients entering the process **in your age group and with your fertility factor(s)***. For example, 1,000 patients, aged forty with tubal blockages and normal male factor, divided into 110 live term births equals an 11 percent success rate.

Among ART programs, today's actual success rates range from about 10 to 35 percent, depending on patients' ages, fertility factors, and the type of ART procedure used — IVF, GIFT, ZIFT, or egg donor IVF. These are ART pregnancies that result in a live, full-term baby. The number of embryos transferred also affects the success rate. When only one embryo successfully divides and is transferred, rates are close to 10 percent. Transferring two embryos increases the chances to about 20 percent, and three or more transferred embryos may result in greater than 25 percent success rates. The chances for success are probably the same with each attempt — up to four to six tries. After six attempts, the chances of a successful ART attempt are low. Boy-girl ratio and Caesarean delivery rates for ART babies parallel those of the general population.

Obstacles to Higher Success Rates. Most ART programs report an 80 to 90 percent success rate for ovum retrieval, fertilization, and cell division. The major obstacles to higher success rates have been proper hormonal stimulation, successful implantation after the transfer, and early pregnancy loss through ectopic pregnancy or miscarriage.

Batches of hMG hormone vary and each woman responds differently to fertility drug stimulation, so some patients are unable to produce viable follicles to aspirate.

Implantation problems and early pregnancy loss may be partially caused by transferring an embryo that is less developed than one normally would be during natural reproduction. Laboratory techniques for ART are still being refined and, at the present time, implanting a two- to eight-cell embryo seems to yield a higher success rate than waiting until it has divided to the body's normal 64- to 128-cell stage.

Early pregnancy losses are also difficult to prevent. In fact, many pregnancy losses occur naturally. If 100 ovulated eggs were exposed to sperm in women twenty-five years of age, only about 30 percent would produce a live birth. This success rate declines as a woman ages. In her mid-thirties, she has only about a 15 percent chance of a successful term pregnancy resulting from unprotected intercourse. These odds decline further as she passes forty. It is doubtful that science will ever surpass Mother Nature, but hopefully a success rate comparable to the body's will be approached as ART technique is further improved.

MEDICAL RISKS OF ART

Hyperstimulation of Ovaries. An ART patient's ovaries and hormonal levels are frequently monitored by sonogram and blood tests during the ovulation induction stage. Many women will experience some discomfort, abdominal swelling, or tenderness while taking hMG or FSH. In most cases, this is annoying but not dangerous. There is a slight risk, however, that the drugs may cause hyperstimulation syndrome. Symptoms include fluid retention, vomiting, and swelling of the ovaries for up to seven days. Less than 5 percent of patients will develop problems serious enough to require hospitalization.

Bleeding or Infection from Aspiration or Transfer. During the aspiration process, a needle must be passed through the vaginal wall to reach the ovary. Although only about 1/16 inch of vaginal tissue is perforated during this procedure, there is a slight chance that bleeding, hemorrhage, or damage to blood vessels can result. The transfer process carries a small risk of uterine infection.

Complications from Surgery. Laparoscopy, performed under general anesthesia, is commonly used during the GIFT and ZIFT procedures to transfer eggs and sperm or embryos to the tube(s). Any surgical procedure and anesthesia carry some risks. (See chapters 5 and 10 for further discussion.)

Fetal Abnormalities. Laboratory fertilization does run a higher-than-normal risk of an egg being fertilized by two sperm. Normally, when the egg and sperm unite, one set of twenty-three chromosomes is contributed by each parent (the diploid number). If two sperm fertilize the egg, three sets of chromosomes are contributed and an abnormal embryo is formed. Such embryos, however, would not be transferred in an ART cycle.

There are six species of mammals in which IVF has resulted in live births. In all six species, the number of normal IVF offspring has been encouraging, and there is probably no significant risk of inducing fetal abnormalities with this process. Because children conceived through IVF are still fairly young, however, the long-term health risks of this procedure are still not known. Several studies of IVF children between five and six years of age have reported normal social, intellectual, emotional, and physical development.

DES-Related Risks. With both natural and IVF pregnancies, DES daughters with uterine abnormalities run a greater risk of miscarriage or premature delivery. Regardless of the method of conception, careful monitoring of pregnancy is advised. Some DES daughters also have an abnormally small cervical opening, which may make insertion of the catheter for embryo transfer more difficult.

Ectopic Pregnancy. With IVF, there is a slightly higher chance (3 percent as compared to 1 percent in the general population) of an ectopic pregnancy. Even though the Fallopian tubes are bypassed during the IVF process, an ectopic pregnancy may occur if the embryos float back into the tube and implant. One theory, difficult to prove, suggests that the force used during the transfer process to inject the embryos may cause one or more of them to wash back up the uterus and into a Fallopian tube.

Multiple Births. In the general population, the chances of a multiple birth (twins or more) are about one in eighty. IVF rates depend on the number of embryos transferred. Most programs try to transfer four embryos to increase the chances for one successful pregnancy. Such a transfer would pose a 20 percent chance of multiple births, with most resulting in twins and perhaps 3 percent in triplets. Several sets of quadruplets have resulted from four-embryo transfers.

PREGNANCY REDUCTION (SELECTIVE TERMINATION)

🍃 We opted for pregnancy reduction when we found out that I was carrying triplets. We had tried for four years to get pregnant and were finally successful with IVF. The specialists told us that with triplets we might not get three live, healthy babies. To increase the likelihood of having healthy children, we chose to reduce from three to two. We had tried so hard to get pregnant and wanted to ensure that our children would be healthy at birth.

I went through the procedure without much emotional turmoil. Even telling people about it didn't bother me much. I felt confident that we were increasing the chances of survival and good health for our twins. The bleeding that had plagued me throughout the first trimester stopped the day following the reduction — a confirming sign to me that we had done the right thing. Some people thought this was a coincidence, but I felt that my body was too stressed by a triplet pregnancy.

The deep sadness didn't hit me until our twins began to be two little people with adorable and quite different personalities. What would the third one have been like? All of the ideas about ill health and death in triplets faded away. I only envisioned a third little child of mine.

I would not have chosen pregnancy reduction if I had been assured that all three would have been healthy babies. No one, however, could assure me of that. The real heartbreaker would have been to birth children who would not live normal lives. I am glad that I prevented that incredible heartache. I could not have withstood raising multiples with health problems. Raising healthy multiples is stressful enough.

The number and viability of fetuses is carefully monitored throughout an ART pregnancy. Most specialists feel it may not be safe, for either mother or off-spring, to carry more than two or three fetuses In such cases , pregnancy reduction will be discussed with the couple. This procedure is usually performed late in the first trimester to reduce the chances of miscarrying the remaining fetus(es). Selective termination of one or more fetuses can be a very stressful, upsetting prospect to many couples. It is best to share your thoughts and preferences with your specialist about this procedure before you initiate a treatment cycle, and to discuss how many embryos you wish to transfer.

Psychological and Emotional Dynamics of ART

❧ We visited Dr. X and his staff a few days after our daughter was born. I asked the nurse what happened to everyone. She told me that I was the only one of the group to get pregnant. The others were still thinking over their options. To this day, I've never contacted anyone, nor have they called me. I think about them all, and especially Isabella, often.

I remember stopping by Dr. X's office to visit one day. In the waiting room there was another group of four women, waiting for their initial interviews and tests. One was knitting a baby sweater. They were swapping stories and sharing their dreams just as we four had — ready to plunge into ART with hope and courage and fear. I cry whenever I hear someone I know is infertile, and I pray for everyone who goes through ART.

Waiting, Watching, and Hoping Against the Odds. *It is important to emphasize that luck, as well as individual fortitude and medical competence, plays a large role in every fertility treatment — especially ART.* Susan and Matt's perseverance and faith resulted in the birth of a beautiful, healthy baby girl. Isabella, Christine, and Cindy, and their mates, equally determined, hopeful, and courageous, did not get pregnant.

Yet nearly all couples entering an ART cycle truly believe they will be among the lucky ones. Indeed, it would be hard to undertake such an arduous experience if they didn't feel this way. They focus solely on the success rate — be it 10, 25, or 30 percent — not on the greater and more probable odds that they will not get pregnant.

This faith is reinforced as they proceed through the protocol. Success at each step — ovulation induction, egg aspiration, fertilization, and embryo transfer — bolsters the conviction that the process is working and they will become pregnant. Positive thinking, visualization, and prayer are evoked daily as blood is drawn and follicles develop. From the initial and often long-awaited interview and through the interminable medical process, the couple's anticipation and hope build, at a feverish pitch, to an almost unbearable magnitude. This Herculean effort culminates in triumph or, in most cases, disappointment and despair, several weeks after transfer with the positive or negative results of one or more hCG tests.

Many couples remark that the first failure is certainly difficult, but not as devastating as subsequent ones. They mourn for awhile, reassess their options, and perhaps try ART once more. Failure becomes harder, they say, with each attempt, intensified by the knowledge that this is the last medical resort.

To complicate matters, modern technology holds an almost irresistible carrot before them. In the 1990s, it is infertile couples, rather than their physicians, who must set the limits and decide "how many tries are too many" and "how old is too old." Ironically, personal qualities such as determination and perseverance, which are assets in many life crises, can almost be a handicap now. Couples with two, three, or more failed attempts may reason that they just might get pregnant on the next one. Sadly, some couples may feel they are unable to stop, convinced, like compulsive gamblers, that they will hit the jackpot on the next try.

Most unsuccessful ART couples, however, reach the point when they realize that "enough is enough." A period of mourning often follows. (See chapter 20 for a discussion of grieving after the cessation of medical treatment.) Afterward, they are able to pursue other resolutions with hope and enthusiasm.

Infertility Feelings Revisited. Those who enter the ART process may also reexperience many old and familiar infertility feelings. They again feel vulnerable and out of control, while coping with a dizzying array of intense emotions. Hope, exhilaration, impatience, excitement, disappointment, devastation, and grief often follow one another in a brief, condensed window of time.

From 70 to 90 percent of ART patients have little difficulty reaching the transfer stage, only to be faced with a negative pregnancy test two weeks later. This is a terrible letdown. One specialist observed that many of his patients "feel pregnant" as soon as embryo transfer is done. When they learn the attempt was unsuccessful, they often experience the emotional aftermath of pregnancy loss. Where unsuccessful laparoscopic or microsurgery is a gradual realization, an ART failure is an immediate and devastating reality. Some patients who do get pregnant will miscarry shortly after and face the intense and complex emotions of multiple loss (see chapter 13).

Impact on the Couple. The couple's life becomes engulfed in the ART process, and it is literally all they think or talk about for a month. Although it brings them closer in many respects, it also creates acute emotion and tension. Husbands often accompany their mates to the laboratory or the clinic, and many also administer the injections. Some women experience side effects from the medications, including physical discomfort, irritability, teariness, or pronounced mood swings. The importance of the husband's love, support and encouragement is critical, yet it is often hard for both partners to understand each other's feelings and to cope with the intensity of their own.

After an unsuccessful try, the woman may worry that she did not lie still long enough, or in some other way rejected the embryo after transfer. The man is often depressed by the entire effort, extremely concerned about his wife's emotional and physical well-being, and equally saddened by the failure.

Couples may also disagree over who to tell about their experience. One partner may wish to confide in friends and relatives about the ART attempt, while the other considers this a private and intimate matter. Both may be concerned about protecting the family's privacy about the details of their child's conception.

This emotional stress is augmented by the considerable expense of ART procedures. The couple must decide how much of their money to put into this infertility resolution. If all of their savings and hope is spent on several unsuccessful ART attempts, they may have little money or emotional energy left to direct toward another alternative such as adoption.

Experts stress the importance of obtaining enough emotional support — through trusted relatives and friends, counselors, or support groups — during the ART experience, and if needed, afterward.

Relationships with the Medical Team and Other Patients. Many of the ART medical team members share their patients' successes and failures. The doctor-patient relationship during this process is one of intense daily interaction for several weeks as they work toward a common goal of pregnancy.

Nonetheless the medical team is *not* equipped to offer the emotional support that most patients need during this ordeal. In many ART programs this vital function is taken on by the patients. Some have traveled far from home and miss the support of family and friends. Sharing joy and sadness with each other fills an important need, yet it is difficult not to feel jealous or competitive. Some ART programs include professional counselors on their staffs to help patients cope with the medical process. Others encourage patients to join a support group during this time.

Some ART patients may also be sensitive about any discussion of their experience with other patients. If you are concerned about this or other confidentiality issues, speak with your specialist and the nursing staff about your feelings.

Single and Gay Women

❦ I feel extraordinarily lucky to be accepted into an ART program in Northern California. I know many programs will not accept single women. This is also a frightening and lonely experience to go through alone.

A single heterosexual or lesbian woman who wishes to undergo ART may experience the same problems encountered in the DI process (see chapter 16). Some programs will accept only a married couple. If she is accepted, she may sense disapproval or judgment from the medical team or her fellow patients for pursuing parenthood as a single woman or gay partner. Feelings of isolation and lack of support are common. Coping suggestions for infertile single and/or gay women are offered in chapters 7 and 16.

Other ART Procedures

The following section discusses variations of the IVF process which have been developed during the past ten years. All ART procedures raise a number of ethical issues that are addressed at the end of this chapter.

Gamete Intrafallopian Transfer (GIFT). GIFT, a medical technique developed in the mid-1980s, is a similar procedure to IVF but has some important differences and advantages. It is only available to women with at least one normal Fallopian tube. While it may be an appropriate treatment for some types of male infertility or sperm antibody problems, most couples who undergo this procedure have unexplained infertility.

The Procedure. GIFT parallels the IVF process in duration, and initially, in procedure. GnRH agonists may be used to suppress the current menstrual cycle and superovulation is usually induced with fertility drugs. Frequent lab work and ultrasound monitoring is also conducted, a number of follicles are retrieved through ultrasound-guided retrieval, and the husband is asked to provide a fresh semen sample.

At this point the process diverges from IVF. With GIFT, the egg and sperm are not fertilized in the laboratory. Rather, up to four eggs are combined with sperm and injected by catheter into the Fallopian tube(s) (up to two eggs per tube) during laparoscopy. (See chapters 5 and 10 for a discussion of surgery.)

Some programs are experimenting with non-surgical GIFT, a technique of transferring eggs and sperm through a catheter into the Fallopian tube(s). Success rates using this method, however, have not been as high as those achieved with laparoscopy. Experts theorize that placing embryos into the wider end of the tube during laparoscopy, as opposed to the narrower end (which occurs during non-surgical transfer) may enhance pregnancy rates. It may also be possible that the non-surgical transfer somehow disturbs or traumatizes either the uterus or tubes, reducing the chances for pregnancy.

Fertilization hopefully occurs in the tube and the embryo travels down to the uterus to implant. GIFT thus allows natural, "in the body" cell division to occur before implantation. Bed rest or limited activity is usually recommended for several days after the laparoscopy.

In some cases GIFT is tried after one IVF attempt in which an ovum was fertilized, to ensure that the egg can indeed be fertilized by the male partner's sperm. In rare cases, the GIFT procedure may fail to aspirate a mature ovum. In that case, the ova may have to be incubated and IVF attempted a day or two later.

Cost. While fewer laboratory charges are incurred with this procedure than IVF, laparoscopy is usually used during GIFT for gamete transfer. Thus, the costs for both procedures are similar. The 1992 cost of GIFT was about $8,000 to $10,000 per cycle. Part of this expense may be covered by some medical insurance carriers as part of infertility diagnosis. In the future, GIFT may be performed during the diagnostic laparoscopy of the infertility workup if ovulation is occurring naturally, unless corrective surgery for pelvic problems is indicated.

Success Rates. GIFT offers about a 10 percent higher pregnancy rate than IVF. Some experts think it may also be a better option for women older than forty. A one- to two-cycle wait is recommended between attempts. For most couples, a maximum of three or four tries is recommended.

Zygote Intrafallopian Transfer (ZIFT) and Tubal Embryo Transfer (TET). With ZIFT or TET, follicles are removed by vaginal aspiration as with standard IVF, and then fertilized and incubated in the laboratory. The viable embryos are transferred the next day (ZIFT) or two days later (TET), usually by laparoscopy, into the Fallopian tubes rather than the uterus.

Unlike GIFT, the ZIFT process verifies that fertilization has occurred, which is beneficial in cases of male-factor infertility. ZIFT or TET may also be recommended in cases of cervical mucus problems or immunological or unexplained infertility. Success rates of 25 to 30 percent, similar to those of GIFT, have been reported.

FROZEN EMBRYO TRANSFER (FET) AND CRYOPRESERVATION

❦ Phillip and Isabella met with Dr. X for their follow-up talk. After three failed IVF attempts, they had tentatively decided to stop treatment. Dr. X explained that sixteen ova were retrieved during Isabella's last IVF cycle and twelve had fertilized. Four embryos had been transferred into Isabella's uterus and the remaining eight, according to the couple's wishes, had been cryopreserved. They now had the option of transferring four of the frozen embryos in a natural cycle, at considerably less physical stress and financial expense.

Sperm cryopreservation (freezing in liquid nitrogen) has been available for several decades now, and frozen samples are often utilized for donor insemination (see chapter 16). During the past few years, impressive advancements have occurred in this technology. Research is currently underway in cryopreservation of ova, which may be especially useful for women undergoing cancer treatment or premature ovarian failure.

Currently, embryos not used in a stimulated cycle can be cryopreserved at the one-, two-, four-, eight-, or sixteen-cell stage and then transferred later during a natural menstrual cycle (FET). Some specialists, however, recommend estrogen and progesterone preparation of the uterus before transfer. This procedure is less physically and emotionally traumatic (no ovulation induction stage) and less expensive (about $1,000) than standard ART protocol.

Between 60 and 80 percent of the embryos survive the thawing process and success rates of 10 to 20 percent have been reported for this technique. Pregnancy rates also depend on the number of eggs initially retrieved and the number of those viable after thawing. The transfer of embryos cryopreserved as long as three years have resulted in the birth of healthy children.

Surrogate Gestational Mothers. Some women may be physically unable to carry a pregnancy because of a hysterectomy, a history of repeated miscarriages, or a congenital absence of the uterus (Rokitansky Syndrome). In some cases, another woman may agree to gestate and birth a genetic child for these couples. The genetic mother undergoes ovulation induction, the ova are fertilized with the father's sperm in the lab, and the embryos are transferred to the surrogate gestational mother. Her uterus may be hormonally prepared for the transfer to maximize the chances for a successful implantation and pregnancy. The ethical, legal, psychological, and emotional issues, unique to both gestational and genetic surrogate mothers, are discussed in chapter 19.

Egg Donor IVF

❦ Rachel was diagnosed with premature ovarian failure, at the age of thirty-three, shortly before she and Brent were married. Both wanted children and were devastated by the news. When they shared their sadness with their families, Rachel's two sisters were especially empathetic. Darlene, however, went a step further and offered to help Rachel in any way she could.

Egg donor IVF is the most recent addition to the burgeoning ART technology. Ova from another (usually younger) woman are aspirated, fertilized with the genetic father's sperm, and transferred to the recipient's uterus for gestation. This procedure was originally developed as an option for premature ovarian failure (POF), a rare condition affecting about 10 percent of infertile women with ovulatory problems. Encouraged by the success of egg donor IVF in women with POF factor (up to a 35 percent live birth rate), many specialists are now offering this option for a wider range of female infertility problems.

Although sperm donation has been a familiar and admittedly controversial option for infertile couples for decades, the advent of egg donor IVF has evoked an even greater flurry of debate about third-party reproductive technology. This section examines both the medical aspects of egg donor IVF, as well as its unique emotional and psychological issues. The chapter concludes with a discussion of some of the ethical issues of all ART technology.

The author gratefully acknowledges the insights, research, and assistance of several egg donor IVF couples, who wish to remain anonymous, to this analysis. They developed and distilled much of the following information. "It is our sincere hope," they write, "that no one faced with this opportunity will have to reinvent the wheel. We are all on the cutting edge of brave new families, and what we do now significantly impacts the choices that will be available in the future."

INDICATIONS

❦ Although Dee Dee had a history of ovulatory problems, she and Chet delayed childbearing while they concentrated on their teaching and business careers. When she was thirty-seven, they decided to try for one child. She wasn't ovulating regularly and underwent a workup. A small amount of endometriosis was diagnosed and surgically removed; Chet's semen analysis was normal. Another five years passed without success. During this time they investigated adoption and considered a permanently child-free lifestyle.

They opted to reenter treatment, and at forty-two, Dee Dee began an arduous three-year course of treatment — numerous fertility drug and intrauterine insemination cycles and, also unsuccessfully, several ART procedures. Her last ART cycle was cancelled at the ovulation induction stage. At the age of forty-five, her ovaries no longer responded to the fertility drugs. Dee Dee still wanted to become pregnant; Chet argued that they had run out of time and medical options. Their specialist mentioned a new ART procedure — in vitro fertilization using eggs from a donor. Both were incredulous. It sounded like science fiction.

The egg donor IVF option may be an appropriate option for the following female fertility problems:

- Premature ovarian failure. In this rare condition, a woman's ovaries cease functioning prematurely, often in her thirties or even younger — years before menopause should naturally occur. Such women do not respond to ovulation induction and may be candidates for egg donor IVF.
- Women aged forty or older who are unable to conceive, or those with a high FSH reading on Day 3 of their cycle. As the reproductive system ages, some women older than forty may not respond to ovulation induction treatment. In addition, these women often experience decreased embryo implantation rates, a higher incidence of miscarriage, and increased genetic abnormalities in their own eggs.

  Recent research suggests that it may be the age of the eggs, rather than the uterus, that influences ART pregnancy rates. With hormonal support, many women in good health can successfully carry a pregnancy through their forties and perhaps even into their fifties. If the eggs are donated by a woman under thirty-five years of age, an amniocentesis is not usually recommended, regardless of the age of the gestating mother.
- Women who have suffered repeated unsuccessful ART attempts. Experts believe that after four, or at the most six, ART cycles, the chances for a successful pregnancy are slim. Using eggs donated from a younger woman increases the live, full-term birth rates for a woman over forty from less than 15 percent to more than 30 percent.
- Women who have undergone radiation or chemotherapy cancer treatment.
- Women who carry genetically acquired health problems.

☐ Women who are unable to ovulate or do not respond to ovulation induction medication.

MAKING THE DECISION

❦ Rachel and Brent spent several months talking with physicians and other couples experienced with egg donor IVF. After lengthy discussion, they agreed to try this procedure, but had reservations about involving Darlene. They wondered whether old sibling rivalries would surface, hopelessly complicating the family dynamics and the sisters' relationship. They shared their decision to undertake egg donor IVF, along with their research and worries, with Darlene.

Recently married, Darlene and her husband Gil were not planning to have children for a few years. Both had concerns about Darlene donating eggs. Gil worried that she might suffer complications or be left infertile. Darlene was afraid of the medical procedures and any pain that might accompany them, and of possibly donating abnormal eggs to Rachel. She also wondered whether she would be comfortable with Rachel and Brent's style of parenting. From the outset, however, she was also committed to, and certain of, her decision to donate eggs to Rachel.

Both couples met with a counselor. In some ways it was difficult and confusing to sort through everyone's feelings. Several of them felt as if boundaries were violated and that, at times, they were "inside each other's marriages." They also met with Dr. X to review the procedure and any medical risks. After a long talk with her mother, Darlene decided that this donation was a gift, and that she would probably have occasional concerns about her nephew or niece's upbringing even if her genes weren't involved.

Slowly and sometimes painfully, each fear was allayed as both couples reached a mutual decision to proceed.

❦ Dee Dee realized as "my birthdays kept coming and the babies didn't," that she still wanted to bear a child and was ready to try egg donor IVF. Chet had deep misgivings about involving a donor in their lives, and about the social and legal ambiguities of the process. At an impasse, the couple saw a therapist to address their concerns.

The egg donor IVF decision-making process is often a complex and lengthy one. Several parties are affected, for a lifetime, by this decision: the couple, the donor, her mate and child(ren), any children born from this process, and to an extent, the extended families of those involved.

Many of the questions regarding standard IVF decision-making and donor insemination (see the beginning of this chapter and chapter 16) are pertinent in this case, along with several unique to the egg donor option:

☐ Why is egg donor IVF a better choice for us than adoption or child-free living?

☐ Have I thoroughly grieved for the loss of my (my partner's) genetic line and for the baby we would have created together? How do I feel about my husband, but not myself (myself, but not my wife) being genetically related to this child?

☐ Have I considered the reality of being medically infertile and pregnant at the same time?

☐ Will we tell our child of this decision? Who, if anyone, among our family and friends? Do we agree about whom to tell and when? If we confide in others, are we prepared for both positive and negative reactions to this unconventional and often controversial fertility treatment?

☐ What will I do if the child has a birth defect? If a multiple pregnancy occurs?

☐ Am I prepared to embark on a path fraught with legal, emotional, social, and ethical ambiguities?

☐ What if this procedure is not successful? How many times would I/we try before considering another option?

☐ Where do we stand as a couple on this issue? Can we manage the stress, and possibly isolation, of this experience? Can we fully support each other through the process?

It is wise to examine feelings and reservations, to carefully consider the consequences that may ensue, and to study the germane ethical and psychological issues before deciding on this option. Partners often disagree or have conflicting feelings about third-party assisted reproduction. Professional counseling, from someone both knowledgable about third-party ART issues and *without a vested financial or emotional interest in your decision*, along with adequate emotional support, is advisable.

FINDING A DONOR

❦ After agreeing to proceed, they consulted a counselor who matched donors and infertile couples. As she studied the resume and picture of each prospective donor, Dee Dee felt uneasy. This was too impersonal for her. She wanted to know her donor, rather than just read a medical history and short biographical sketch. She discussed her feelings with a colleague familiar with the couple's struggle. Eileen thought it over for a few weeks and then offered to donate eggs to Dee Dee. They saw a counselor together. Dee Dee was concerned about future repercussions and wanted Eileen to be sure about her decision. They agreed to proceed and drew up a written agreement.

Four embryos were transferred during the first unsuccessful donor attempt and five were frozen. The frozen embryos were transferred in a subsequent ZIFT try. This attempt also failed. Dee Dee was devastated and stopped treatment.

Six months later, Dee Dee at forty-seven, and Chet, nearly fifty, again entered counseling and decided to try again with a different donor.

Jessie, a twenty-four-year-old mother of three, had known Dee Dee for several years and greatly admired her. She thought about how being a mother had enriched her own life and how Dee Dee had missed that experience. Their infertility problems had saddened Jessie and she seriously considered donating some of her eggs to the couple for another try. Jessie discussed it with her parents and husband. They also knew Dee Dee and were supportive of the idea. Jessie also saw a counselor.

A week later she met with Dee Dee. "If you're in need," she said, "I'd love to be able to do this for you." Both women began to cry.

Once a couple opts for this process, they must decide whether to seek a known or an anonymous egg donor. Specialists recommend that donors be under thirty-five years of age, in good health, and have no history of genetic disease. In addition, they should undergo a thorough medical and psychological screening.

Known Donors. Some couples pursue this option with the help of a sister, relative, or close friend. The advantages of a known donor include a complete and easily accessible genetic history, a more involved, empathetic and perhaps dependable third party, and, if desired, future involvement with the child. Disadvantages may include complication of present relationships and obscuring of established boundaries, a rekindling of old rivalries or jealousies, and increasingly complex family or friendship dynamics.

Anonymous Donors. Although they may not obtain as extensive a medical and genetic history, other couples prefer to work with an anonymous donor — someone outside their immediate circle of family and friends.

ART clinics will also sometimes match prospective candidates with cryopreserved gametes or embryos donated by other couples who have successfully conceived. Genetic health histories of both partners are usually available. Some donor and recipient couples also choose to meet each other. Other ways of finding donors include advertising in college newspapers or other youth-oriented publications, and working with a counselor or facilitator who matches women wishing to donate ova with infertile couples.

As with all infertility options, one should approach this process as an educated and cautious consumer. Carefully investigate the screening procedures, cryopreservation techniques, and relevant success rates of a prospective clinic, as well as their policies regarding gamete donations. Many donors prefer to meet the prospective couple; others do not. If all parties decide to maintain anonymity, ensure that a permanent record will be kept by the clinic of the donor's identity and health history. If you both wish to meet, each must consider the degree of involvement both before and after the baby's birth. Some couples may also have concerns about the donor providing ova for another couple in the future. It is best to confront these issues beforehand.

Similarly, check the credentials and references of any third-party facilitator you are considering. A conflict of interest, for example, may arise if a therapist engages in both counseling infertile couples and donors, and also acts as a broker between them. Subtle or even overt pressure may be placed on either party to participate in the process. *A counselor should never have a vested interest, emotional or financial, in a client's decision.*

Fees. The Ethics Committee of the American Fertility Society recommends that donors be exactly that, and that no fee, excepting reimbursement for travel and lost wages, be paid to gamete donors. In reality, both sperm and egg donors are frequently paid, egg donors often receiving between $1,500 and $2,500 per cycle. Additional costs of $2,000 or more may be charged by a third-party facilitator.

Consentual Agreements between Donors, Recipients, and the Clinic. Many couples and donors sign agreements before treatment is begun. These contracts may include provisions for the expectations of each party, disposition of unused eggs or embryos, informed consent and termination of parental rights of the donor, and perhaps future visitation. Currently, there are no statutes or court rulings regarding egg donation, and it is unlikely that such contracts are legally enforceable.

ART clinics have designed consent forms to clarify the conditions of donation, treatment, and if preferred, anonymity, to be signed by donors and patients. Donors are asked to keep the clinic apprised of their current address and any on-going or newly developed health problems.

MEDICAL PROCESS

❧ They started with GnRH agonist shots for both sisters. Then Darlene began the ovulation induction phase. About a week before Darlene's egg retrieval, Rachel received a series of estrogen and progesterone injections to prepare for the embryo's implantation. Twelve eggs were aspirated from Darlene, seven fertilized with Brent's sperm, and three embryos were transferred to Rachel's uterus. The remaining four embryos were cryopreserved. By mutual agreement, Darlene withdrew from the process after the aspiration.

Five weeks later, Rachel and Brent viewed the single fetus, heart beating, on the ultrasound screen.

❦ Jessie responded well to the hMG and developed, the nurses joked, "too many follicles to count." Everyone was excited and optimistic. Fourteen eggs were aspirated and fertilized; six were transferred through ZIFT to Dee Dee. She did not become pregnant. The remaining unused embryos were frozen, but did not survive the thaw for the next attempt. Both women were sad and disappointed when the first cycle didn't work.

The medical process of this procedure closely parallels that of standard IVF. Some programs recommend an "evaluation" cycle for the recipient to perform any necessary tests or lab work prior to the actual egg donor IVF attempt. Natural cycle IVF, where the donor does not undergo ovulation induction, may also be offered by some programs.

In most cases, both donor and recipient undergo GnRH agonist treatment, with injections or nasal spray, to halt their current cycles. Then ovulation induction of the donor is attempted with hMG and/or FSH. (See IVF discussion above and chapter 9.) The recipient often undergoes estrogen and progesterone treatment, monitored with blood tests and ultrasound scans, to prepare her endometrial lining for the transfer.

After retrieval, the donor's eggs are fertilized with the male partner's sperm and transferred to the tubes or uterus of the recipient through either IVF, GIFT, or ZIFT. After transfer, the recipient receives progesterone supplements until an hCG test is administered. If pregnancy occurs, some programs continue progesterone treatment for the first eight to ten weeks of gestation.

SUCCESS RATES

❦ They waited two months and tried once more. This time six embryos were transferred. Dee Dee felt she entered the process with more serenity than usual. She had prepared herself physically and emotionally, and yet was equally resigned to another disappointment. This time she became pregnant with twins.

Some programs achieve egg donor IVF pregnancy rates close to 40 percent, but statistics must be adjusted to reflect subsequent ectopic pregnancies and miscarriages. In patients older than forty, live, full-term birth rates of 25 to 35 percent have been reported with egg donor IVF, as opposed to 5 to 10 percent with standard IVF using their own eggs. Although GIFT and ZIFT offer about a 10 percent greater pregnancy rate for women older than forty using their own eggs, success rates are about the same with all donor egg ART procedures.

To avoid exposing the donor to the stresses and risks of ovulation induction, some programs will offer a natural donor egg IVF cycle. If the recipient undergones hormonal uterine preparation, success rates of 15 to 20 percent are predicted with this method.

Experts believe that the higher success rates of egg donor IVF can be attributed to both the use of younger donor eggs and an ideally receptive recipient uterus. In biological terms, eggs under thirty-five years of age are less likely to carry genetic abnormalities, and more apt to easily fertilize and implant than "older" ones. At the same time, the recipient has both avoided the ovulation induction protocol and its effects on her body, and has hormonally prepared her uterus for the transfer of the embryos.

Specialists recommend a maximum of three tries at donor egg IVF, and sometimes suggest using a different donor after the second unsuccessful cycle. For donors, most experts recommend *no more than four stimulated cycles*.

Cost. Donor egg IVF is an expensive undertaking, involving the cost of standard IVF plus charges for donor screening, recruitment and donor fees if applicable, medical treatment, and counseling for all parties. Total cost will vary in each case.

For a couple who has a sister or close friend donate without a fee, pays for medical screening and counseling for themselves and the donor, agrees to a medical "evaluation" cycle for any necessary tests, and undergoes one egg donor IVF attempt, an approximate cost breakdown might be:

Medical screening	1,000
Counseling	500
Evaluation cycle	500
Egg donor IVF cycle	8,500
TOTAL	$10,500 PER CYCLE

Another $2,000 to $4,000 may be added if donor and/or facilitator fees are incurred — upping the tab to a staggering $12,500 to $14,000 or more per cycle. Depending on their coverage, a couple's insurance may pay for part of the medical protocol and perhaps counseling costs. Many couples, however, pay for all costs themselves — some affluent enough to afford several attempts, others borrowing and depleting all savings to finance one try.

PSYCHOLOGICAL AND EMOTIONAL ISSUES

❧ Rachel and Brent met privately with their parents and extended family to discuss their decision. They patiently answered questions and provided information, believing it was important to squelch rumors before they started. A few relatives reacted with disbelief, dismay, or criticism. Most were supportive and noted the similarities of their situation with divorced and blended families.

Physically, the pregnancy progressed normally while Rachel's emotions seesawed wildly. On one level, the whole experience seemed strange and surreal. She was often asked, by those "in the know," how it felt to be carrying her sister's child. And like many infertile women, she couldn't quite believe she was finally pregnant. It wasn't until she felt those first kicks that bonding began, and she truly believed that this was HER baby.

The sisters' relationship has become more complex. Although Rachel feels that she is the baby's mother, a small part of her realizes that this child does not carry her genes. Darlene regards herself as "just this baby's aunt," yet also feels a very special tie to the child. She also feels very close to both Rachel and Brent. Although Rachel is deeply grateful for her sister's gift, she acknowledges that old sibling rivalries occasionally surface. Most times, the sisters can accept their feelings with humor and equanimity.

The egg donor IVF process is a complex psychological, emotional and ethical one that profoundly impacts the infertile couple and their child(ren) and the donor and her family.

The Couple. The donor egg IVF option parallels donor sperm insemination in several ways. One mate will be the genetic parent of the child; the other will not. Both resolutions may result in an imbalance of power between the partners as one remains medically infertile and the other does not. Old infertility issues such as depression, inadequacy, and grief for one partner may reemerge in a different and more complicated context.

With donor egg IVF, however, the infertile woman is the gestating mother of the child, and is thereby both medically infertile and pregnant. Most women feel that, even though they are pregnant, an enormous loss is still experienced. For many, grieving for the loss of their lineage and their genetic union with their mate, continues through the pregnancy and beyond.

As with DI, this pregnancy often seems surreal or strange. Several women said that the process sometimes seemed like "high-tech group sex" and that they didn't truly "bond" or "feel pregnant" until their babies began kicking.

It can also be difficult to separate egg donor issues from common post-infertility or "normal" pregnancy emotions. Regardless of how they ultimately conceive, many women often experience strange, ambivalent, or frightening, as well as joyful and exhilarating feelings during their pregnancies.

Thus it is crucial that the partners are able to support and communicate with other, and obtain enough emotional and psychological support. They must face considerable challenges and make a number of difficult decisions together, including their criteria for the donor and her involvement, if any, in their life; whether to tell their child about his or her genetic origins; and who, if anyone, among their family and friends, to tell and when.

The "who to tell?" question is complex and partners often disagree over who should know. One mate may feel closer to certain relatives and friends than the other. He or she may view the circumstances of their child's conception as a technological feat, and want to share it with those who have supported their infertility struggle. Other partners feel that the conception and pregnancy, albeit medically assisted, is a private, intimate matter. "We wouldn't share the juicy details with anybody if we conceived this baby the old-fashioned way," argued one father-to-be. "Why should we 'tell it all' with a high-tech conception?"

Achieving pregnancy is also another step in the bonding and maturation of the partners, as a couple and as parents-to-be. For many, protecting the privacy of their new family becomes the priority as the pregnancy advances. As the birth approaches, expectant parents prepare in many ways for their new role. They often feel extremely protective of the child's physical and emotional well-being, as well as privacy. Many also realize that their child will live with the legacy of their decisions. If they tell others about her genetic origins, they lose control over how and when to tell their child. Others will know the details of her genetic history before she can understand them. (See chapter 18 for further discussion of parenting after infertility issues.)

If a known donor is involved, her feelings are another factor to consider. Does she want her involvement with the child's conception discussed? If so, with whom and when? How does she feel about future contact with the family? How does her mate and children feel about sharing this information?

THE DONOR

🐦 Being a mother meant a lot to Jessie and she expressed deep compassion for Dee Dee: "If I could give her the opportunity to experience a child's love, it would be worth any trouble to me."

But Jessie also wondered how she'd feel toward the baby if this worked. She thought she could separate herself emotionally, but realized she wouldn't know until it actually happened. Jessie didn't care what other people thought, but wanted to be sure within herself of this decision. After careful reflection, Jessie concluded that this was a gift and any babies created would be Dee Dee and Chet's, not hers. She feels the woman who gestates and nurtures these babies is their mother.

She has gone to the pre-natal appointments with Dee Dee and feels like an honorary aunt. "I know these kids will be raised in a wonderful home and that they will have good and loving parents," she says.

Her mother is excited that Jessie could help an infertile couple. One of Jessie's aunts and her grandmother, however, don't approve at all. They think the twins are Jessie's babies and can't imagine how she could do such a thing.

Jessie was paid for her donations and used the money for college expenses, but insists she would have done it for nothing. She is very proud of her role: "Besides saving a life, it's one of the only ways you can give the gift of life."

🐦 Darlene arrived at the hospital just a few hours after Elana was born. Seeing her for the first time, and recalling the love, pain, and struggle that resulted in the miracle of Elana's creation and birth, moved Darlene to tears. "My pride, happiness, and joy that day were indescribable, and grow each time I see her."

She visits often and helps feed and care for Elana. Like Rachel and Brent, Darlene feels Elana should know the truth, as she is ready, over time. Most of all, Elana's well-being, happiness, and privacy come first.

Why do women consider egg donation? For many donors, a love of motherhood, commitment to family, and compassion for the infertile are key motivating factors. As with sperm donation, this altruism may also be tempered with narcissism and financial incentive. Some donors undoubtedly consider this gesture a lovingly and freely bestowed gift, as well as a life accomplishment. Others may feel subtly pressured or obligated to be "a good friend, sister, or cousin."

Beside examining, and feeling comfortable with, their motivation, potential donors should also consider the time-consuming and often stressful IVF medical procedures involved with this decision. In most cases, daily injections and frequent ultrasounds and blood work will be required for several weeks. Ovulation induction with either hMG or FSH involves exposure to large quantities of drugs, and the risk of immediate side effects or medical complications. The long-term effects of these medications and procedures is still unknown.

This experience may also affect her partner and any child(ren) they might have. Will she meet the couple, and if so, maintain contact with them and the child in the future? Does she have a preference for the marital status, sexual orientation, or lifestyle of the recipients? Will her mate feel jealous or uneasy about any child(ren) resulting from this process? Will her children be frightened by the medical procedures or confused about their relationship with the child?

Donors may also encounter criticism or judgment from their relatives, friends, acquaintances, and even society at large. These are new and largely uncharted social waters. Many people have already formed strong opinions about the ethics or wisdom of third-party assisted reproduction.

In addition, prospective donors must clarify their expectations about whether they expect a fee and how many times they wish to undergo the medical procedures. Suppose the first cycle or two doesn't work? Other dilemmas may also arise. What if the donation results in a multiple pregnancy? How would she feel if the recipient couple should opt for pregnancy reduction or abortion of a fetus with a birth defect? What if extra embryos are frozen for later use or donated to another couple?

These are all complex and difficult issues which require careful thought before a final decision is made. Many donors find it helpful to seek counseling with their mate and, in some cases, with prospective recipient couples to clarify their feelings and expectations.

The Ethical Challenges

🍃 Dee Dee views herself as both a social and medical pioneer who willingly sought treatment, though at times, she also felt "experimented on." She thinks technology has reduced the pressures of the biological clock for many women, and objects to either society or the medical profession arbitrating maternal age. She believes this is a personal choice.

She is concerned about having enough energy to raise her children, joking that the kindergartners may mistake her for the kids' grandmother. While she reflects that she may not live long enough to see her own grandchildren, she also says with a smile, "There are plenty of tired twenty-year-old parents and my grandparents lived to be ninety!"

❦ Looking back on the experience, Rachel, Brent, Darlene, and Gil are glad they faced the tough questions beforehand. Thorough research, emotional support, and counseling were a great help. Having Elana here is a joy to them all and interacting with each other feels natural.

They think egg donor IVF is a wonderful, but very different way to parent and, like themselves, those who choose this path will face the challenge, triumph, and controversy of being a social pioneer.

For decades, Americans have passionately debated the ethical and moral ramifications of technologically-assisted reproduction. For so long an abstract, science-fiction concept, the term *test-tube baby* has evoked, over the years, images of Aldous Huxley's frightening, futuristic society of *Brave New World*, along with concerns about how such technology, if ever developed, would be applied, regulated, and controlled.

In the 1990s, the technology to create ART babies, with a variety of possible gamete combinations, is available, advancing at a rapid rate, and being offered to patients in clinics around the world. The media is filled with reports of the latest scientific breakthroughs, and the moving human stories of triumph and devastating disappointment inherent in their application. Everyone seems to be talking about ART these days, and the ethical implications of these procedures are hotly debated by politicians, psychologists, theologians, scientists, feminists, philosophers, social workers, physicians, and infertile patients.

In response to the debate surrounding the proliferating ART technology, several groups have formally examined, discussed, and in some cases, developed professional or social policy recommendations. In 1988, the Office of Technology Assessment issued its compendium, *Infertility: Medical and Social Choices*, which includes an excellent discussion of the germane social, ethical, religious, economic, and women's issues of ART and surrogacy from a variety of traditions and perspectives (see Bibliography).

The Ethics Committee of the American Fertility Society has met periodically since its inception in 1984, and has issued a number of recommendations, papers, and policy statements regarding application of the evolving technology. In its 1990 report, the Committee examined the medical, social, and ethical considerations of several ART procedures, advising that they:

> ... be performed in accordance with the recommendations contained in that report, as well as any future reports from the Ethics Committee. At the present time, IVF, GIFT, ZIFT, and the use of donor oocytes and donor preembryos, and embryo cryopreservation are recognized as clinical, i.e. non-experimental, procedures. Examples of procedures which are currently considered experimental include oocyte freezing, "ovum transfer" (or embryo flushing from the uterus and transfer to another woman), and oocyte and embryo micromanipulation techniques. Procedures considered experimental must be conducted under the supervision of an Institutional Review Board or equivalent committee.

Most recently, the Canadian government has appointed a Royal Commission on New Reproductive Technologies, with the mandate:

> ... to inquire into, evaluate, and make recommendations about new reproductive technologies in terms of their social, legal, ethical, economic, research, and health implications for women, men, and children and for society as a whole.

For several years, the Commission has gathered data, initiated research projects, and solicited testimony from a broad segment of Canadian citizens and interest groups. Interim updates and summaries are now available; publication of their final report and recommendations is expected in late 1992 (see Resources).

Caught in the midst of this spirited, often heated, and frequently confusing debate, are the infertile women and men — most veterans of a long, discouraging, and emotionally painful medical struggle — who are considering ART. Often bewildered, frustrated, or angered by the controversy surrounding these options, these couples and single women may also feel ambivalent themselves. The high-tech, clinical aura surrounding ART, and the physical, social, psychological, and legal aspects of these practices may conflict with their values, cultural traditions, and expectations about procreation. At the same time, ART may indeed be their last hope for a biological child.

Society as a whole, and infertile women and men as individuals, face the considerable challenge of obtaining reliable and accurate medical and legal information, examining the complex ethical implications of these options, and instituting social policies and making personal decisions that carefully consider and weigh the needs, rights, dignity, and physical and emotional well-being of all involved parties.

This section presents some of myriad ethical, social, women's, religious, moral, legal, and economic issues, many overlapping and intersecting, that have been raised about ART. (Discussion of the ethical issues of genetic and gestational surrogate mothers is presented in chapter 19.) Among concerned individuals and groups, there is a wide spectrum and divergence of opinion about relevant issues, appropriate recommendations for policy and regulation, and acceptable solutions to the social and medical problem of infertility.

ART in a Pronatal Culture. For millions of years, pregnancy, childbirth, and parenting one's biological children has been lauded, encouraged, and inculcated in nearly every culture — a value system often referred to as pronatalism. For most of human history, pronatalism has served the vital and necessary purpose of perpetuating the species. Through the present day, children have been taught that biological parenthood is an important and perhaps necessary part of adult development, and to varying degrees, integral to individual status and feelings of self-worth. Although our world is now, many would argue, dangerously crowded with 5.5 billion people and consequently facing a multitude of resource and environmental problems, pronatalism persists. Despite the sweeping social changes of the past thirty years and the advancement of the women's movement, many women and men still feel pressured to reproduce, and stigmatized when a fertility problem occurs. For the infertile, this problem may be, and often is, both a medical and social affliction.

Although the development of ART has created more medical options and hope for infertile couples, there is also concern that many will feel obligated or pressured to use this technology once, or repeatedly. Will women, who must undergo the procedures in cases of either female- or male-factor infertility, feel that they must birth a child — regardless of the emotional, physical, or financial cost — to be valued by themselves, their mates, their families and friends, and our society? With the tempting carrot of a possible ART pregnancy hovering a cycle away, can a woman "just say no" to one try, or two, or five? One couple, who adopted a child shortly after their second unsuccessful ART attempt, were asked by several incredulous acquaintances: "You gave up after only TWO tries?"

Many also wonder how the availability, and continued refinement, of ART will affect society's and infertile couples' view of adoptive parenting and child free living. Will adoptive families be accorded the respect and status they deserve? Will all the children already born who need loving homes find placement? Will the choices of child-free women and men who seek other ways to contribute to society, and to relate to children, be honored and respected?

Issues of Health and Well-Being. Questions have also been raised about the safety of prescription drugs and procedures used for all infertility treatment — for both women and men. Are patients able to make informed choices? Are they receiving accurate information about medications and procedures? Are they being quoted realistic success rates, derived from accurate, unskewed data?

Citing the increasing medicalization of infertility, pregnancy, and childbirth, and the current social and judicial debate about women's reproductive rights, concerned groups also worry that ART may further distance women from the personal and private sphere of reproduction. They ask whether this technology will adversely affect women's self-esteem, feelings of power, emotional health, and sense of well-being.

And what of the children born from these technologies? Are there any long-term effects from medications taken by their mothers prior to conception or during early gestation? Will they be physically or emotionally affected by the way they were conceived or gestated? Should they be apprised of gamete donation or the involvement of surrogate gestational mothers? How will they make sense of their origins? Will society regard and treat these children with respect and dignity?

And Donor(s) Make Three, Four, Five. Now that egg donation, involving drug stimulation and vaginal egg retrieval, is being utilized, along with donor sperm, with ART, questions arise regarding donor motivation and treatment.

Are these women making informed choices? Is this decision based, as with sperm donors, on a combination of altruism, ego gratification, and financial incentive? Or will women feel pressured to donate eggs, or, in cases of surrogate gestational mothers, the use of their wombs, out of feelings of duty or responsibility, to infertile relatives or friends? Will some be tempted or pressured, by themselves or others, by financial incentive to donate?

Is it acceptable for an egg donor to undergo medical treatment when she does not have a fertility problem? Do donors understand the possible side effects or risks involved? Have limits been established as to how many times a donor may give eggs or gestate a pregnancy for others? What about inter-generational or inter-familial donation — between mother and daughter, aunt and niece, brother and brother, sister and sister? How will this decision affect existing family relationships and the children born from such donations?

Unplugging the Biological Clock. Egg donor IVF has extended the possible window of pregnancy for some women through their forties and beyond. On the one hand, many consider this a wonderful gift — an opportunity to circumvent the unalterable schedule programmed into our bodies, and birth a child later in life. Others question the wisdom of birthing after nature's suggested deadline. Should society or the medical establishment determine the limits of maternal age beyond menopause? How old is "too old" for a woman to undergo pregnancy and birth? No age limit, by nature or society, has been placed on fatherhood. Yet do women and men contemplating parenthood in their forties and beyond realize how much stamina and energy is required to raise a child to adulthood? And have they considered the exhausting responsibilities of the mid-life "sandwich generation," who may have to care for young children and aging, perhaps ailing, parents at the same time?

Religious Perspectives. Depending on their religious orientation and present commitment, ART couples may encounter support, censure, or perhaps confusion from their clergy and fellow parishoners. The Roman Catholic Church has voiced strong objection to any artificial assistance with conception or gestation, or the use of donor gametes, stating its rationale and intent in the

Instruction on Respect for Human Life in its Origin and on the Dignity of Procreation. Opinion about the appropriateness of ART or gamete donation, the point at which life begins, the moral status of the embryo, and the issue of selective termination in cases of multiple pregnancy, differs among, and within, other religious denominations.

Some theologians have also raised concerns about separating the act of conception (baby-making) from the intensely personal, private, and sexually loving expression of mutual marital commitment (lovemaking). Some wonder whether the utilization of donor gametes, or involvement of third parties in a child's gestation, may threaten or challenge the integrity of the family unit. Others worry that the increasing medicalization of conception may also separate or alienate the couple from emotionally and psychologically critical spheres of kinship, such as extended family, friends, church, and community.

Embryo Status and Cryopreservation. At the present time, both the moral and legal status of embryos is ambiguous. Concerns have been voiced about the ethics of freezing embryos (cryopreservation) and for how long, their disposition (donate to other couples, to research, or discard), the "ownership," "custody," or "inheritance rights" of embryos in cases of death or divorce, and screening of embryos for genetic disorders. In addition, the number of parties — sperm donor, egg donor, surrogate gestational mother, and rearing parents — who may possibly be involved in the creation of these embryos will probably pose complex legal issues for years to come.

To Regulate or Not, and by Whom? Individuals and interest groups have expressed concern over the lag between technological advancement and the development of a social and legal framework to assimilate, sanction, and regulate the application, commercialization, and accessibility of these practices. Should ART services be regulated, monitored, or controlled? If so, by whom and in what manner?

Economic Issues of ART. Among those who support the development and use of ART, many are concerned about the availability of these services. Is ART accessible to those low-income couples, the disabled, single women, lesbian couples, or women of color who wish to try it? Should ART be available only to those with sufficient funds or medical insurance coverage? Should insurance companies be required to cover all fertility costs, including high-tech and third-party assisted procedures? Should society underwrite some of these costs through research grants or funding of fertility clinics?

There is also concern over what drives the technology — a sincere interest to help infertile women and couples become pregnant, or a furthering of commercial enterprise, medical research, and the technology itself?

The debate of these provocative and complex questions will undoubtedly continue for years to come, while more ART programs open around the world. Spurred by hope, faith, and their dream of a baby, couples like Susan and Matt, Christine and Joe, Cindy and Hal, and Isabella and Phillip will enter their programs. The technology will continue to race forward, leaving joy, disappointment, ambiguity, uncertainty, and bewildering ethical, legal, and moral conundrums in its wake. And the pioneers of ART — the patients, their medical teams, and those who donate gametes — will continue to be studied, praised, admired, and criticized by an ambivalent society.

CHAPTER 15

Diagnosis, Causes, and Treatments of Male Infertility

❧ Eight years ago my doctor told me that I had a fertility problem. This was like telling me that elephants quack — it didn't conform to my ideas about how the world works. Women are the ones who have fertility problems; men are simply around to comfort them and accompany them to their doctors.

I said to myself, "Well, if her doctor just used the right procedure she would get pregnant, ending any nonsense that I might be part of the problem. I can still get it on as well as any nineteen year old. I don't need to waste money on a doctor's opinion when no male in my family has ever had fertility problems."

Thank goodness my wife prevailed in getting me to see a specialist. After years of laboratory visits (which now make for great party stories) and one varicocele operation, I have a four-year-old son who is the light of my life. Having Adam is so wonderful that I have gone through a second varicocele operation, fertility drugs, and a round of those 7:30 A.M. races to the doctor's office with my sperm in a plastic bag, just for another chance at fatherhood.

Robert Bookman

❧ My wife's gynecologist phoned me and simply said, "You have no sperm. None." When I heard this news, I felt like someone had kicked me in the nuts.

A MALE INFERTILITY PROBLEM is diagnosed in about 40 percent of couples seeking treatment. In another 20 percent or more of cases, problems in both partners will contribute to their infertility. Experts now think the combined fertility of both partners is a critical factor. Some men with low sperm counts easily impregnate their mates, and some women with known fertility problems become pregnant within a few cycles — while other couples with similar factors encounter years of infertility. In addition to the chemistry between the partners, the ages of both may also significantly affect their combined fertility. A woman's fertility naturally declines through her late thirties and forties, and such male-factor problems as varicocele may increasingly affect sperm count or motility over time.

Some experts, however, do think that the incidence of male infertility may be increasing in the United States. One study has suggested that there has been a decline in sperm count among American men over the past several decades. Although many urologists dispute the validity of this study, others suggest that the increasing incidence of sexually transmitted diseases such as chlamydia and mycoplasma, environmental pollutants, alcohol and drug abuse, exposure to X-rays or workplace toxins, and perhaps our modern, stressful life-style may be affecting male fertility.

Over the last twenty years, the field of andrology has evolved to study and treat disorders of the male reproductive system. Andrology has lagged behind gynecology in its research and understanding of physiology and reproduction. This is because of both a reluctance of many men to be tested and prior assumptions by both society and the medical establishment that a couple's infertility was always caused by a problem in the female partner. Thus a discussion of the causes and treatments of male fertility problems is regrettably shorter than that of female infertility. With further research in andrology more infertile men may be treated successfully.

To facilitate understanding of the physiology and hormonal chemistry of the male reproductive system, which is discussed throughout this chapter, refer to "Human Reproduction," pages 103 to 112.

The Urologist

❦ For six months I listened to the anguish my wife was going through. I was the good husband. Then she suggested that I have a sperm count done. It was just a suggestion, not a strong request, for she knew instinctively that my male psyche could handle only the vaguest hint at such an idea. With the grace and statesmanship of a Mahatma Gandhi, she said, "Dear, perhaps you should see a urologist so we can eliminate any possibility that the problem may also be with you."

This delicate suggestion fell on me like a ton of bricks. I couldn't believe my ears. I staggered to the couch trying desperately to catch my breath. After some more unnecessary theatrics, hurt feelings, and three-year-old behavior, I went off to see the urologist. And life hasn't been the same since.

Stop worrying about what the urologist is going to do to you. I promise he won't examine you with a lawn mower. You will hardly feel a thing. One word of advice, though. I have seen several urologists and after comparing notes with the men in the couples' support group my wife and I attend, I find we are in agreement on the importance of going to a urologist who specializes in male fertility problems. Usually these urologists are connected to a hospital-sponsored fertility clinic.

Robert Bookman

❦ One of my patients was told by a number of internists that nothing could be done with his zero sperm-count problem. I discovered he really didn't have a zero count. An X-ray revealed a cyst behind the prostate gland. Both ejaculatory ducts came into the cyst, which had no connection to the urethra. The whole system was dilated. The sperm were being produced and going into the cyst instead of the urethra — a fairly rare condition. In this case, it was simple, under anesthesia, to go in through the urethra and make a slit in the floor of the prostate. His sperm count rose to 30 million a few months later.

A urologist is a physician who specializes in disorders of the urinary system of both men and women. Some urologists are also andrologists and treat male reproductive problems. A physician with this specialized training is best qualified to interpret test results, prescribe treatment, or perform surgery for male infertility.

Such a specialized urologist should be consulted when the semen analysis reports a low or zero sperm count or a problem with movement, shape, or volume of sperm, or when an abnormality such as obstruction, varicocele, or hormonal imbalance is suspected.

Optimally the couple, the urologist, and if appropriate, the infertility specialist or gynecologist, work as a team, discussing tests and findings, and coordinating possible treatments as they progress through the workup. The couple should feel comfortable discussing their questions and concerns at any time. They are also strongly encouraged to educate themselves about the diagnosed problem and suggested treatment and to seek adequate emotional support.

Your gynecologist or infertility specialist may be able to refer you to a qualified urologist. Other sources of referral are RESOLVE and the American Fertility Society (see Resources), or your local medical association.

The Male Infertility Workup

❦ The semen analysis revealed a low count with no motility. A blood test showed a low level of testosterone. My initial reaction was shock. I felt my very masculinity was being challenged. All kinds of fears about my sexuality, losing my beard, even developing cancer filled my mind. Was my entire system out of whack? Finally I calmed down and began to ask questions: What does this mean? Can you fix the problem? Is surgery necessary?

A man's initial appointment with a urologist is similar to that of a female infertility patient. The specialist will first meet the couple in his or her private office and take a detailed medical history of both partners. They will review any

TABLE 15.1 MALE INFERTILITY WORKUP TESTS

Procedure	Purpose	Benefits, Risks, and Inconveniences	Approximate 1992 Cost*
Initial Visit— interview, physical exam	To gather medical history of both partners, detect obvious anatomical or physical abnormalities that may be impairing fertility	May reveal causes of infertility without necessity of more costly, invasive testing	About $100– $150, plus any lab work ordered
Semen Analysis	To evaluate number, motility and characteristics of sperm	Repeated analysis may be embarrassing, inconvenient and stressful	$75–$100
Sperm Anti body Test	To test for antibodies to sperm in both partners	May give indications of fertility impairment in cases of long-term or unexplained infertility	$75–$100
Scrotal/Rectal Ultrasound	To detect varicoceles or possible duct obstruction	Simple office procedure that may detect problems not found with physical examination	$100–$200 for scrotal $200–$300 for rectal
Vasography	To evaluate structure of duct system and locate any obstructions	Patient is exposed to risks of anesthesia and surgery	Usually included in charges for testicular biopsy
Fructose Test	To determine whether fructose from seminal vesi-cles is reaching the semen	An absence of fructose may suggest a congenital abnormality or absence of the seminal vesicles or vas deferens	$25
Hamster Egg Test	To provide information not available from semen analysis; assesses sperm's ability to penetrate a ham-ster ovum	Useful before costly IVF attempts. Cannot predict positively how sperm will interact with human egg	$250–$400
Hemizona Assay (Sperm Binding)	Assesses sperm's ability to penetrate split, non-viable human egg	Better indicator for IVF suc-cess than Hamster Egg test; currently only available in a few research centers	$250–$300
Testicular Biopsy	To determine whether low sperm count is caused by testicular or duct problem	Patient is exposed to risks of anesthesia and surgery	$800–$2,000 depending on whether proce-dure is done in physician's of-fice or hospital

*Costs vary in different geographic areas. These charges are based on an average of the fees of several West Coast hospitals, specialists, and laboratories.

past surgeries (such as hernia repair) and exposure to drugs (including alcohol, cocaine, marijuana, and nicotine), current medications, occupational or environmental toxins, specific childhood illnesses (such as mumps), and past illnesses or diseases (such as viruses, infections, or sexually transmitted diseases). The specialist will ask about the frequency of intercourse and whether the couple has experienced any sexual problems.

PHYSICAL EXAMINATION

The history taking is followed by a thorough physical examination of the patient, including a careful examination of the penis, testes, prostate, and scrotum. The physician will check that each testicle is at least one and a half inches in length and will look for a varicocele, which can often be felt in the scrotum while the patient is standing. They then meet again in the office to review the course of the workup and discuss physical findings, such as hernia or varicocele, and relevant medical history.

A METHODICAL INVESTIGATION

To ensure accuracy, the urologist repeats and personally interprets the semen analysis. It may provide some clue to the fertility problem. If not, the specialist and couple decide on other appropriate laboratory tests such as urinalysis, ultrasounds, X-rays, blood testing of hormonal levels, and testicular biopsies to detect infections, hormonal imbalances, obstructions, diabetes, or retrograde ejaculation (See Table 15.1). At the end of this workup both the physician and the couple should have more information and can work toward a resolution.

THE SEMEN ANALYSIS

❦ I have lots of great stories on this subject. Once I received a standing ovation from a construction crew. I arrived at the hospital parking lot at 7:05 A.M. (For some reason all the labs that I have visited do a semen analysis only between the hours of 7:30 and 8:30 A.M. There must be some prestigious research that suggests that the male homo sapiens finds this the most conducive time frame in which to ejaculate into a plastic bag or cup.)

I parked my yellow Volkswagen in the most secluded part of the large empty parking lot. I taped newspaper all around the windows and then proceeded for about ten minutes to do what I had to do. Apparently the rollicking motion of the car alerted a group of about twenty guys wearing hard hats that some folks were having a mighty good time. As I opened the door, I was met with approving male smiles and appreciative applause. My shock probably equaled their disappointment when they soon realized that my conquest was completed single-handedly!

Robert Bookman

🐝 The experience is just plain embarrassing. You are given a glass jar, sent to a bathroom (a totally asexual environment), and expected to produce a sample of semen — right now. If you can do it, you hand it to a nurse or technician, and they always seem to be females. The first couple of times they didn't even give me a bag or covering for the jar, so the entire waiting room audience could see it too! It seemed like everyone looked up from their magazines when I approached the desk. I also worried whether I'd pass the test: Were there enough sperm? Were they swimming fast enough?

A semen analysis should be routinely performed at the onset of both the female and the male infertility workups. It is essential to rule out any sperm abnormalities before extensive testing is done on the female partner (See Table 15.2).

Although the semen analysis is an important part of the workup, a single specimen may not be an accurate indicator of male fertility. Fevers, viruses, diet, heat exposure, or stress can affect sperm count for months afterward. Rather than relying on one test, most urologists prefer to obtain several semen analyses to observe the range of the patient's semen quality. Many personally perform the lab work on a fresh specimen obtained in their office. Otherwise, the sample should be analyzed by a reputable laboratory with good quality control. At least three samples should be analyzed before a diagnosis of male infertility is confirmed.

Collection Procedure. A precise collection procedure is essential to ensure accuracy and validity of the sample. The *entire* ejaculate should be collected in a clean, clear glass jar. In 90 percent of men, sperm are heavily concentrated in the first half of the ejaculate, so the second half is usually sperm poor. If the entire ejaculate is not collected, the count may be misleading.

The specimen is usually collected at the laboratory or clinic where the analysis will be done. Many men find this a difficult and embarrassing experience. Sensitive to these feelings, some labs provide a more private setting. Some men prefer to obtain the sample at home. In this case, it should be kept at room temperature and delivered to the lab within an hour of collection. At least two to three days of abstinence is necessary before the test.

If personal or religious beliefs prohibit masturbation, your specialist may have suggestions for obtaining a specimen without violating religious decrees. Recently a special silicon condom has been devised to collect a sample during intercourse. A few researchers, in fact, argue that semen ejaculated during intercourse varies markedly — in count, motility, and volume — from that collected during masturbation from the same man. They believe that the former is a better indicator of the male's fertility. Other experts disagree with this theory. In any case, if a collection condom is used, the sample must be brought to the lab within two hours for analysis.

Counting and Evaluation. After collection the ejaculate is drawn into a white blood cell pipette. It is diluted with a special solution that immobilizes the sperm and is placed in a blood cell counting chamber, which is divided into several large grids, each containing sixteen smaller squares. The semen now has a volume one cell layer thick. Under the microscope, the number of sperm in five large grids are counted. This number is multiplied by one million. The process is repeated with another set of five grids and the two numbers are averaged. This sperm count is obviously a rough estimate, with at least a 10 percent margin of error. For this reason semen analyses done by some general pathology labs are sometimes inaccurate or unreliable.

Some experts utilize computers to analyze the sample, a technique known as Computer Assisted Semen Analysis (CASA). Some urologists favor this technology and predict it will be increasingly utilized in the future. Other experts are skeptical, arguing that computers have difficulty differentiating debris and other matter from sperm, and that the resulting data is often inaccurate. And, although a great deal of information can be gathered in this way, they aren't sure how to interpret it. They favor the traditional method of analysis performed by knowledgable and experienced technicians.

Sperm counts can vary considerably between men, and more important in the same man day to day. A sperm count of 20 million or more per cubic centimeter (cc) of semen, however, is usually considered normal (especially in the presence of good motility), although 60 to 100 million per cc are optimal counts.

Motility, or movement, of the sperm is also carefully observed within two hours of collection. Some scientists now believe that motility is more critical to male fertility than sperm count. A sperm cannot fertilize an egg unless it reaches the Fallopian tube and finds and penetrates the ovum.

To assess motility the percentage of moving sperm in ten random high-power microscopic fields is estimated. Ideally at least 50 percent of the sperm cells should be moving two to three hours after ejaculation. The quality of motility refers to the degree of forward progression, and is graded from zero (no movement) to four (excellent forward movement). Grades one and two are considered poor motility; while Grades three and four are rated good. Asthenospermia is a condition where less than half the sperm are motile.

The *morphology*, or shape and maturity, of the sperm cells is also examined. A smear of semen is placed on a slide, air-dried, and then stained. Approximately 100 cells are classified in six categories: (1) normal (oval) shape and maturity; (2) amorphous (irregular or immature shape and size); (3) tapered; (4) double-headed (or duplicate); (5) micro (too small); or (6) macro (too large). At least 60 percent of the sperm cells should be normal in shape, contour, and maturity.

Normally the semen is liquid when ejaculated, coagulates quickly, and then reliquifies within twenty to thirty minutes. As part of the semen analysis the ejaculate is evaluated for its liquidity (viscosity). After ejaculation it should easily pour drop by drop.

The *volume* of the ejaculate varies among men, but about one teaspoonful, or between two and five cubic ccs, is considered normal.

Results of the Semen Analysis. The results of the semen test are generally categorized in one of four groups: (1) normal; (2) azoospermia (lack of any sperm); (3) abnormalities in several categories such as density, motility, morphology; or (4) isolated problems of one type (e.g., low sperm count).

The semen analysis should be repeated periodically during long-term infertility because acquired problems can reduce fertility during adulthood. These include hormonal imbalances, ejaculation abnormalities, exposure to drugs or toxic chemicals, and sperm antibodies.

TABLE 15.2 SEMEN ANALYSIS FACTORS

Factor	Method	Evaluation Criteria	Reported Results
Sperm Count	Semen diluted and placed, one cell layer thick, in a counting chamber that is divided into grids	The number of sperm in five large grids is counted and multiplied by one million. A similar area is also counted and the two numbers averaged — a rough estimate with a 10% margin of error	A count of 20 – 100 million sperm per cc of ejaculate is reported "normal"; below 20 million is reported as "low sperm count"
Motility	Two to three hours after ejaculation, the percentage of moving sperm in 10 random high-power microscopic fields is estimated	Degree of forward progression is rated on a scale of 0 – 4 (none – excellent)	Grades One and Two are reported as "poor motility"; Grades Three and Four as "good motility"
Morphology	A smear of semen is air-dried on a slide and under the microscope 100 cells are studied for shape and maturity	Sperm cells are categorized: (1) normal (mature with oval shape); (2) amorphous (immature shape or size); (3) tapered; (4) double-headed; (5) micro (too small); (6) macro (too big)	If 60% or more of the cells fall into category 1, a "normal morphology" result is reported. Less than 60% indicates abnormal sperm morphology
Viscosity	The liquidity of the sperm 20 – 30 minutes after ejaculation	Should pour easily drop by drop	If semen remains gelled, poor viscosity is reported
Volume	Measuring the amount of semen that is ejaculated	2 – 5 cc is considered within normal range	Less than 2 cc is considered low volume; greater than 5 cc is considered excessive volume

SPERM ANTIBODY TEST

A male workup may also involve testing of both partners for antibodies. Like viruses and bacteria, sperm are a foreign substance and have the potential to engage the body's immune system.

A small percentage of women have antibodies to sperm similar to the immunity developed to a particular disease. The antibodies occur in vaginal or cervical secretions and kill the sperm or cause them to clump together. Men may also develop antibodies to their own sperm, especially after a vasectomy is done.

Indications for sperm antibody testing include a normal sperm count with poor motility, clumping of sperm, a poor postcoital test result, a good count with poor motility after a vasectomy reversal, and unexplained infertility.

The immunobead binding test is usually performed to check for the presence of sperm antibodies in either partner. (See chapter 12 for further discussion of sperm antibody testing and treatment.)

ULTRASOUND

In recent years, ultrasound has been increasingly utilized for male fertility testing. The technique has been useful in both detecting varicoceles and duct obstructions. When the instrument is placed gently against the exterior of the scrotum, the testicular veins can be visualized on a screen. A somewhat more invasive but painless procedure, where a slender probe is inserted rectally, may reveal duct obstructions.

HORMONAL BLOOD TESTS

In most men, the levels of FSH, LH, and testosterone fluctuate. However, blood tests that reveal unusually high or low hormonal levels may indicate endocrinological or testicular problems that merit further investigation.

FRUCTOSE TEST

When working properly the seminal vesicles add fructose to the semen. A negative fructose test suggests a congenital absence of the vas deferens or seminal vesicles. In such cases, surgical removal of sperm for use in Assisted Reproductive Technology (ART), may be an option. (See chapter 14.)

SPERM PENETRATION ASSAY (SPA)

The Sperm Penetration Assay (SPA), also called the Hamster Egg Test, assesses the capacity of the sperm to penetrate a hamster ovum — a function not measured by the standard semen analysis. The gelatinous zone surrounding the hamster egg is removed, and about a million sperm are prepared in the lab and incubated adjacent to the eggs to attempt penetration. Experts recommend using fresh sperm and at least thirty fresh hamster ova and running a control test, using donor semen from a fertile male. If the sperm have less than a 10 percent penetration score, a male fertility problem is suspected.

Before a couple undergoes the expense and stress of in vitro fertilization, the SPA is often used to confirm the sperm's ability to fertilize. It may also reveal male fertility problems in cases of unexplained infertility; when a varicoele is detected, the test can help physician and patient to decide if surgery is indicated.

This test, however, cannot assess motility or predict how the sperm will react to the zona pellucida (outer covering) of a human egg. In fact, there may be 18 percent or higher false negative results reported, and some men whose sperm fail the SPA test successfully fertilize their mate's ova during in vitro fertilization. For this reason, experts disagree about the reliability or efficacy of the SPA. In conjunction with other fertility tests, however, it can provide useful information during the workup. (See chapter 14 for additional discussion of the SPA and Assisted Reproductive Technology.)

HEMIZONA ASSAY

Also called the sperm binding test, this recently developed technique tests the ability of the sperm to adhere to the zona of a split, non-viable human egg. It is still in the experimental stages and in use in only a few research centers.

VASOGRAPHY

Vasography (or vasogram) is another test that checks the structure and patency (openness) of the duct system and locates any obstructions. Some urologists perform a vasography, which clearly defines the affected area, at the same time as corrective microsurgery. During this outpatient procedure the scrotum is opened under local or general anesthesia, a dye is injected into the duct system, and X-rays are taken to reveal any blockages. Microsurgery may then be immediately performed, or rescheduled at a future time.

TESTICULAR BIOPSY

If the semen analysis shows a very low count or no sperm at all and hormonal levels are normal, a biopsy can be performed to determine whether the problem is caused by a blockage or impaired sperm production.

The biopsy is performed in either the specialist's office or the hospital as an out-patient procedure. After administering local or general anesthesia, the urologist makes a small scrotal incision and takes a tissue sample from the testicle. The procedure is usually accomplished within fifteen to thirty minutes. Because it is easily destroyed the tissue must be handled carefully and preserved in a special solution. The tissue is stained and examined under the microscope for the presence of sperm-generating cells. Absence of these cells indicates a testicular problem and, sadly, permanent infertility. If sperm production appears to be normal, the urologist can then investigate obstruction problems.

In most cases, no adverse effects are experienced. Rarely, swelling, bleeding, or infection may occur. The patient is advised to wear a scotal support for about a week. Work and most other normal activities can be resumed in two to three days.

Diagnostic Categories of Male Infertility and Their Treatment

For decades low sperm count was blamed for all male-factor problems. There is now increasing evidence that other factors such as varicocele, duct obstruction, ejaculation abnormalities, and hormonal imbalances can also contribute to male infertility. Unfortunately, there is little knowledge of how such problems specifically affect it. More research is needed in the areas of sperm production and motility, infection, immunology, and characteristics of seminal fluid. The following section discusses the various causes of male infertility and current modes of treatment.

LOW SPERM COUNTS AND POOR MOTILITY

Fevers, illnesses, infections, and stress can temporarily affect sperm count for up to three months. Before a low sperm count is diagnosed, three or more semen analyses should be performed over at least three months. Sperm motility can be affected by a varicocele, prolonged periods of abstinence from ejaculation, and exposure to heat from saunas or hot tubs.

Problems with persistent low sperm count (oligospermia) or poor motility account for 60 to 70 percent of male infertility complaints. A low sperm count usually refers to less than 20 million sperm per cc of ejaculate. Poor motility is diagnosed when half or more of the sperm are not swimming properly.

In half or more of these cases the cause of the problem is unknown. This condition is termed "idiopathic oligospermia." In other instances low sperm counts may be caused by varicocele, duct obstruction, undescended testicles, retrograde ejaculation, workplace toxins, surgery, drug use, hormonal imbalances, some medications (especially cancer treatments), in utero exposure to diethylstilbestrol (DES), or neurological disorders.

Treatment. Treating a low sperm count problem is a difficult task. There is no known "cure" because the abnormality itself is not fully understood. In fact, about 25 percent of couples with this problem will conceive with no treatment at all! Good motility and an especially fertile female partner improve the odds for a pregnancy.

Many couples, however, wish to investigate some form of treatment, despite the fairly low chances for success. Options for low sperm count or poor motility currently include:

☐ **Sperm washing with Intrauterine Insemination (IUI).** In cases of low sperm count, some specialists will recommend IUI. During this procedure, the semen is concentrated, "washed" and centrifuged to a fraction of the original volume and then artificially inseminated into the women's uterus. Success rates for IUI run between 5 and 20 percent. (See chapter 16 for further discussion of IUI.)

☐ **Fertility Drug Treatment.** The Federal Drug Administration (FDA) has not approved the use of fertility drugs for males, and they are not available for routine clinical use. However, such drugs may be prescribed by a specialist — with the patient's informed consent — to study and test their value in fertility treatment.

Use of fertility drugs probably offers only about the same chances for success as the spontaneous pregnancy rate (25 percent) achieved with no treatment at all. Individual successes, of course, depend on both luck and other fertility factors in both partners. In many instances pregnancy rates are much lower. Most couples conclude that drug therapy is not worth the stress, risk of possible side effects, and bother.

Many medical experts also argue that investing time in drug treatments for male factor fertility just delays the resolution process — especially a concern for older partners — and prolongs frustration and emotional stress. Instead, they suggest immediate consideration of other resolution alternatives such as donor insemination, Assisted Reproductive Technology, adoption, or child-free living.

In some cases, however, drug treatment will increase sperm count, through chemical stimulation of the pituitary, testes, or hypothalamus, to 20 million or more. Patients with extremely low counts consider these tremendous increases. Unfortunately, since the technique for counting sperm is inexact, changes of a few million are usually not significant. A few couples, however, opt for fertility drug treatment because they have been trying unsuccessfully for a pregnancy for years and want to at least try this option.

At this time the drugs used to treat specific types of male infertility are: clomiphene, hCG (human chorionic gonadotropin), hMG (human meno-pausal gonadotropin), and bromocriptine. Each has specific uses and indications (see chapter 9 for more detailed discussion):

□ **Clomiphene** is a synthetic estrogen commonly prescribed for ovulation induction. In the male it blocks the estrogen receptor site in the hypothalamus, which results in secretion of GnRH, and eventually, LH, and FSH. The LH prompts the Leydig cells in the testicle to increase testosterone production, and the FSH stimulates the production and maturation of germ cells. Sperm counts theoretically may increase.

Low dosages of clomiphene are usually prescribed for up to six months. A common therapy begins with 12.5 mg daily. Dosage is monitored and possibly increased or adjusted. Hormonal levels are usually checked after two months, and treatment may be continued for up to a year if hormone levels remain normal.

Side effects vary among men but can include temporary visual disturbances and slight enlargement or tenderness of the breasts. Liver damage is a rare side effect.

Improvement in sperm count varies between patients; motility is not affected. Some studies claim a 20 percent or even greater pregnancy rate after male clomiphene therapy, depending on whether other fertility problems are present in either partner.

☐ *hCG and hMG.* The hormone hCG has been used to treat undescended testicle problems for several decades. It has also been prescribed in some cases of low sperm count. In cases of abnormal
hypothalamic activity hMG (Pergonal) may also be prescribed with
hCG. Some experts feel that hMG use is appropriate only in men with
abnormally low FSH levels.

There isn't any scientific evidence that either drug is effective for
improving sperm count, unless there is a specific hormonal imbalance.
These drugs, which should be considered only in cases of long-term,
repeatedly low sperm counts, are administered by intra-muscular injections, two to three times per week, in carefully monitored and adjusted
doses.

The side effects may include temporary breast enlargement and
weight gain. The drugs are expensive, and no advantage has been
shown in using them instead of clomiphene when no hormone problem exists.

The use of hCG alone or with hMG may improve sperm count in
idiopathic oligospermia cases. The pregnancy rate, however, is only
about 20 percent.

☐ *Bromocriptine.* The role of prolactin hormone in the male is not fully
understood. In rare cases, however, some men develop elevated prolactin levels and bromocriptine (Parlodel) may be prescribed. To date there
is little data on success rates.

ASSISTED REPRODUCTIVE TECHNOLOGY (ART)

Initially such ART options as in vitro fertilization (IVF), gamete
intrafallopian transfer (GIFT), and zygote intrafallopian transfer (ZIFT) were
offered only to couples whose infertility was caused by tubal or other problems
in the female partner. Now, many couples with male-factor infertility are
accepted in these programs.

Carefully investigating ART programs and their success rates by age group
and fertility factor(s) is extremely important. With careful laboratory technique, success rates for male-factor couples, (which are usually lower than
female-factor ART pregnancy rates), can be improved.

In recent years, micromanipulation techniques have been developed to
enhance chances for pregnancy in male-factor couples. These procedures, Partial Zona Dissection and Subzonal Injection are still in their experimental stages
and may not be available in all ART programs. Partial Zona Dissection is a process that creates a minute opening, mechanically with a tiny needle-like device,
in the outer covering of the ovum (zona pellucida). Sperm are then placed near
the opening so one can enter and fertilize the oocyte. Subzonal Injection
involves literally injecting sperm into the subzonal space surrounding the
nucleus of the ovum. After fertilization, standard ART techniques are followed
(see chapter 14).

VARICOCELE

A varicocele is a mass of varicose veins of the scrotum. Between 10 and 15 percent of all men — and perhaps 40 percent of infertile men — have a detectable varicocele. It may, however, affect fertility in only about half the cases. It is also thought that some men may have a varicocele that cannot be clinically diagnosed.

A varicocele forms when the valves of the vein fail to close behind the retreating blood. The blood backs up and pools, and the vein swells. Varicoceles nearly always occur unilaterally on the left side of the scrotum, or bilaterally. Rarely do they occur only on the right. The blood travels through the renal vein and empties into the vena cava at an angle on the left side; the right side empties directly into the vena cava. The angle encountered on the left side causes more opportunities for reflux (backing up) of the blood.

Effect on Fertility. In about 30 to 40 percent of infertile men, varicoceles cause variable sperm count, motility, and morphology problems. They are the most easily identifiable and surgically correctable cause of male infertility, ranging from large (visible through scrotal skin), to moderate (easily palpable), to small (difficult to detect). There is no relationship, however, between the size of the varicocele and the sperm count.

It is not known exactly how a varicocele reduces sperm count, although one popular theory suggests that the accumulated blood in the vein increases scrotal temperature and slows or reduces sperm production.

There are two clues that the varicocele is actively reducing fertility. The first is atrophy of the testicle, usually on the same side as the varicocele. The second is impaired semen quality (count, morphology, or motility) after all other abnormalities are ruled out.

Treatments. Every year, as many as 30,000 American men seek treatment for variocele — either by surgery or with an occlusive radiological procedure.

Surgery. A quick and fairly simple operation can be performed under general or local anesthesia. An incision is made in the lower abdomen or groin, and the internal spermatic vein is tied off rather than removed. This method prevents the backflow of blood into the scrotum. Many urologists now perform this surgery on an outpatient basis, and normal activity can be rapidly resumed. In addition, some urologists are now utilizing laparoscopy for some types of bilateral varicocele surgery. Although general anesthesia is required, recovery from laparoscopic surgery is usually faster. (See chapters 5, 8, and 10 for further discussion of the emotional effects of surgery and a discussion of laparoscopic surgery.)

Sperm count and motility improves in about 65 percent of cases, although this percentage varies between individuals depending on their count before surgery. The pregnancy rate is 30 to 50 percent after surgery if no other fertility problems are present. If surgery is not successful, an occlusive radiological procedure or drug therapy with either clomiphene or hCG may be suggested.

OCCLUSIVE RADIOLOGICAL PROCEDURES: THE MINI-BALLOON AND COIL

These radiological procedures are nonsurgical treatments usually accomplished in one to two hours. They should be performed by a radiologist specially trained in these techniques.

The patient lies on the X-ray table and his genitals are covered with a lead protective covering. A small amount of hair is shaved from the groin area. After administering local anesthesia, the radiologist inserts a small, thin catheter into the femoral vein in the groin, guides it through the interior vena cava and down into the spermatic vein, and permanently positions a detachable, silicon balloon or coil in this area to block the flow of blood. Flouroscopy, which emits radiation equal to that of a chest X-ray, is utilized to guide the balloon or coil into the vein. Within three weeks, scar tissue forms around the coil or balloon and permanently blocks the blood flow.

After two to four hours of recovery, the patient can go home and most normal activities can be resumed in a day or two. These procedures are similar in cost and success rates to surgery. The patient is exposed to radiation, however, and the physician does not have the direct view of the varicocele that would be possible in surgery. And not all radiologists have sufficient training to perform this procedure. This technique may be more appropriate for men who have a recurrent varicocele problem that has not responded to surgical treatment.

DUCT OBSTRUCTION

A small number of men with persistently low sperm counts (10 million or less) have an obstruction that inhibits the sperms' journey to the urethra. A zero sperm count may also suggest an obstruction if a testicular biopsy has ruled out problems with sperm production. Diagnosis is made through sonograms, testicular biopsy, X-rays, or surgical exploration of the scrotum under anesthesia. During surgery an incision is usually made into the vas deferens or epididymis to identify the location of the obstruction.

Obstructions, which most commonly occur in the epididymis, may be caused by congenital problems, scarring, surgery, infections (particularly from sexually transmitted diseases), or other traumas to the scrotum.

Congenital problems can include epididymal scarring or an absence of part of the vas deferens. (If the vas is absent, surgical removal of sperm — Microscopic Epididymal Sperm Aspiration [MESA] — for use in IVF or GIFT is an option. See chapter 14.) Secondary damage following an initial infection may cause blockages in other areas of the duct system. Either a complete or partial obstruction of the epididymis may prevent sperm from reaching the urethra.

Treatment. If the male evaluation, including the biopsy, shows that an obstruction is present, microsurgery is indicated. If the biopsy results are not definitive, drug treatment to elevate sperm count may be recommended.

Surgery is performed under general, local, or regional anesthesia, usually on an outpatient basis. A scrotal exploration is done to locate, and hopefully bypass, the obstruction. As with varicocele surgery, limited activity is required for several days or longer. Subsequent pregnancy rates range from 35 to 40 percent for epididymal obstructions to 50 percent or greater for those located in the ejaculatory duct.

EJACULATION ABNORMALITIES

A small percentage of men have a problem either with the volume or viscosity of their ejaculate, or with an absence of semen. Retrograde ejaculation, a condition where the sperm spill out of the urethra into the bladder, can occur as a result of previous surgery, high blood pressure medication, nerve damage caused by diabetes, or for no apparent reason (idiopathic). In some cases, sperm may be recovered from the urine after ejaculation and cleansed and prepared for an IUI attempt (see chapter 16).

Excessive Ejaculate. In most cases ejaculation problems involve an excessive amount of semen. This dilutes the sperm concentration in the seminal fluid. In many cases, however, this still does not affect fertility. An evaluation of the postcoital test (see chapter 8) is important to ascertain whether treatment may be appropriate. If the PCT shows few sperm, there may not be a great enough concentration to form the phalanxes necessary to penetrate the cervical mucus.

Treatment is sometimes attempted with sperm washing, in which the sperm are concentrated in less semen and artificially inseminated.

Too Little Ejaculate. Too small an amount of ejaculate may indicate a blockage in the ejaculatory duct, which contribute fructose sugar and most of the seminal fluid. A simple laboratory test can check the semen for the presence of fructose. An absence of this sugar suggests a blockage.

Inability to Ejaculate Because of Spinal Injuries. In recent years, an electro-ejaculation procedure has been developed to help paraplegics and other men unable to ejaculate because of spinal injuries. A probe is gently inserted rectally and a mild current is activated which usually prompts ejaculation. The semen is gathered, processed, and artificially inseminated into his mate's vagina or uterus.

Viscosity Problems. Ideally enzymes produced by the seminal vesicles coagulate the semen shortly after ejaculation. Other enzymes produced by the prostate gland cause it to reliquify five to twenty minutes later.

Sometimes the ejaculate remains coagulated and does not reliquify. In some cases the sperm may be trapped within the coagulated ejaculate and unable to swim through the cervical mucus.

Treatment. If the postcoital test reveals favorable cervical mucus with a low sperm count in the volume, sperm washing and intrauterine insemination may be tried.

ENDOCRINOLOGICAL ABNORMALITIES

❦ Several of my hormonal levels are quite low. We eventually traced this to a congenital problem with my testicles. For years I didn't know about it, and I actually found a bit of humor in this ignorance. I thought back to fumbling around in the dark for prophylactics. The humor took a bit of the pain away.

Hormonal abnormalities occur in 3 to 5 percent of infertile men and may result in low or even zero sperm counts. These imbalances are sometimes caused by head trauma, pituitary tumors, infection, drug use, chemotherapy, or Klinefelter's syndrome (a hereditary condition that causes a complete absence of sperm).

In most cases, however, the imbalance is caused by reduced function of the pituitary gland. In cases of a high FSH reading, there is currently no available treatment. If the FSH levels are low, fertility drug treatment may be effective.

DIETHYLSTILBESTROL (DES)

Unfortunately there have not been as many studies of DES sons as of DES daughters, and little medical information is available. It is known that DES sons may develop anatomical abnormalities, such as epididymal cysts or smaller testicles, or have problems with low sperm counts.

DES sons should inform physicians of their exposure, and those who suspect reproductive problems should seek the advice of an urologist knowledgable about DES effects on males. DES Action USA is also a good resource for readings, referrals, and emotional support (see *Chapter 10* and *Resources*.)

VASECTOMY REVERSAL

❦ I got married when I was twenty-two years old. My wife and I promptly had two boys in four years. We were happy, didn't want to have any more kids, and figured we'd be married forever. I had a vasectomy to simplify birth control.

Our marriage fell apart about five years later. We shared custody of the boys and I had no interest in marrying again until I met Tina. We were both in our mid-thirties when we decided to get married.

This is Tina's first marriage and having a child was very important to her. Although my sons were ten and twelve, I decided I'd also like to have another child.

Since it was ten years since my vasectomy, the specialist warned me that a reversal might not be successful. Even if it was, it could take years for the sperm count to rise high enough to get Tina pregnant. I wanted to try anyhow.

The reversal was done under a local anesthetic, so I was conscious but pretty groggy. The doctors told me this was a better route to go than general anesthesia, only I had to promise not to move. No problem: There was no way I was going to move during that surgery!

I was pretty sore for about a week. My sperm count rose steadily over the next six months. About a year later Tina got pregnant, and my third son was born nine months later.

Every year about 500,000 American men who believe they have finished fathering babies elect to be sterilized by vasectomy. This simple surgical procedure, performed under local anesthesia in the doctor's office, severs the vas deferens and thereby prevents any sperm from reaching the urethra. Sex drive, performance, and quantity of seminal fluid are not affected.

Each year several thousand of these men regret their decision. They may divorce and remarry or tragically lose one or more of their children. In any case they consider restoring their fertility through vasectomy reversal.

Surgery. The surgery is performed under general, spinal, or local anesthesia (see chapter 5 for a discussion of surgery and anesthesia). Fine microsurgery techniques are used to realign the severed vas exactly. This is painstaking work as the inner canal of the vas is only about 1/64 inch in diameter. The ends are carefully sutured with a microscopic material only three times as thick as a red blood cell. Vasectomy reversals are often done on an outpatient basis and typically take about two to three hours. Patients are advised to wear a scrotal support for about two weeks. Soreness usually persists for about a week and mild analgesics may be prescribed for discomfort. A semen analysis is done about six weeks after surgery and repeated monthly to monitor increases in sperm count.

Success Rates. The success of a vasectomy reversal depends on several factors. The first is the amount of time that has elapsed since the original sterilization was performed. The vasectomy can cause pressure to build within the epididymis, which may rupture the duct. The longer the duct is under this pressure, the greater the chances of rupture, although it is possible that epididymal damage can be repaired through microsurgery. Other key factors are the skill of the microsurgeon and the quality of the surgical equipment.

One study reported a 3 to 4 percent decline in pregnancy rates for each year after the vasectomy. Experts, however, have performed successful reversals ten or more years after the patient's vasectomy. In general, normal sperm count is often restored in 80 percent of patients within a year after reversal surgery, and the pregnancy rate is about 50 to 60 percent.

The incidence of birth defects or other abnormalities in children fathered after vasectomy reversal is no greater than in the general population. Some men do develop sperm antibodies after a vasectomy that may affect fertility after the reversal. (See chapter 12 for further discussion).

Psychological and Emotional Impact of Male Infertility

❦ My sperm count was very low, and the sperm were immature — without tails. For some reason, my testicles didn't mature and my testosterone level is low. It was quite a shock to find this out. Although I was grateful that my equipment worked, I also worried whether I would be more susceptible to cancer. The doctor evaluated my beard and voice, and suggested hormone shots. I felt almost embarrassed. I wondered if I was smaller than other men. Did I last as long or ejaculate as much?

❦ We were somewhat annoyed when our doctor requested that my husband have a hamster egg test before my laparoscopy — another delay and $250 down the drain, I thought. No one else had ever even mentioned this test. The end result was that my husband scored 0 percent penetration, twice. The news of his infertility hit us like a loaded log truck on a hill. We had always assumed that the problem lay with me, especially since I'd had a troublesome IUD years ago. Between the first and second tests my husband was in a state of denial and I was sure it was true and went around weeping and mourning the loss of his genes, funereally.

Infertility raises many intense emotional and psychological issues for men and women as individuals and as couples. Part One examines many of these dynamics in detail. A few issues unique to male infertility are briefly discussed in this section.

The Couple. When a male-factor problem is diagnosed, the anger, shame, and grief commonly experienced with any fertility problem are focused on the husband. The wife often feels angry and sad that she cannot conceive her mate's child. She may feel he has let her down in one of the most important ways she can imagine. She wants very much to be pregnant. At the same time, she often feels deep concern and compassion for her husband. Usually she also feels it is unacceptable to express these strong, conflicting emotions to her partner.

The male is trying to cope with a gamut of feelings: fear that he has disappointed his wife; shock, inadequacy, and perhaps shame that he is infertile; and grief for the loss of a biological child. This is a devastating experience for both partners and requires time to absorb and grieve. (A man's perspective on male-factor infertility is discussed in further detail in chapter 2.)

TO GO PUBLIC OR NOT?

🐛 After finally seeing a fertility specialist to help my wife with her problem, it was determined that I did have a low sperm count, and that possibly a varicocele operation six inches above each of my testicles might produce the desired results. I am an extrovert, who likes to share what is going on in my life with a rather wide assortment of people. I usually find them insightful, comforting, and helpful.

But when I mentioned my upcoming operation, I found that my male friends were distant. A common response was something like, "Do you need a little help?" Just in case I missed the joke, the person often followed up with a wink and an elbow nudge. For the past six years I have endured such offers of help from males in every walk of life. Many times this "DO YOU NEED A LITTLE HELP?" line is delivered within full earshot of my wife.

Does the sender of this remark expect her to say, "Great idea, Harry. I would love to be with a real man! Oh, Bob dear, would you make Harry and me a Bloody Mary?"

It is as if there is a chromosome in the male make-up that is wired to respond to another male's infertility problem with the sophistication of a drooling three-month-old.

Robert Bookman

Many couples, fearing just such a reaction, shroud a male fertility problem in secrecy. Both partners suffer, often isolated from any source of emotional support, in different ways. Men, often devastated by their infertility diagnosis, often withdraw in an angry silence. At the same time, many women grieve as if it were their physical problem. Many often state they wish they could undergo some of the procedures themselves, or share the burden emotionally by providing more solace and support to their mates. Rather than trying to cope alone, consulting with an experienced and empathetic counselor or joining a male infertility support group can be of tremendous help while you work toward resolution.

Other couples, tired of secrecy and hoping for support and empathy, may "go public" about the man's problem and share details about tests or treatments with colleagues, friends, and relatives. They are often surprised and dismayed by the resulting reactions. Even though they now realize it is the man's problem, most relatives and friends will continue to question the woman about the treatment and prognosis. Meanwhile, the male may be teased or ridiculed about his problem. Neither partner may receive much support. Many people also associate male infertility with impotence. While listening to their friends' cruel jokes, many infertile men secretly worry either that they will lose their masculinity and sexual potency or that others will think they have.

During this time, the couple may also be considering options for resolution, including donor insemination (DI). Whether to confide in others about undertaking DI is a complex issue further discussed in chapter 16.

ETHNIC HERITAGE

❦ I have had patients from the Middle East and Africa who have been completely devastated by their fertility problem and have told me they would consider suicide if they could not father a child.

America is a mixture of diverse subcultures and ethnic traditions. Some of these heritages place an extraordinary emphasis on fertility and siring children. Just as some women from different ethnic backgrounds feel especially inadequate when told of their infertility, many men from a variety of "macho" backgrounds may feel inferior, demasculinized, or worthless.

It is often difficult for these men to ask for or receive emotional support from their peers or family. Even worse, many of these cultures also attach a stigma to seeking professional counseling or therapy. Fortunately there is support available to all infertile men and women from RESOLVE and other support organizations (see Resources).

CULTURAL CONDITIONING

❦ I had to ask myself if there was something missing in my relationships with male friends that inhibited them from dealing with my pain. Or was it that they confused male infertility with impotence? Or was I simply communicating my pain within the tacit rules of male conversation that require that you mask real feelings through an exchange of crude one-liners, to be followed up with loud laughter and several punches in the arm? I believe all these things were in operation. I pondered over the nagging questions of whether I had developed good male friends or had simply confused friendship with patter about sports, stocks, and sex.

Eventually, I decided to talk to my male friends about my feelings of not being able to have a child, in a very open and frank way. I talked about the sadness of seeing my wife go through painful operations and procedures; I lamented that this should happen to me, and I asked for their understanding if at times I was withdrawn when they talked about their children.

Not surprisingly everyone I spoke with in this way proved to be a genuine friend. They gave me hugs and listened to my sadness; they celebrated wildly when Adam was born, and they are there for me now as I have gone through another round of treatment in the hopes that I can be the daddy to a second child.

Robert Bookman

From a young age many American males are taught to hide their feelings and, above all, not to acknowledge or express pain. When infertility is diagnosed, many men revert to these patterns and refuse to discuss their reactions or grief. Our society reinforces this behavior by approaching the woman about the couple's fertility problem, which allows the male to further recede into his isolation.

A man may also react differently to an infertility problem than his wife. Women usually grieve longer and more deeply over fertility loss, mainly because many are taught to define their identity through their relationships (e.g., wife and mother) rather than an occupation or career. Men, on the other hand, generally derive more identity through career status. One urologist observed:

> ❧ Many of my patients treat their infertility with the same rational, businesslike approach that they would use on the job. They want to define the problem, consider their options, make a decision, and move on.

Although his problem is painful, an infertile man may channel his frustration and anger into his work.

Eventually, though, most men experience grief and a deep sense of loss after a male-factor diagnosis (see chapter 2). They find they must confront and mourn their infertility in their own way, and if they cannot father a child, the loss of biological offspring. It is especially difficult for men to acknowledge and express grief in our culture. Many, however, find that support and understanding from their mate, a few caring friends or relatives, a compassionate counselor, or other couples facing this issue, helps them finish their grief and heal.

CHAPTER 16

Artificial Insemination

❦ Because we had a combination of fertility problems, our specialist suggested we try inseminating my husband's sperm directly into my uterus. Although we were glad there was a treatment that might work, we were also reminded that we couldn't seem to get pregnant the "normal" way.

❦ After I learned I was sterile, I was angry and bitter for months. I wouldn't discuss it with my wife and didn't want her talking to anyone else about it.

After a while, though, I began to consider donor insemination. I finally convinced Nina I was serious. From my perspective, the child would be half ours and we could control the pregnancy. Because I was the advocate, I felt powerful rather than useless.

ARTIFICIAL INSEMINATION IS THE PROCESS by which sperm are inserted by syringe or catheter into a woman's vagina or uterus. There are two types: insemination with husband's sperm, usually performed through intrauterine insemination (IUI) and donor insemination (DI), a process that uses donor sperm to hopefully achieve pregnancy.

Intrauterine Insemination (IUI)

❦ At first we did natural cycle intrauterine inseminations using my BBT chart. When four of those tries didn't work, we moved to clomiphene with ultrasounds to monitor the follicle development, and then an hCG shot to trigger ovulation. As soon as I got the shot, I called Mike at work and told him to make time tomorrow because we would need that sperm. By then, he felt so pressured about producing the sample that we couldn't go to the doctor's office together. So he went on his lunch hour and left the sample to be processed. I came in two hours later for the insemination.

I lay on the examining table and they reclined it a bit. The insemination itself just took a moment and I never felt any discomfort when they inserted the catheter. Then I lay there for at least twenty minutes, praying.

I was always by myself. They often gave me a magazine, but I never read it. I remember one kind doctor who looked back at me

as he left the room, and turned out the light before he gently closed the door. I used that time to pray, think, and visualize about the baby planting, and think about what good parents we would be.

IUI is usually used to bypass cervical mucus problems (see chapter 9). In the past few years, IUI (often with the use of ovulation induction drugs) has also been adapted as a type of "pre-ART" (Assisted Reproductive Technology) option for couples with low sperm count, poor motility, sperm antibodies, or unexplained infertility who have completed workup testing, tried other recommended treatments, and have not become pregnant within a reasonable length of time. (To utilize IUI, the woman must have at least one normally functioning Fallopian tube.)

Although some specialists question whether this method increases the chances of conception for these couples as opposed to spontaneous pregnancy rates achieved without treatment, others argue that three to six IUI cycles are worth trying before ART is considered. IUI is less expensive (about $400 per cycle in 1992 if clomiphene is used) and less stressful than standard ART, and offers a 5 to 20 percent pregnancy rate, depending on the age and fertility factors of both partners. If ovulation induction medications are used, the woman is exposed to the possible side effects of clomiphene or hMG. (See chapters 9 and 14 for discussions of ovulation inducing drugs and ART.)

The insemination is timed to the female partner's ovulation, through the use of a basal body temperature (BBT) chart, ovulation predictor (LH) kit, or perhaps by ultrasound imaging of the developing follicle(s). When ovulation is imminent, a semen sample is collected. The semen is diluted with a saline solution and repeatedly centrifuged, a process that washes the proteins, prostaglandins, chemicals, and bacteria from the ejaculate and condenses it into a small pellet. This pellet is incubated for about an hour at body temperature, and then inseminated into the uterus through a slender catheter. The sperm-washing process reduces, but does not eliminate, the small risk (less than 1 percent) of cramping, allergic reaction, fever, shock, or infection from this procedure.

For most couples, using the husband's sperm for artificial insemination poses few moral, ethical, or legal questions. IUI treatment, however, may be emotionally stressful. As with the postcoital test and many ART procedures, timing is a critical component of an IUI attempt. The male has to produce a semen sample, through masturbation, usually at the lab or physician's office, on fairly short notice. Conflicts with religious traditions or decrees may engender guilt and confusion, magnifying the couple's feeling of alienation or isolation. And like so many others undergoing medical treatments, IUI couples are trying to conceive a child in a clinical, strictly scheduled, sometimes hurried, and definitely unromantic atmosphere. Feelings of unreality and loss of control and spontaneity are common. Again, these women and men are reminded that their path to pregnancy is not the "natural" one that most others travel.

Donor Insemination (DI)

❦ At a symposium panel discussion, we listened to a couple who had resolved their infertility with DI. It brought tears to my eyes and I remember feeling wistfully that it was such a nice solution. We had been dealing with our infertility for two years and were ready to come to a decision. It's true that the news of my husband's infertility was a death knell for Steve's biological contribution, but at least we finally knew *why* and could move out of that never-never land of "unexplained" infertility. And while I was grieving, I still felt a joyful renaissance of hope: Maybe I wasn't infertile! Maybe I could get pregnant!

❦ Although I shared by wife's monthly roller coaster ride of hope, disappointment and frustration, and our sexual relationship was sorely tested by scheduling and the stress of procreational failure, I maintained throughout an unassailed sense of completeness as a male. We considered adoption as a last resort — my wife longed to be *pregnant*. If we did decide to adopt, I felt the potential loss of my genetic line, yet could accept it. It did not call into question my "manhood."

When I received the news of my own untreatable infertility, our lives suddenly took a fundamental shift. We were no longer dog-paddling in the swamp of unexplained infertility. We now had resolution staring us in the face. Yet at the same time I suddenly felt in a sense immasculated. I suspect that every man, myself included, has a visceral reaction along these lines upon awakening to their infertility. And why not? It is in some sense the essence of the human condition that men and women beget babies. To be suddenly out of that fabric of life because of some deficiency of my body is bound to take its toll.

For me, though, this visceral reaction was shortlived. We felt renewed hope that my wife could achieve pregnancy, and at least her genetic contribution to our children would remain.

The DI procedure, in which donor sperm is used by a fertile woman for artificial insemination, has been practiced for more than a century, and commonly used to treat male infertility for the last forty years. An estimated 5 percent of couples encountering male infertility, genetic or inheritable disease problems, or unsuccessful vasectomy reversals will try DI. About 10 percent of DI patients are single women, both heterosexual and gay. Although there are no available statistics of the actual number of DI attempts, experts estimate between thirty and eighty thousand babies are conceived annually in the United States by this process.

DI has always been, and remains, a controversial social and legal issue. Many people in our society disapprove of the practice, and couples undergoing

DI often do not tell friends or family about their treatment. The laws regarding DI vary from one state to another. Only twelve have legitimized DI, while about thirty states have specific laws addressing DI for married couples. A number of states have adopted some form of Section V of the Uniform Paternity Act, which deals exclusively with DI. In these states, a husband consenting to a DI pregnancy is considered the legal father. Other states address the paternity issue via other statutes or court decisions. In a few states, the law is vague or silent about paternity in DI offspring. Questions of child support, for example, may remain at issue. To further complicate the issue, a California appellate court ruled in 1986 that, in cases where donor sperm was inseminated by someone other than a physician, the donor has paternity rights. Whether this ruling will be adopted by other state courts remains to be seen. No state addresses the issues of single women and DI, nor is there a national record-keeping system or data registry of sperm donors or DI births at this time.

If you are considering DI, obtain legal advice from an attorney familiar with the laws of your state. Before performing the procedure, specialists, fertility centers, and sperm banks require all parties involved with DI — patients, their husbands, and donors — to sign consent forms that clarify rights and responsibilities.

Despite its controversy, DI can also be a joyous, life-affirming process. For thousands of infertile couples who cannot be medically treated, and for single heterosexual or lesbian women who desire a child, it creates a path to pregnancy and parenting. One prominent infertility specialist, who has facilitated and monitored more than five hundred DI pregnancies, considers this "the happiest, most positive part of my infertility practice."

DECIDING ON DI

❦ The decision was easy for us. My husband was sterile and we wanted kids. He wasn't worried about the other man's sperm. He said, "If it grows within you, it's part of me."

❦ I preferred adoption to DI. I felt I couldn't participate in DI at all, and that gave me feelings of impotency.

❦ The decision to pursue DI came almost immediately and without serious reservation by both of us. My biggest difficulty was to accept that I could not be a biological father. For me this problem had no bearing on our decision to pursue DI. ("I can't be a biological father, so you can't be a biological mother?") I have subsequently come to terms with it, largely with the help of my beautiful son. I've discovered that being a father to a child has nothing to do with genetics.

Initially, most couples move through a process, often progressing at different paces, of confronting and grieving the painful issues of their infertility. (These intense emotions and reactions are discussed in chapters 1, 2, and 15.)

Over time, they seek information, validation, and support from health professionals and others facing the same challenge, perhaps informally or through
support groups. Some also obtain professional counseling. Eventually, most
couples reach a point of healing, strength, and perspective that enables them to
consider a variety of resolution options, including DI.

Many factors enter into a couple's decision to pursue DI. First they must
believe that it is unlikely the woman will get pregnant by her partner. This is a
logical conclusion if he has a zero sperm count or a congenital absence of the
vas deferens where nature has permanently impaired fertility. A low sperm
count or poor motility, however, is involved in most cases of male infertility.
The husband is not clinically sterile and there is a chance, albeit an increasingly
smaller one as time passes, that he can father a child. Most couples with male-factor
infertility first try a number of IUI cycles or perhaps several ART attempts (see
chapter 14).

If such treatments are unsuccessful and the couple accepts the unlikeli-
hood of pregnancy with the husband's sperm, they may then consider the
options of donor insemination, adoption, or child-free living. All three of these
resolutions involve the loss of one or both partner's genetic lines, and often precipitate a period of mourning. (See chapter 20 for a discussion of grieving the
loss of biological children and child-free living decision-making issues; adoption issues are presented in chapter 17.) For couples interested in DI, the following questions may help clarify goals and feelings.

- ☐ Have we acknowledged and grieved the loss of a child of our genetic
  union? Of my genetic line?
- ☐ Have we faced the shame and stigma of male infertility? Does the male
  partner retain feelings of inadequacy or guilt?
- ☐ Does the husband feel that his wife values a pregnancy and a biological
  child more than his feelings or their relationship? Does he feel obligated to consent to DI out of guilt or fear that she will leave him?
- ☐ How do both partners feel about the wife being impregnated with
  another man's sperm?
- ☐ Does either partner fear that the husband may not bond with, or feel
  close to, the child? That the child will not bond with his or her father?
- ☐ Will either of us feel an imbalance of power within the family because
  our child will be genetically related to mother, but not father?
- ☐ Will we tell our child(ren) about their DI origins?
- ☐ Will we tell others of our decision, or do we prefer to maintain our privacy and let others assume the child is genetically ours?
- ☐ If told, how would our extended families and close friends react to this
  decision and regard our child?
- ☐ Do we prefer an anonymous, identity-release, or known donor? (See
  section below.) If we choose a known donor, how will this affect that
  relationship, future contact, and our family's privacy?

☐ Will we have enough emotional support during the pregnancy and after our child's birth?

The couple (or single woman) may also wish to balance the pros and cons of a DI pregnancy. The advantages are: The woman can experience pregnancy, birth, and breastfeeding; both are assured that the baby receives good prenatal care and nutrition; the child will carry his or her mother's genes; and they can have a baby without the red tape, wait, or possible rejection involved with agency or private adoptions. On the other hand, DI poses a number of unique challenges to the family, such as religious, legal, or moral considerations; anonymous, identity-release, or known donor issues; and perhaps subsequent identity or search issues for the child.

BEING IN ACCORD AS A COUPLE

❦ **I had a hard time believing Jim wouldn't mind the DI. It took quite a while for him to convince me and for both of us to agree that DI was the right option.**

Partners commonly have conflicting or ambivalent feelings about DI. Although being in agreement about DI is crucial, few couples initially concur about pursuing this option. The wife often pushes for DI treatment soon after her husband learns he is infertile. She wants a biological child, and this is a way to get pregnant. Initially, her mate is usually less comfortable with this option; DI won't give him a genetic child.

During this stage, each mate faces a number of difficult issues that often take some time to answer. To facilitate this process, it may be helpful to study literature about DI, speak with health care professionals and other DI couples, and seek private or infertility support group counseling.

Experts stress the importance of partners acknowledging, confronting, and, to their best ability, resolving feelings before beginning DI. As with high-tech assisted reproduction, egg donor IVF, and surrogacy, partners must look within themselves and ask whether they can manage and weather DI as individuals and as a couple, and support each other through it.

Pursuing DI while in conflict is not advisable; after the fact is *not* the time to decide that this was the wrong decision. It takes time, honest and open communication, grieving, and patience to reach a mutual decision. Physicians and counselors find that couples who have spent months of careful consideration do best with this process. Mary Rodocker, Ph.D., studied the reactions of twenty-six DI couples and found a high degree of partner satisfaction with the decision, that prior concerns about bonding with the child did not materialize after the baby's birth, and that 85 percent of the couples would choose DI again to enlarge their families.

DONOR SPERM

The couple or single woman who has opted for DI is naturally concerned about the health, genetic history, and physical and mental characteristics of the donor. In most cases, sperm donors are either college or medical students. Their motives are usually a mixture of altruism, ego gratification, and financial reward.

Matching can be done for general physical characteristics such as race and hair and eye coloring, but the child may still have very different physiological characteristics from the husband. For example, blood can be matched for a general type such as O, but there are more than fifty characteristics for which blood is typed. There may also be a scarcity of donors from certain ethnic groups, or of those willing to be identity-release donors.

Screening Donors. Over the years, donor screening practices have varied considerably among physicians and sperm banks. In 1986, the American Fertility Society (AFS) established screening guidelines that are updated annually. In response to these guidelines and the increasing severity of the AIDS (HTLV-III/LAV virus) epidemic, reputable DI programs and sperm banks have established thorough (or refined existing) screening procedures. Many now require medical examinations, complete three-generation health histories, several initial semen analyses, and comprehensive and periodic blood testing for the presence of AIDS, gonorrhea, herpes, ureaplasma-mycoplasma, chlamydia, syphilis, hepatitis B and C, cytomeglaovirus (CMV), Group B strep, staph aureaus, and if appropriate, Tay Sachs disease and Sickle Cell Anemia.

When considering a DI program, ask how donors are selected and what information is available about them. Some physicians or sperm banks encourage the recipient(s) to select the donor from a file or catalog that usually contains an identification number and general physical characteristics such as height, weight, race, hair and eye coloring, and ethnic heritage. In some cases, more detailed information about interests, talents, hobbies, and personal messages to potential offspring may also be available. Other specialists select the donors themselves, after an extensive interview with the couple. Some couples and single heterosexual or gay women choose to use a donor known to them — a close friend or relative.

Guidelines Regarding Frozen Sperm. Both the Reproductive Council of the American Association of Tissue Banks and the American Fertility Society now recommend the exclusive use of frozen semen for DI. Although pregnancy rates are often higher with fresh sperm inseminations, most experts feel that using frozen sperm is necessary in order to protect recipients and offspring from exposure to serious or fatal disease through insemination.

Guidelines suggest that prospective donors, no older than forty years of age, be tested for AIDS and other sexually transmitted or genetic diseases. If these initial tests are negative, a semen sample is collected, frozen in tiny vials in liquid nitrogen at -324 degrees Fahrenheit, and quarantined. If the donor again tests negative six months later, the frozen sample may then be used for DI.

Donors should be re-tested every three to six months, resulting offspring should be limited to fifteen per donor, and frozen samples should be used within ten years.

ANONYMOUS, IDENTITY-RELEASE, AND KNOWN SPERM DONORS

❦ I don't know anything about the donors, really. Just that they are students and little chance remarks made. I don't have a picture in my mind. It's more like a place of utter gratitude and a prayer for the well-being of the anonymous person who gave me the gift of my child's life, and the gift of (I'm sure) a little girl who did not make it here. I hope these men know this. I wish I could thank them. I guess I can do that only by loving my children well.

❦ Steve had an interesting insight yesterday. He had always felt comfortable with the fact that the donors are completely anonymous and we know virtually nothing about them, nor is this a possibility. I personally would have liked more information, and also support the idea of identity-release donors — men who agree to be reachable by their offspring when they reach a certain age, if they so desire. In our case, this was impossible, and I could sense that there was some element of emotional self-protection in Steve's position that I didn't need to challenge, because there was nothing we could do about it anyway.

After watching a videotape with Reuben Pannor and Annette Baran, authors of *Lethal Secrets,* Steve said he could see that his satisfaction with total anonymity came from a sense of competitiveness with the donor. He felt that if Tyler ever met his biological father, he might find some aspect of fatherhood fulfilled by the donor that Steve did not. He also acknowledged that it might be valuable for a child to be able to do that.

For decades, the practice of DI has been surrounded by secrecy within the family, and anonymity concerning the donors. In many cases, records were either not kept regarding the identity of the donor and any resulting offspring, or destroyed a few years after the child's birth. Many parents never told their child(ren) about their DI origins. Some DI offspring learned the truth later in their lives from parents or relatives, sometimes in a hurtful way. Others sensed that something was wrong between their parents, and after a number of discussions or confrontations, were told about their DI conception.

The movement toward openness about identity, which has greatly impacted adoption in the United States over the past decade, has sparked debate in other types of alternative family-building, including DI and egg donation. With most agency and independent adoptions today, the identities of the birthparent(s) and adoptive parents are known to each other. Some type of contact by letter, phone calls, or visits, before the child's birth and after, commonly occurs. The degree, frequency, and duration of contact varies with each adoption.

Many couples and single women considering either DI or egg donor IVF are similarly interested in some type of openness with the donor. One IVF specialist estimated that up to 75 percent of his program's egg donors and recipients choose to exchange identifying information; some meet prior to the treatment cycle, and others continue contact afterward. Permanent records are kept and maintained of the egg donor's identity, resulting offspring, and continuing health history.

Semen from anonymous donors, who do not wish to be identified at any time, is currently used by most DI programs and sperm banks. Many specialists and recipient couples favor the continued practice of anonymous, non-identified donors for several reasons. Some recipients fear that the possible involvement of identified or known donors — either now or in the future — would be intrusive to their family, or confusing to their child(ren). There is also concern that if anonymity is not preserved, or if future identification or contact from the offspring is possible, there will be a scarcity of men willing to donate sperm.

An identity-release donor agrees to the release of identifying information to his genetic offspring, if they desire, when they reach the age of eighteen. The Sperm Bank of California, now in its tenth year of operation, currently offers both identity-release and anonymous donor sperm. Before joining the program and beginning the screening process, potential identity-release donors agree that identifying information may be released *only* to the offspring at age eighteen, upon receipt of a written petition. This option does not involve, or in any way facilitate, interaction between donor and recipients, nor does it create any donor rights or responsibilities toward the offspring.

The known donor option involves using the carefully screened and tested semen of a friend, or perhaps relative, for artificial insemination. In these cases, the parties already know each other and, in many cases, will continue contact after the child is born. As with cases of open adoption or egg donor IVF with ongoing contact, issues about the degree of involvement and delineation of boundaries may arise for all parties.

Experts estimate that 250,000 to 500,000 or more children have been conceived by DI. To date, there has been little research about the perspectives and feelings of, or long-range effects of DI upon, donors, recipients, or offspring. One study has recently been published by Kris Probasco, LSCSW, and Patricia Mahlstedt, Ed.D., regarding the attitudes of seventy-nine donors from Houston, Texas, and Metairie, Louisiana, about providing identifying information. The authors, who state that their findings were consistent with studies previously published in Australia and New Zealand, found that 96 percent were willing to share non-identifying information; 90 percent would provide personal, medical, and psychosocial information; 47 percent from Houston and 25 percent from Metairie favored openness between donor and recipient families; 72 percent wrote personal messages to potential offspring; 60 percent would agree to some form of personal contact when the child reached eighteen; and 41 percent would like to be informed if pregnancy occurred. If anonymity was not guaranteed, 19 percent of Houston and 42 percent of Metairie donors said they would not donate.

THE MEDICAL PROCEDURE

❦ When I saw the syringe, I almost jumped off the table in last-minute panic. But, once again, my desire for a child kept me in place and I watched the "stranger's" semen enter my body. The procedure itself is not painful, but the emotional turmoil is quite strong.

❦ At first I viewed DI almost as a rapelike act, perhaps because once again I was not in control of the situation. But by the time I started the inseminations, it felt like just another medical procedure.

DI, a relatively simple medical procedure, is usually done in a doctor's office, medical clinic, or sperm bank, although some couples and single women choose to perform the inseminations at home. Insemination is generally tried one or two days a month, timed to coincide as closely as possible with ovulation. Although some physicians use sonograms or hormonal blood tests to pinpoint ovulation, others rely solely on an ovulation predictor kit or basal body temperature (BBT) chart. Women's reactions to the medical procedure of insemination vary considerably.

During the insemination procedure, the woman lies on the examination table and a speculum is inserted into her vagina. Using a syringe, either the physician or her mate inseminates donor sperm at the cervical opening. Some programs, however, may process the sperm and use intrauterine insemination. At the couple's request, most specialists will allow her mate to perform the insemination, including him in the process and perhaps easing his feelings of inadequacy or isolation. The woman then rests on the table for fifteen to thirty minutes to give the sperm time to reach the Fallopian tubes. Some women experience slight cramping after the procedure.

Some clinics, if requested, will mix small amounts of the husband's sperm with the donor's for psychological reasons. In such cases there is a slight possibility that the child may be fathered by the husband. Some men also feel that in this way they are at least symbolically participating in the conception of the child. On the other hand, some therapists caution that a desire to mix the sperm may indicate that the male partner, or couple, has not reached a comfortable decision about using DI.

Success Rates. Overall success rates for inseminations with frozen sperm are 50 to 75 percent within twelve months. The ratio of male infants born is 55 to 45, probably due to the timing of insemination. If the fertility drug clomiphene is used to stimulate ovulation, this ratio changes to an even 50/50 chance for a boy or girl.

DI is usually tried with a healthy woman who has no known fertility problem. It is traumatic and expensive to investigate female infertility if there is no reason to suspect it. However, if pregnancy does not occur after six tries, the physician will usually recommend a female infertility workup. Attempts to inseminate are usually halted after a year, although the couple may determine how long to continue treatment.

It is not unusual for the stress of DI to cause irregular menstrual cycles for the first few months. This usually corrects itself. Fertility drugs are not used unless indicated by an ovulatory problem.

DI Siblings. When trying to become pregnant for the first time with DI, many couples or single women don't consider the issue of second or additional children. In retrospect, some parents wish they had discussed obtaining and freezing additional samples from their first child's donor for future insemination. As one woman remarked:

> ❦ I love my child so dearly, he is so beautiful and sweet; I'd fallen in love with his genes and come to think of them as family. I wanted to recognize the new baby and had thought it might mean something to them to be full-blooded siblings. Now I have to give that up and again cast myself into the unknown with a different donor.

If you may want to conceive another child(ren) in the future, perhaps using the same donor's sperm, discuss this with your physician before beginning DI.

EMOTIONAL AND PSYCHOLOGICAL ISSUES OF DI

Although DI is a fairly routine medical procedure, it is a complex psychological and emotional process. Couples undergoing periodic inseminations commonly experience a number of reactions.

ISOLATION

> ❦ We felt estranged from even other infertiles. We were "in the closet" and missed the recognition and sympathy they were getting.

> ❦ We've been very open about DI with people and will, of course, tell Tyler. We could never live with a secret just because "society" has a negative opinion about DI. My parents adore Tyler, but I think they are uncomfortable with DI. They are against my having another child, for idiotic reasons (in my opinion), and my "singlemindedness" in pursuing this "upsets" them. It is a sorrow that of all the people who know about our struggle to have a family, my parents and sister have been the least empathetic, supportive, and kind.

During the DI process, a couple may feel an even greater isolation than with other types of infertility. Because many people, including relatives and friends, are critical and unable to understand their decision, many couples do not tell anyone they are involved in DI. Sometimes women may wish to confide in family or friends, but their husbands feel uncomfortable or embarrassed about discussing it with others. Others who do share this information encounter negative or judgmental responses. Few DI programs require or provide counseling, and many physicians find it difficult to deal with their patients' emotional reactions.

Some couples cope with this isolation by confiding in a few trusted friends or relatives. Others join a DI support group and discuss their feelings only with those experiencing the same issues. Often couples find that sharing their feelings is an enormous relief and find empathy, understanding, and support at these meetings. If a group situation is not comfortable for you, private infertility counseling, or meeting or corresponding with one other DI couple may provide a welcome outlet. Such networking is offered by some infertility specialists and many RESOLVE chapters (see Resources).

Guilt or Shame. A woman may feel guilty about getting pregnant with a donor's sperm or for being fertile, while her partner is not. Either partner may feel ashamed about pursuing this path to pregnancy.

STRESS

❦ After the insemination, my emotions changed back and forth from happy and optimistic to frightened and unsure.

DI is an invasive medical procedure and a highly stressful experience. The sperm of another man is inseminated into the woman, and both partners may experience conflicting emotions. Couples may find the insemination treatment a weird event, and not the "natural" conception they had envisioned.

As a woman begins DI, the worry about both the process itself and about whether pregnancy will occur can sometimes affect her first few menstrual cycles. Stress itself, however, has not been found to be a significant factor in infertility, especially for women. Often couples create even more stress by worrying that their anxiety is preventing pregnancy! It may help to reduce tension in other, more manageable areas, such as work or social obligations.

Fantasies and Nightmares. This is a time of intense emotion, as well as transition, and fantasies and nightmares often occur during the DI process. Residual guilt, ambivalence, or anger may surface, and sometimes the only safe way to express such emotions is through dreams. One woman recalled "nightmares about some strange being growing in my abdomen." As these feelings are resolved, the fantasies and nightmares usually decrease and then stop.

SEXUALITY

❧ DI brought up feelings of somebody else sleeping with my wife, but I knew how desperately she wanted to carry a child of her own. It was important to her concept of herself as a woman and a mother at that time.

A loss of sexual interest may occur in either or both partners during the first few cycles of DI. A husband may feel superfluous or unnecessary at this time. His wife is receiving donor sperm to become pregnant, reinforcing his belief that he is inadequate or not needed. Trying to cope with her own complex feelings, the woman may also feel overwhelmed and not desire or seek intimacy with her partner.

Old infertility feelings may also resurface during this time, such as the woman's anger at her husband's inability to impregnate, and his guilt, frustration, and inadequacy about his infertility. Feelings of infidelity and jealousy are common when a woman is being impregnated by another man's sperm, and either or both partners may liken DI to adultery.

Anger, depression, shame, guilt, or jealousy can certainly affect sexuality, and some infertile men may experience temporary impotence during the resolution process. It is important to remember that this problem is *quite common* and *only temporary*. There may also be misunderstanding about when, and how often, couples should make love during a DI cycle. Other than the few hours preceding or following insemination, most specialists encourage intimacy throughout the DI cycle.

This is a time when women and men need love, patience, and understanding from each other. Touching, warmth, caring and loving conversations and gestures, and spending time together are important expressions of love. Having the husband attend, and perhaps assist with, the inseminations is another way to remain close during DI, if that is comfortable for both partners.

FEELINGS DURING PREGNANCY AND BIRTH

❧ We were lucky and my wife conceived with the second DI cycle. I felt somewhat estranged from the developing embryo. I cannot say if this was totally due to my not being biologically connected. I imagine this could also be a common reaction for any father-to-be, since at this time the pregnant woman is the star of the show. I took it on faith that once the child was born we would connect. Indeed, it is not possible for someone who is not a parent to comprehend the magnitude of the bond that begins to form at birth between father and child. Here is the real miracle of continuity from generation to generation.

Many couples find pregnancy after infertility an alternatively joyful, frightening, ambivalent, and surreal experience (see chapter 18). In cases of DI and egg donor IVF, there may be times when sadness and grief about a partner's

infertility resurfaces. With either mate, attachment or bonding to the developing baby may occur gradually, or be delayed until later in the pregnancy. Some
women may not "feel pregnant," or truly believe they are expecting, until the
baby begins kicking and moving. (Fertile couples, however, may also experience similarly detached or ambivalent feelings during pregnancy.)

By the third trimester, most couples acknowledge and process these feelings, address any residual grief, and excitedly prepare for their child's arrival.
Birth and early parenthood are powerful times of transition, and all new parents
commonly experience a variety of intense feelings. During this normally cha-
otic and emotional time, DI parents also hear well-meaning comments — especially from those not "in the know" — that may hurt and perhaps re-open old
wounds: "Boy, is he a ringer for his Daddy!" or "She sure has her father's eyes!"
Like adoptive parents, DI couples try to handle these awkward moments with
humor or a knowing wink or smile between them.

SINGLE WOMEN, LESBIAN COUPLES, AND DI

**❦ I strongly feel the judgment of others about my decision to try
DI. Single women who adopt are considered selfless angels. I
think that those of us who attempt pregnancy through DI are
viewed as tainted or promiscuous.**

An estimated 10 percent or more of DI patients are single women or lesbian
couples, who often encounter disapproval from family, friends, and society, as
well as discrimination from the medical profession. Many physicians will not
treat unmarried women, or if they do, convey a cool or judgmental attitude
toward them.

A single woman may experience a wide range of reactions during the DI
process. On the one hand, she has the freedom to make the decision alone without coping with a male partner's infertility. Conversely, this freedom can create
a sense of isolation and lack of support throughout this experience. And some
women may not be able to afford monthly inseminations, which may cost
between $150 and $250 per try. Since DI is a hit-or-miss process, an infertility
problem can go undetected for some time, especially if the inseminations are
done infrequently.

Some women's health clinics offer DI to interested women of all sexual ori-
entations and marital or single statuses. Available services, donor policies, and
pregnancy rates may vary among clinics, so research potential clinics or sperm
banks carefully. Many medical specialists are also sympathetic and respectful of
single and/or gay women, and provide access to DI. Some programs also facilitate support groups for women both during the DI process and after their
children's births.

FAMILY ISSUES

❦ We have two children, aged four and six, who were conceived by DI. We have already told them that we needed help to get pregnant. When they are ready, we'll tell them about DI and what we know of the donors. We want them to hear it from us and think they should have this knowledge for medical, as well as psychological, reasons. We have been *very* selective, however, in telling friends and relatives.

❦ We've been advised to share our feelings about Steve not being able to biologically father them with our children, when they are mature enough to understand this. That way they can share THEIR sense of loss as well, in a kind of closing of the circle. The families in which this happens all felt much closer afterward.

Several religious denominations do not accept DI as an ethical, moral, or legitimate resolution to male infertility. Many in our society share this bias, and do not approve of family-building through DI. Given this reality, DI couples often wrestle with two issues about openness: whether to tell their child only, at some point, about his or her DI origins; and whether, during the pregnancy or after the birth, to confide in relatives or close friends.

Some argue that the "closed" adoption experience has shown that, in most cases, it is a mistake to conceal a child's genetic origins. They feel parents should discuss DI with their child, beginning around age three, in language appropriate to his age, and continue this dialogue throughout his childhood. In cases of anonymous or identity-release DI, search questions may arise later in the child's life. If a known donor is involved, all parties may need to discuss boundary and privacy issues.

Other couples believe that DI is the private, loving, and intimate way in which they created a child, and not a shameful secret. They do not feel it is desirable or appropriate to tell their child, or anyone else, about DI at any time.

Regardless of their feelings about telling children about DI, many couples feel this information should not be shared with extended family and close friends. They are concerned about judgment, criticism, or ostracism being directed toward themselves or their children, as well as blood-relative challenges to inheritances — particularly in states where laws are vague or unclear. Many also wish to protect their child's privacy. If they plan to discuss DI with their child, they want to control how, when, and by whom she is told.

Others wish to be open about their choice, and seeking understanding and support, may confide in those they trust. Family therapists advise potential parents to consider whether they want others to know about their child's genetic origins before he or she is able to understand this information. If the couple does plan to tell relatives or friends, experts advise being selective in who you tell, to request confidentiality, and to be prepared for negative, as well as positive, reactions. Those who may have been compassionate during your infertility workup or early treatment, may not be accepting or supportive of a DI resolution.

COPING SUGGESTIONS

❦ RESOLVE has been a lifeline to me. I correspond with four DI moms around the country, met as a result of my letter in a national newsletter. Their support as well as that of other friends met through RESOLVE as a volunteer for the Telephone Assistance Program (TAP), have buoyed me up and carried me along. RESOLVE has also given me the opportunity to play an important part in helping other couples decide to go through with DI. My husband volunteers as a network person also. It's a wonderful way to help.

The following coping suggestions are offered by DI couples and infertility professionals:

□ Before starting DI, be sure this is a mutually agreeable decision and that, to your best ability, you have both worked through lingering anger, jealousy, and grief.

□ Throughout the decision-making and treatment process, seek information, advice, support, and counseling from those with first-hand personal and professional experience with DI.

□ Maintain your sense of humor. It is a great tension reliever during DI treatment.

□ Make this a special bonding time. Go to the inseminations together if you are both comfortable with that. Plan special outings, treats, and rewards for yourselves during this time.

□ There can be on-going stress after pregnancy and birth, especially if the DI remains secret. This is a lifelong experience that requires continuing patience, love, and understanding. (See chapter 18 for further discussion of parenting after infertility.)

❦ Part Three
Resolutions

CHAPTER 17

Adoption

🐦 *The Answer (To An Adopted)*

Not flesh of my flesh
Nor bone of my bone
But still miraculously my own;
Never forget
For a single minute
You didn't grow
Under my heart
But in it.

Fleur Conkling Heyliger

THE PRACTICE OF ADOPTION is as old as humankind. Since prehistoric times, people have informally adopted children — often within the extended family or tribal unit — who needed nurturing and parenting. In some agricultural societies, including the United States, orphaned children were sometimes placed with families to help with the ceaseless and arduous labors of farming. Over the millenia, and among families within different cultures, adopted children have experienced love and acceptance, as well as resentment and cruelty.

Adoption, an important and essential social institution, continues to be practiced in various forms around the world. In many countries, most children are still adopted by relatives. In the United States, adoption has been formalized, and during this century, regulated by both licensed agencies and state statutes. The practice and character of adoption, however, has changed dramatically in this country during the past fifty years. For many decades, most adoptions were handled by public or private agencies that had more babies available for adoption than families willing to parent them. Since the 1970s, the broad and sweeping social changes of our times have also impacted the nature of adoption. Bearing a child outside of marriage, once a social stigma, is now widely accepted, and many single women who become pregnant decide to keep and raise their babies. More effective and increased use of birth control, as well as liberalized abortion laws, have also significantly reduced the number of unplanned infants who might be placed through adoption.

A growing movement toward openness has further altered the way adoption is practiced. Many birthparents now actively participate in the selection of adoptive parents and the placement of their babies, through agency or, in some

states, independent (private) adoption, and in many cases, maintain some type
of contact with them. There also continue to be many children of color, sibling
groups, older, and foreign-born children, as well as handicapped and other
special-needs kids who need loving adoptive homes. In 1986 (the latest statistics available), the National Committee for Adoption reported that 114,000
children were adopted in this country, 51,000 of those by non-relatives. Among
these adoptions, about 20,000 children were placed through public or private
agencies, 16,000 through independent adoption, and about 10,000 adopted
internationally.

In contemporary, industrialized society, adoption provides an opportunity
for individuals and couples to love, nurture, and parent a child. Those considering this option may include "fertile" families who wish to adopt in addition to,
or perhaps instead of, bearing biological children, as well as infertile couples or
singles who consider adoption after unsuccessful medical treatment.

While adoption is indeed a wonderful and joyous path to parenting,
experts emphasize that it is *not* a "cure" for infertility. Although couples or individuals may parent through adoption, their infertility and its emotional aftermath remains, to varying degrees, with them for the rest of their lives. Further,
adoption by its nature involves and tremendously affects a triad of parties —
birthparents, adoptive parents, and adopted children (and their extended families) — for a lifetime. Adoption, which involves both loss and triumph, is a
highly personal and often intense lifelong process.

Dozens of adoption triad members and professionals have contributed
their experiences and perspectives to both editions of this book. Each had their
own feelings and philosophy about the impact and legacy of adoption, along
with recommendations for the way it should be practiced. This chapter offers a
sampling of their insights, along with brief discussions of the evolution and
meaning of "open" adoption, relevant decision-making issues, grieving for the
loss of and inability to conceive biological children, adoption's lifelong issues,
and some practical aspects of agency, identified agency, special-needs, international, transracial, and independent adoption. Refer to the Bibliography and
Resources sections for expert analysis and advice regarding the "how-tos," and
emotional and psychological complexities of adoption.

The Evolution of Open Adoption

   ❦ When we first heard of Rosie, our child's birthmother, she was
trying to decide whether or not to have an abortion, keep her child,
or place him for adoption. At this point we could do nothing but
wait for her decision. Again we had no control and felt vulnerable.

     Our attorney called asking if we wanted to speak with Rosie
and her mother on the phone. He would introduce us over a
conference call and then allow us to talk privately. I have never
felt so many butterflies, and a million fears surfaced within

minutes: What if she didn't like us? What if we didn't like her? What would we talk about? After the initial hellos, there were laughter, tears, and a strong sense of love that I never would have thought possible between virtual strangers.

We all felt strongly that God had brought us together. That helped seal the bond that began that day and continues with each day of our child's life. We talked again a few days later and decided to meet. Rosie would fly up to spend several days with us in our home.

She made the trip when she was seven months pregnant. When she stepped off the plane, we embraced and then fumbled shyly with words while retrieving her luggage. We were in the car for about five minutes when she began to sing along with the radio and then giggled that she must not be nervous anymore. We all relaxed. We had a wonderful visit, a time for us to get acquainted that will always be fondly remembered. She was reassured about the home her child would be raised in; we were able to express our gratitude for her wonderful gift. When she left, we agreed not to meet again before the birth. None of us knew if she would be able to go through with the adoption.

We left for her hometown the day the baby was due. Rosie had become more and more emotional, and we tried to brace ourselves for another disappointment. We met her parents, and this was another beautiful experience: They weren't much older than us! Her mother gave us a letter for the baby to read as an adult — a letter from Rosie explaining her reasons for the adoption, along with pictures of Rosie and her family to give our child some sense of his biological roots.

The day our son was born was truly one of mixed emotions. We were so happy for ourselves, but felt Rosie and her family's pain. We held him in our arms when he was four hours old and spent as much time at the hospital as they would allow. When we left, there were hugs, tears, and that same inexpressible love that we had felt before. Rosie did not look at her son at birth, but held him in her arms and said her goodbyes before she went home. When we left the hospital with that tiny bundle, we knew he was ours.

We have heard from Rosie twice since Kevin's birth: once when he was about a year old and again before his fourth birthday. I do feel fear when I see the envelope in the mail, but it is only fleeting because of the openness of our adoption. When we visited with Rosie we told her that the door would always be open to her. If she ever wanted to inquire about our son's health and happiness, we would reply. If it weren't for her, we wouldn't have our wonderful son. How could we deny her? She, in turn, assured us that she would never try to intrude and we trust her in that. Her letters were written to let us know that she is happy and to request some pictures, which we sent along with news of Kevin. Her sister has told us the pictures and letter have brought great comfort to Rosie.

Open adoption is relatively new, so it's hard to know how it will affect our children as they become adults. We discussed the possibility of Rosie meeting Kevin when he is an adult and have assured her that we would not be opposed to it if he chooses to do so. We do not feel threatened: We may not have given birth to him, but he is our son in every way and no one can ever take that away. Our love is too secure.

I think closed adoptions will soon be a thing of the past and the fears and myths will be put aside where they belong. By being sensitive to one another, expressing fears and expectations, and understanding each other, I believe that all members of the adoption triangle can emerge as happy and whole beings.

Postscript, 1992: Kevin is now eleven, and our feelings about open adoption have not changed. We have heard from Rosie by letter about once a year, and, of course, we have responded. She has never married, and two years ago had a hysterectomy. Our hearts ache knowing that Kevin will be her only biological child.

Our promise to each other that we would respect a "distance" has been difficult at times. We have not heard from Rosie this past year and we hope that she is well. We hesitate to write because she may be trying to break away for her own emotional well-being, and yet we worry about her. Likewise, we have had to hide my treatment for cancer from her because we do not want her to worry about us. (I hasten to add that I am seven years past treatment and doing well.)

We have shared our pictures of her with Kevin and have answered all his questions, but we have not yet shared her letters. His interest is more of a curiosity at this point, and we want to be sure he is mature enough to understand her gift of love when he reads her letters. We still believe that some day we will all be reunited.

For decades, most adoptions in the United States were "closed" and enveloped in secrecy. Birthmothers relinquished their babies to agencies or other intermediaries who screened and selected parents to legally adopt these children. An amended birth certificate was issued by the state naming the adoptive parents as the birthparents. Neither party knew the identity of the other, and agency and court records were "sealed," their contents and identifying information permanently unavailable to birthparents, adoptive parents, or adoptees.

Adoption experts trace the origins of the closed system to several factors. The transition of our society from a primarily rural to predominately urban one, which occurred during the first half of this century, separated and fragmented family members from their communities and each other. The isolation of, and lack of support for, pregnant, unmarried women, together with the pervasive middle-class stigma of illegitimacy, resulted in the relinquishment of their babies for adoption by "strangers" — people unrelated and unknown to the mother, who often lived in other cities or states. Public and private agencies, together with subsequent state and federal legislation, were created during this time to formalize and regulate the adoption process. It was decided, by those in control, that secrecy was necessary to "protect" all involved parties.

Several myths, which caused considerable anguish to many of those involved, were developed to reinforce the secrecy integral to closed adoption. Birthmothers were often told that their pregnancies were shameful and that they would "forget" and "get over" the relinquishment of their babies. In reality, thousands of women grieved deeply and continually, year after year, not knowing where their children were, how they fared, or whether they were even alive. For many, the aftermath of closed adoption greatly affected the course and quality of their lives.

> ❦ Birthmothers of closed adoptions have only a loss, a loss that is difficult to grieve because their children aren't dead, but rather living with strangers. It presents a life-long problem, one that society chooses to ignore.
>
> We had no choices then . . . no sex education, no birth control, no legal abortion, no support for keeping our babies. We were told that we would forget about the loss of a child to adoption. Many older birthmothers have avoided intimate relationships and never had other children and many, like myself, have experienced secondary infertility.

Adoptive parents were often told that adoption would "fix" the pain of their infertility, and that adoptive families were the same as biological ones. They also received the message that it was somehow wrong or dangerous to know or have contact with the birthmother.

Adopted children often felt curious about their birthparents and the circumstances of their adoption, confused about their identity, and perhaps guilty that these feelings might be hurtful to their parents. Some adoptees, who didn't have any identifying information or pictures of their birthmothers, describe an eerie feeling that they weren't really born.

Philip Adams, a pioneering adoption attorney, questioned the notion of secrecy fifty years ago, when he first began faciliating independent adoptions in San Francisco. "It made no sense to me why people should be so afraid of this 'phantom birthmother,'" he recalls. "Why not have the parties meet each other and assure themselves that they are making the right choice?" Starting with a few cases in the 1940s, Adams has facilitated several thousand open adoptions to date.

As the effects on the triad members became apparent, more professionals began to question the wisdom of continuing closed adoption. Annette Baran and Reuben Pannor, longtime adoption social workers and authors, were among the first to challenge the entrenched system. They argued that children, as a birthright, are entitled to know the identities of their birthparents; that birthparents have a right to know where their children are placed, how they are faring, and to let them know, especially on birthdays and holidays, that "even though they couldn't care *for* them, they care *about* them"; and that adoptive parents have a right to know the identities of their children's birthparents and share that information with them. Over the past decade, increasing numbers of adoption professionals, birthparents, adoptive parents, and adoptees have agreed that secrecy spawns shame, guilt, unresolved grief, and unfounded fears and fantasies. The number of closed adoptions has steadily decreased.

What Is Open Adoption?

In the 1990s, there has been an increasing trend toward openness in both agency and independent adoptions. Although precisely defining an "open" adoption is difficult, adoption expert and author Sharon Kaplan-Roszia offers this "bottom-line" interpretation:

> ❦ The identities of the involved parties are known to each other and, consequently, the child will never have to "search" for his or her biological parents. The birthparents are acknowledged as such to the child. The adoptive parents are indisputably the child's rearing parents, and should absolutely feel "entitled" to the parental role and responsibilities. The relationship of all the parties is founded on truth. In this way, losses can be grieved openly and a foundation of honesty and trust is established between parents and children.

Beyond these parameters, the application of open adoption varies widely among families. In many cases, contact continues throughout the birthmother's pregnancy. Many adoptive parents attend the birth and bring the baby home from the hospital. Communication in some form may continue between the birthparents and the adoptive family after the child's adoption. Most often this involves an exchange of letters and pictures or phone calls several times a year. In some families, occasional or frequent visiting occurs. As with all on-going relationships, the degree, frequency, and duration of contact varies and may be modified throughout their lives.

> ❦ We have three adopted children. Over the years our understanding of adoption has changed enormously. We have been taught by our children, their birthparents, and other birthparents and adoptees that we have met in support groups and workshops, and by becoming aware of our own beliefs about adoption.

We adopted our oldest child, Jed, in a closed agency adoption. We told him, at a very young age, that he was adopted. When he was about three, he began asking questions about the person who had given birth to him. I could see he was hurt and confused about this "phantom birthmother" who gave him up out of love, but was not a real person he had met. I told him he might be able to meet her when he was eighteen. I knew by the look of confusion and pain on his face that this was the wrong solution. It felt as if we were keeping something from him.

By this time, we had adopted our second child, Sarah, through an open independent adoption. We met Sarah's birthmother just a few weeks before her birth. Our mutual agreement was to exchange letters and photos after the birth, but have no personal contact until Sarah reached adulthood. At that time, we still believed that contact would be confusing for the children.

Now we wanted to open up both adoptions more. The adoption agency facilitated an exchange of letters between Jed's birthmother and our family. Eventually they allowed us to meet face to face when he was about four. She is a wonderful person — our lives have been made richer by knowing her. Jed's feelings have been mixed about his birthmother, Joan, but he seems comforted by knowing who and where she is. Now he has a real person in mind when he thinks about her — someone to direct his feelings toward.

When Sarah was a year old, we wrote her birthmother, Carol, and asked if she'd be willing to resume contact with us. She agreed and we have been seeing each other occasionally. Her willingness to visit seems in part determined by how well her life is going at the moment. She shies away from contact when things are difficult. And we don't seem as compatible with her as we are with Jed's birthmother. This probably has to do with re-negotiating the original agreement. In an ideal situation, perhaps you choose each other on the basis of whether you can form a relationship that will be comfortable and mutually supportive. Still, we love this young woman who looks so much like Sarah and has her warm, gentle personality. It is great to pick up the phone when we have a question about past medical history or developmental milestones. Sarah's response to her birthmother has changed over time. Now, at age seven, she thinks fondly of her, misses her if a long time passes between visits, feels briefly sad when we separate, but is strongly connected to us and has no confusion about who her "real" parents are.

Our third adoption was unexpected and seemed to be a culmination of all we had learned in the processes of the other two. Our daughter, Carrie, is a relative of mine — the child of my first cousin's son. She contacted us wanting advice for her son and his girlfriend who were seeking a traditional, closed adoption. They didn't really know of any other kind. We sent them some books and articles and a long letter offering to adopt the baby ourselves. From that point, four months into the pregnancy, the process developed in what I have come to view as a nearly ideal open adoption: counseling for all parties, early involvement with an experienced attorney, frequent contact and visits, and if possible, the presence of the adoptive parents at the child's birth.

Seeing that small pink body emerge and the looks of amazement and love on the faces of her birthparents was a gift I will be able to share with Carrie. The deep trust we had developed enabled us to face, together, a frightening week of tests and uncertainty. Carrie was diagnosed with a medical problem which required surgery at three weeks of age. We found ways to share this baby and communicate with each other through the whole ordeal. This was one of the most challenging and rewarding experiences of my life. I came out of it with lifelong friends.

It seems there are rules and myths about adoption that are based more upon tradition than on the actual need for healthy experiences on the part of the people involved. Perhaps the rules have always been written, in part, by adoptive parents, whose interests lie in preserving denial about their infertility, and hiding doubts about their entitlement to their children. I feel that knowing their birthparents will help my kids cope with the painful identity issues that accompany adoption. I also think both adoption and infertility are parallel lifelong processes. By openly addressing one, I am acknowledging the other.

Marc and Bonnie Gradstein, an adoption attorney and counselor and adoptive parents themselves, surveyed 775 families who adopted through their practice between 1980 and 1990 and received the following responses regarding open adoption: 63 percent had met their children's birthmothers, 18 percent had met both birthparents; 32 percent had no further contact with birthparent(s) after the child's birth (termination of contact was mostly initiated by birthparents), while 68 percent continued contact; 61 percent communicated through letters and pictures, 39 percent by telephone, and 14 percent visited each other. Most parents supported future meetings between child and birthparents. Virtually no adoptive parents felt intruded upon by birthparents.

Making the Decision to Adopt

❦ My marriage was only two months old when I had my first surgery. An emergency removal of a badly diseased right ovary and tube was done. I was consumed with the need to get pregnant right away. This has been my year and a half for acting upon, and diligently concentrating on, what is so terribly wrong with me that no child can be realized through my body — being torn apart physically to probe for a cause and mentally trying to adjust to my sorrow and despair.

Now I see a light growing brighter at the end of this tunnel of infertility. Adoption is my chance to believe again in, and concentrate on, what is good and strong about myself and my marriage. I am out of practice, but am again learning to dwell on what I do have to offer a baby. I am rising above the realization of imperfect physical being, and the suffering this brings, to view myself through adoption as whole again — as the mother of someone who needs me. I am again seeing myself with much to give — if not my uterus to grow in, then my arms to lie in, my love to have, my life to share.

Childlessness is not me. And now I know it does not have to be. I have resolved myself to adoption in mind and heart, and welcome the love it will bring to me. I will be a mother — the realization of a dream.

Most couples who wish to parent assume they will bear one or more biological children. Those who want a large family might plan to adopt additional children after they experience childbirth. Infertile couples, however, often realize that adoption may be the only way they can have children and approach this option with a great deal of frustration or grief. Adoption may seem like a last resort to these couples: "If we can't get pregnant, or get too old, then we'll have to adopt."

At the same time, they may also receive a lot of unsolicited advice from friends and relatives who *know* how "awful, stressful, expensive, risky, and impossible" adoption is, who *guarantee* they will get pregnant as soon as they adopt, or who *warn* them to adopt quickly before it is too late.

Making the decision to adopt under these circumstances can be a long, painful process. It may be helpful to speak with adoption experts: adoption attorneys, facilitators, and counselors, and a variety of parents who have recently adopted. They can give you accurate information and reassurance about both the stresses and joys of the adoption process. Many RESOLVE chapters also sponsor pre-adoption meetings where adoptive parents share their insights and experience.

After gathering this information, you can individually and collectively consider the issues involved with adoption. The following questions are offered as a starting point. Both partners (or a single individual considering adoption) might read them over, think about their reactions for a few days, and then compare their feelings.

- ☐ Do I feel inadequate, inferior, or incomplete because of my infertility?
- ☐ Have I thoroughly grieved for our inability to have a biological child, for the loss of our genetic line(s), and for a child of our union?

- ☐ How will our extended families react to our decision to adopt and how would they treat our child(ren)?
- ☐ Can I love and parent a child who may have quite different looks, temperament, personality, talents, strengths, or weaknesses?
- ☐ Do I wish to continue to try for a pregnancy while pursuing adoption? Suppose I become pregnant while awaiting an adoption?
- ☐ Do I feel as excited about adoption as I did about trying to get pregnant?
- ☐ Are we ready, financially and emotionally, to become parents tomorrow, next week, or next month? As a single woman or man, do I have the resources and support to undertake adoption?
- ☐ Are we aware that adoption is a lifelong process, a fact that our family must always cope with?
- ☐ Am I prepared for the emotional stress of the adoption process and to again feel "out of control" and vulnerable to disappointment and possibly loss?
- ☐ Can we afford the costs of agency or independent adoption?
- ☐ How do I feel about open adoption? About on-going contact or visitation with the birthparent(s) during pregnancy or after the child's birth?
- ☐ Do we wish to adopt only an infant? Would we be comfortable with an older child, one with a handicap, or a child of another race or culture?
- ☐ What are our reservations? Why haven't we adopted already?
- ☐ Where do we stand as a couple about adoption? How committed am I to this decision and to supporting my partner through the process?

Considering and discussing these issues often elicits, or intensifies, anger and grief in one or both partners. Couples may disagree on a number of issues and feel irritated or impatient with each other. Both may already be distressed and exhausted from their infertility experience. At this time it may be difficult to communicate honestly and objectively about adoption until the grieving process is completed.

Grieving for Your Biological Child

❦ I had been unable to admit that I couldn't get pregnant through my own force of will; I could not accept defeat. After this realization, I gradually began to feel more comfortable with the notion of failure. And I could begin to separate failure to get pregnant from failure as a woman or as a person.

It was at this point that, for the first time, I was able actively to pursue my goal to become a parent. Today my husband and I are the parents of a beautiful, bright, loving two-year-old son whom we began parenting on the day of his birth.

❦ The sadness of not birthing a child still occasionally surfaces. It is, however, not the same wrenching pain as before we adopted Tracy.

I've made my peace with what happened. The sadness has been put in its place.

Some infertile couples realize that parenting, rather than pregnancy, is their primary goal, and after a number of months or years, stop medical treatment. With enormous relief they end this frustrating quest and turn toward adoption. Before making their decision, however, most grieve for the loss of the biological child they had hoped to birth and raise. This is often a devastating loss, perhaps compounded by guilt that they waited too long, or by anger at the unfairness of their infertility. Accepting adoption as an equally exciting alternative may be a difficult process.

Inherent in the decision to wholeheartedly pursue adoption is an acknowledgment of the losses of infertility and one's genetic children. (See chapter 20 for a discussion of grieving after medical treatment is stopped.) Partners commonly move through their grief at different paces; in some cases, one may prefer another resolution, such as donor insemination, surrogacy, or child-free living, to adoption. During this time, a consultation with an infertility therapist may be helpful to sort through feelings and reach a decision. Most experts feel it is essential to take the time to mourn the considerable losses of infertility before entering the adoption process.

Our Fantasy Child

For many couples, the pregnancy and birth of a child of their union is a life's dream. Most also assume that their biological offspring will be perfect specimens with all their best qualities. Few fantasize about a child with a disability or even a disagreeable personality. There is also a natural curiosity about one's biological child. Would she or he have my nose, your dimples, our artistic bent? Humorously posing an alternative fantasy can put things into perspective.

> ❦ It hit me that there was no reason to assume that this fantasy child was going to get all our good qualities. While playing roulette with these genes, those of our relatives might get the upper hand. I started to laugh right on the freeway. I pictured a little cousin Henry!
> The flip side became apparent. Some pregnant young lady might have all kinds of good things connecting inside her. In our case it was true. We got a cute, wonderful kid. I take the credit whenever he does anything good!

Certainly, everyone would like to pass their physical traits and emotional chemistries to their children. But when pregnancy is not possible or likely, consider the other qualities you have to offer.

> ❦ What do you really want to pass on to your kids? I feel most grateful to my own parents for emotional, rather than genetic, heritage. I would like to pass on values, love, and feelings to my children, rather than the shape of an ear. I'm not belittling

pregnancy. If you can do it, fine. But if you're having problems and shying away from adoption because of the fact that this is not your biological child, it's important to question what you fear.

Parenting is about having a child. This can be done without a child coming out of you. You don't have to be related to people by blood to love them.

For some couples, the loss of having biological children remains, to some degree, throughout their lives. Jed Somit, adoption attorney and adoptive father of three, suggests that this loss be acknowledged, accepted, and gently let go because it is unrealistic and unfair to apply that image to one's adopted children. They deserve, in their own right, their parents' love, pride, and enthusiasm for the unique people they are.

❦ I think the gain of parenting through adoption exceeds the loss. The diversity among my adopted children is a source of great delight, and even exceeds the differences between my brother and myself, although I thought we were night and day. Like the entire recorded Somit bloodline, we were naturally unathletic; my son Hal is a natural athlete, and I can only marvel, and be both proud and jealous, of his achievements. Jake is most like me temperamentally, but can draw — again, a trait lacking on either side of my ancestors' family charts. And Julia — well, she is so unlike anyone I know from my own experience, I don't even know what I know about her. All this is compounded by their own sibling dynamics. If you want the challenge and experience of parenting, adoption is sure to test your skills!

Friends and Family

Because our society tends to favor biological parenting over adoption, infertile couples often think that their relatives and friends consider pregnancy the only real way to have a family. As potential grandparents confront their own mortality, they often yearn for biological descendants and may convey this message, subtly or not, to their own children. Couples considering adoption often fear their child won't be treated "like blood" by their extended family. It is often helpful to discuss these concerns with adoption professionals, other adoptive parents, and your extended families and friends before you start this process so fears and misunderstandings can be aired. In many cases, those who have helplessly witnessed your infertility struggle will enthusiastically support, and perhaps assist, with your adoption and accept and, even before he arrives, embrace your child.

❦ Sean is so special, not only to us but to our friends and family who now understand what we went through to have him. He is a special blessing resulting from our infertility. We could not love him more if he were our biological child. He is truly a miracle. Although

he will learn that I didn't carry him, he knows I am his mother —
the one who feeds him, cares for him, and loves him.

After working through their losses and fears concerning infertility and adoption, the couple or individual can approach this process with renewed energy and love —a commitment their adopted child needs and deserves.

❦ Don and I had never considered adoption because we had endless hope I could get pregnant. When our treatment ended, we felt great relief that the stress and tension were over; yet we were in limbo about our lives. Weren't we five years ago trying to enlarge our family? Had we forgotten our original goal of wanting to give love and security to our child? This haunted us for some time.

We started talking to adoptive parents, adopted children, and doctors. We phoned friends, read books about adoption, and had long discussions. One evening Don said, "Let's go for it."

From that moment on we worked 110 percent for an adoption, just as we had with our infertility, and there were never any regrets, remorse, or skepticism. We knew it was only a matter of time before we would start our family, our original goal.

Five years is a long labor that a fertile woman will never understand. Three years ago, Don and I were blessed with our adoptive baby daughter, and you can't bring us down from the clouds yet!

Pursuing Both Adoption and Pregnancy

❦ We went to an agency group meeting and were told that the wait for an infant may be quite long. However, I was only thirty, John was thirty-four, and we could still try for a pregnancy. We were just covering all the bases and felt we were taking positive steps forward.

Some couples may decide to begin the adoption process while continuing their infertility treatment, willing to parent either biologically or through adoption. Others want a larger family and adopt one or more children while trying for a biological child. Whatever your reasons for pursuing both options, experts emphasize the importance of putting the same careful consideration, soul-searching, energy, and heart and soul into adoption as you did to getting pregnant. To do otherwise, they argue, is unfair to both yourselves and your adopted child. This can be difficult under any circumstances, but particularly if you are pursuing such intensive medical treatment as Assisted Reproductive Technology (ART). These procedures are emotionally, physically, and financial draining in themselves (see chapter 14).

Couples who wish to have only one child, or children spaced several years apart, should also weigh this decision carefully. A common myth predicts a pregnancy for every couple who adopts. Actually there is only about a 5 percent chance of such an event, and most likely this spontaneous pregnancy would have happened anyway. But it does happen. Are you both willing and able to raise two children closely spaced, one biological and the other adopted? How would growing up in such a "blended" family affect your children? Would your adopted child feel "left out" or "second best"? Would your biological child feel guilty and possibly "favored" by you or your extended families? How would you handle these challenges?

If you feel medical treatment is consuming most of your resources and energy, or uncomfortable about creating a blended family, you may wish to postpone one option while pursuing the other.

Adoption as a Lifelong Process

❦ When I was in my early twenties, I suffered from severe endometriosis, which required surgery to remove my ovaries, tubes and uterus. My husband and I wanted children very much. Fortunately in those days, many couples were able to go to an adoption agency and, if they qualified, request a little girl or boy. We were so lucky to adopt two girls and a boy all in their infancy.

At first we encountered the usual well-meaning but thoughtless remarks from friends and relatives. But most irritating was the comment, "How lucky those children are that you adopted them!"

Why, from the very first John and I have felt that we are the lucky ones, and we still do! Our children are wonderful people who have given us such joy. Neither of us has ever regretted their adoption or the fact that we did not birth them. They are our children in every way that matters.

When they were each about three years old, we matter-of-factly told each of them that we were unable to have children and that we adopted them. After that, we rarely discussed it. We didn't consider them "special" because they were adopted. From the very beginning, we thought of and treated them as our own children.

As my children grew up, each experienced different emotions about adoption. I remember my little boy, at just five or six years old, being very angry with his biological mother for giving him up. When I explained that she just couldn't afford to raise him, he muttered, "Well, she could have got a job!"

We have been the happiest of families. I never thought much about adopting my children until my oldest daughter got pregnant. When she first told me the wonderful news, we looked at each other and cried. I realized that the birth experience was one thing we couldn't discuss and compare notes on. This daughter is also quite adamant about not ever meeting her biological parents. She requested that the adoption agency put a letter in her file that states her desire not to be contacted by either party. She told me of this decision one Mother's Day, saying that she feels I am the only mother she has.

At one time, my youngest daughter was curious about her birthparents. She told me, "Mom, I don't really want to meet them, or have them in my life. I would just like to see what they look like." I told her that I was secure in her love and understood her curiosity. I would help her locate her birthparents if this is what she wanted. Since then, she has changed her mind. She now feels searching for her birthparents would complicate her life.

All three of my children are now married and two are parents. Looking back, I wish we had been given more genetic and medical facts. This information would be useful for both my children and grandchildren.

I also see that extended family support and understanding is critical throughout our lives. There is still a lot of fear and misunderstanding about this subject and we've had to educate potential in-laws about adoption. Many people fear the unknown background of adopted people and worry about their children becoming involved with them.

And it's been a challenge deciding whom to tell about our children's adoption and when. My daughter's step-children, for example, were quite hurt to learn about her adoption years after they met her. We just never thought about mentioning it until the subject came up one day. They felt they had a right to know from the beginning and had been left out! As we age and our family grows, I am continually learning about the impact and legacy of adoption.

I have never felt less of a woman because I did not bear a child. My husband and I have had a very happy marriage of forty years. For those who are infertile and wish to have children, I strongly recommend adoption. For us, it has been a joyous and wonderful experience.

Adopting a child is the first step of a lifelong experience. Like biological parenting, adoption brings the laughter, tears, and exhaustion of raising a family. It also carries unique joys, stresses, and losses.

The adoption triad consists of the birthparents, adoptive parents, and the adopted child. All three parties, and their extended families, are affected by this adoption for the rest of their lives, although the intensity of feelings varies with each individual.

For the infertile couple, adoption brings the joy, love, and fulfillment of parenthood. Yet the couple is parenting the birthchild of others, not one of their bodies. Those who do not have biological children may grieve for that loss and carry residual feelings about their infertility throughout their lives.

> ❦ I don't think it is easy for a woman to accept the fact that a life may never grow within her. But it is harder to imagine never experiencing the joy and pleasure of raising a child. I will always wish that I had actually carried my son and given birth to him. I feel the loss of those nine months even while I cherish the blessing of having him as my son for the rest of my life. But I have come to realize that pregnancy lasts a very short time; raising a child lasts a lifetime.

Some parents, still vulnerable and wounded from their infertility, may not feel they are "entitled" or, on some level, deserving of parenting their adopted child. It may take some time, and perhaps counseling, to heal these wounds and develop a sense of entitlement. Regardless of whether the adoption is closed or open, and the degree of that openness, adoptive parents may also feel uncomfortable with, or fearful of, birthparent contact. Some may feel it is a painful reminder of their infertility; others may worry that their child will feel closer to, prefer, or perhaps love her birthparents more.

The birthparents, and often their families, are struggling with the loss of a child and part of their genetic line. In many cases, the birthmother is a single teenager or young woman, and her baby may be both families' first grandchild or great-grandchild. Some birthfathers run away from the problem, or refuse to acknowledge the baby; others, along with their families, share feelings of love for the child and take an active role in the adoption process.

Often birthmothers are without financial resources, high school or college educations, or job skills. Some have been rejected or abandoned by the child's father and perhaps their own families. One therapist described many of the birthmothers she counsels as "floundering, frightened, and overwhelmed by their circumstances." Throughout their pregnancies many of these women are ambivalent about their decision to relinquish their babies. Indeed, birthing is such a powerful transition that it is hard to predict how any woman will feel until she delivers her baby. Many have great feelings of love toward their unborn child and have continued their pregnancies because of it. Because they feel unable to parent at this time, relinquishing the child is usually a painful, wrenching decision that may leave a lifetime of ambivalent feelings. Some later suffer the added pain of not bearing other children.

> ❦ Like me, I think most birthmothers never get over relinquishing their child. After carrying your baby and feeling that life bounding within you, you can't just forget about your child, or stop wondering how he is doing throughout his life. This is particularly painful if this choice is made from family pressure or economic necessity.

As their lives progress, many birthparents come to terms with their relinquishment decision, although feelings resurface over the years. Those who relinquished children through closed adoptions, although fearing rejection from the adoptive parents and their birthchild, may, at some point in their lives, attempt a "search." The increasing incidence of open adoption has helped many birthparents and their extended families better cope with their loss. They are assured that their child is healthy, happy, and growing up in a secure home. Adoption attorney Diane Michelsen observes that this pregnancy and relinquishment is often the lowest point in birthmothers' lives. Planning and participating in open adoption is often the catalyst that turns their lives in a positive and fulfilling direction. Despite these assurances and comforts, however, feelings of loss remain.

❦ I got pregnant, at twenty-two, while working in the mountains during summer vacation. I knew I wanted to go through with the pregnancy, although I had ambivalent feelings about placing my baby for adoption. I knew, on the one hand, that it was a good decision, but I also felt guilty and selfish. I joined a birthmothers' support group and realized these feelings were common. I was also lucky that my parents and brothers were behind me and supported my decision.

I met a facilitator who showed me some letters from couples wanting to adopt a baby. I picked out three, read them over and mentally ordered them 1, 2, 3 in preference. I showed them to my parents and, without discussing it with me, they also came up with the same ordering.

I met Sherry and Kip and liked them immediately. We had a lot in common and I trusted them as I would friends. They met my whole family and everyone hit it off. As the birth approached, we went to the hospital and talked to the social worker and nurses about how we wanted things handled when my baby was born. We left the future of the relationship open. We realized that it was impossible to predict our feelings after the birth.

The day of Brett's birth was incredible. My parents, brothers, and Sherry and Kip were there. My mom and best friend helped me through the labor and birth. Brett was absolutely perfect, with lots of hair like me and his birthfather. We spent the night together and everybody took turns holding him.

I asked Sherry and Kip not to see me the day they brought Brett home. Even with all the support, it was unbelievably painful. I went to my parents' home and stayed for about a month. I thought I would never stop crying. I remember taking a shower one morning and hearing "Teach Your Children Well" on the radio. I cried like my heart would break. My friends and family stayed right by me and let me grieve. I also kept going to my birthmothers' group.

Sherry and Kip said they would respect my privacy after the birth and wait for me to contact them. About four weeks later, though, a letter came. It was so like them. On the back of the envelope, Sherry had written, "Kip thinks this is intrusive, but I couldn't help myself. If you're not ready to hear from us, just put this aside until you want to read it." Of course I opened it and it was so loving. Sherry had written little notes almost every day, like "Today we went out and Brett wore that cute hat you bought him," or she would let me know how much he had grown and the weight he had gained. That letter meant so much to me.

Over the past six years, our relationship has naturally grown and changed. All of us — their extended families and mine — get together for occasions and, of course, Brett's birthday. It is really a wonderful situation.

Not long ago I bought Brett some glow-in-the-dark stars for the ceiling of his room. Sherry told me he put one in the middle and then lots of others surrounding that one. Each stands for someone in his life. The two closest to his star are Sherry and Kip. A little further away are me and my boyfriend. And my parents and brothers are up there too.

But there's still loss and pain with adoption. When Brett skins his knee, he runs to Sherry. She's his mom. I realize that both Sherry and Kip and I lost babies — I lost parenting Brett and they lost the baby they worked so hard for during all that infertility treatment.

As they grow up, children experience a variety of emotions about adoption. Depending on the age and temperament of the child, the way adoption has been discussed in the family, and the amount, if any, of contact with the birthparent(s), the fact of being adopted can evoke a number of feelings: acceptance and love, as well as fear, confusion, or identity questions. As with blended families, children growing up with open adoption will probably face similar issues and form uniquely individual impressions of, or relationships with, birth relatives.

Identity issues often come into focus or resurface during adolescence and may be compounded if the child does not physically resemble his adoptive family. If the adoption was closed, he or she may lack a "birth story" and connections to his genetic background.

❧ My adolescence was quite painful. Along with the normal identity issues all teenagers experience, I also wondered why I carried one family's name and another's heredity; why my biological parents didn't want me; whether I looked like them.

Such questions may eventually lead some children of closed adoptions to search for their birthparents (and genetic heredity) and perhaps arrange a reunion. This meeting can raise many feelings: hope of discovery and reconciliation, fear of another rejection by the birthparents, and pain that this decision is hurting the adoptive family. Experts emphasize that the decision to search should not be equated with a loss of love for the adoptive parents. Instead the child is looking for a tie to her genetic origins, which may or may not result in an emotional bond.

Some triad members report little emotional turmoil about their adoption experience and don't pursue on-going contact or searches, while others experience continuing feelings of anger, love, abandonment, gratitude, and sadness. These emotions are unique to each individual and cannot be quantified, universally applied, or deemed right or wrong. A number of organizations, included in the Resources section, have been created to support the lifelong needs and issues of all triad members.

Public and Private Agency Adoption

🐛 My first call was to an adoption agency that told me my husband was just at their cut-off age for applications and that if we applied that day and were accepted, it would probably take some time to adopt a healthy infant. I hung up totally discouraged.

🐛 Just a few months after we filed our application we were surprised by a call from the county adoption service. They had a baby girl who needed a home. Were we still interested? Were we!! We madly scrambled for clothes, crib, and diapers and brought her home a few days before Christmas.

Adoption agencies are licensed, state-regulated private or public organizations that coordinate the adoption process between birthparents who wish to relinquish their child (or those whose children are removed from their homes by the state) and couples or individuals seeking to adopt a child. The process includes the birthparent's relinquishment of legal custody (and if necessary, termination of the birthfather's legal rights) of their child to the agency, careful screening of prospective parents, and placement of the child with an adoptive couple or individual. The final stage of agency adoption occurs with the transfer of legal custody by a court to the adoptive parent(s).

There is usually less risk of a child being reclaimed by the birthparent(s) with an agency adoption because, in most cases, they have surrendered their legal rights upon relinquishing the child to the agency. Unless they can prove the relinquishment papers were signed under fraudulent conditions, incapacity, or duress, it is highly unlikely (but in a small percentage of cases, possible) that a court would return the child to them after placement.

In most instances the child is not placed with an adoptive family until he or she is legally free. However, in some cases the child has not been legally freed by both birthparents. For example, the agency may have been unable to locate the birthfather and obtain his signature for relinquishment. In these cases, the child may be placed in a fost-adopt or foster home arrangement until the legal procedures are completed. There may be a small chance of a court hearing for custody. Before placement, the agency will notify the adoptive parents of the situation and any risks involved.

IDENTIFIED AGENCY ADOPTION

Identified agency adoption is a fairly new practice that incorporates elements of both agency and independent adoption. In these cases, the birthparents and adoptive parents select each other and ask the agency, who is committed to their decision, to provide a home study and to assist with counseling, facilitation, trouble-shooting, creating a hospital plan, and the legal steps necessary to finalize the adoption. As with agency adoption, the birthparents relinquish the baby to the agency. Adoption attorneys may also be involved with parts of this process. Birthmother and newborn expenses are paid through either an agency or attorney trust account. Identified agency procedures and fees vary among agencies and in each state, so check with any adoption agencies you are considering, as well as your state's Department of Social Services.

FEES

Adoption agencies charge a fee for their services that varies depending on whether the organization is public or private. Most reputable adoption agencies conduct informational meetings to discuss their operating procedures and fees. Fees may range from a few hundred dollars to $4,000 or more. Sliding scale fees are often available, and some employers and insurance companies may cover all or part of the adoption expense. Experts caution prospective adoptive parents to study all proposed charges and be suspicious of excessively high, unidentified costs. Sources of referral to reputable agencies include your specialist, state or county department of social services, or local RESOLVE chapter.

QUALIFYING AS AN ADOPTIVE PARENT

❦ The agencies willing to work with us had long waiting lists. We would also have to expose ourselves body and soul in order to qualify. Before considering us, they wanted a reason for my infertility. I was unwilling to discuss it; after three years of tests, I had no medical reason. I was just "different" and I was angry. This stage of anger has been the most difficult for me to face and resolve. I'm sure it has impacted our subsequent attempts at adoption.

❦ We had heard that it was difficult to adopt through an agency and that the social workers were veterans of the system who really put you through the wringer. We had, however, made up our minds to go through whatever was necessary; we really wanted to be parents. From the beginning, though, the county staff made us feel comfortable. They wanted to know about our family backgrounds and occupations. Our initial meeting lasted more than two hours, but the time flew by. We passed through the first screening and two more appointments were made: one with only my husband, the other in our home.

Before you can adopt a child through an agency, you must meet their requirements as suitable parents. The criteria for qualifying varies with each agency. While long waiting lists were once common, agencies are increasingly screening couples and then letting them know whether they will be placed on a waiting list or not, and for how long. If you are not accepted, try not to take it personally. There just aren't enough infants available through agency adoption to meet the demand.

The qualifying process itself can be stressful. Many individuals and couples are not accustomed to the amount of scrutiny and investigation required. In addition, anger about infertility may resurface as one realizes that biological parents do not have to "qualify" to become pregnant or to parent.

Many agencies call this qualifying or screening procedure the "home study process," which begins with a detailed questionnaire regarding your income level, age, medical history, living environment, and reasons for wishing to adopt. In addition, one or more informational meetings, several interviews at the agency, and a home visit will be required. A social worker will work with you during your home study.

Most couples fear that the social worker has a great deal of power and may make subjective judgments about their ability to parent and provide a good home. Understandably they want to make a good impression and "pass" the test. The infertile couple is also being evaluated at a time when they feel quite vulnerable. This is a tense situation where misunderstandings may occur.

❦ Sessions with our worker were emotional and not always positive or productive as I tried to deal with my anger. I was trying to accept my own incapabilities, but angrily refused to let go of the hope that I might solve my infertility without help from an agency. I resented the power our worker had over us, the fact that I was not in control, the questions we had to answer, and the degree to which we had to expose ourselves. After all, most people didn't have to go through all this; they just got pregnant. We had to deal with our own feelings and doubts while being judged suitable or unsuitable to be parents.

Each social worker has an individual perspective and every agency has its criteria for "good parents." Most agree, however, that emotional maturity, stability, a loving home, and a strong desire to parent are most important. The social worker will observe how the couple has accepted their infertility and whether they feel inadequate because of it.

❦ Our worker, Jenny, talked with us at length about our infertility. We were very honest and told her of the medical treatment and futile months of trying to conceive. She also asked about my background, upbringing, and family history. We felt good about her: here was a person sincere in her questions who would help us find a child.

The social worker will also note whether a couple is entering the adoption process while still in grief, and will question their intentions if they get pregnant while awaiting adoption or shortly thereafter. Many couples panic when they suspect a fertility problem and rush into the adoption process without careful thought. Although few social workers expect couples to permanently give up the idea of becoming pregnant, most look for an enthusiastic, realistic, and sincere present commitment to adoption.

The agency is also interested in the couple's marital relationship. Are they open and flexible to the changes parenting will bring? How do they settle differences? Most workers also want to ensure that couples are well informed about adoption, and aware that it is different from biological parenting. They will ask how the couple would cope, over the years, with the child's curiosity about adoption and birthparents, and about their feelings about openness among the parties.

In most cases, prospective adoptive parents and their social workers like and respect each other. It sometimes happens, however, that the entire interview process is unpleasant and upsetting. You may have a personality conflict with your worker, feel overly investigated, or receive an unfavorable evaluation. In this event you might discuss your feelings with other agency personnel and perhaps request that another social worker be assigned to your case, or consider working with another agency or facilitator.

THE HOME VISIT

❦ The days before the home visit were filled with anxiety, happiness, and a great sense of relief. We had finally done something positive for ourselves for a change. We cleaned, cleaned, cleaned! Our case worker was a warm, wonderful woman, and soon we were all laughing and talking. She asked to see our home. I showed her all around, including the room we were saving for our child. It had not been painted, wallpapered, or cleaned since we moved in a year before. We couldn't bear to fix it up until we really had a child. We adopted a little boy soon after and remain grateful for our worker's kindness and help.

The agency screening process usually involves a series of interviews with at least one "home visit." The social worker is interested in the living environment, as well as how the prospective parents interact at home. Most couples are, naturally, nervous before this visit and worry that their home may be judged inadequate. Once the interview has begun, however, most find that the visit goes smoothly.

A home visit will also be required in cases of independent, identified agency, or international adoption. In these cases, the parties have already selected each other and the agency provides the home study to meet the legal requirements of the process. In most cases, this process is more informal and relaxed, and serves to confirm and approve the choice of the birthparents.

PLACEMENT

❦ We called the final set of papers the "soul-searching" set. The questions asked what kind of child we would accept into our home, which handicaps and medical conditions we could handle, and what racial backgrounds were acceptable. We had to dig deep into ourselves and ask, for the first time: What kind of child could we see ourselves parenting?

After completing the interview process, accepted couples or individuals are placed in a waiting pool until a child is available. At this point, you must decide which race and age of child, and which, if any, physical, mental, and emotional handicaps are acceptable. Most agencies can immediately place older or handicapped children and sibling groups. The wait for a Caucasian infant is usually longer. For many years, agencies have preferred to place children with families of the same ethnic heritage. Today many families of color can be ethnically matched with children within a few months. In addition, there are increasing numbers of transracial adoptions, among families of all races, facilitated through both independent and international adoption (see sections below).

Length of wait may also depend on the preferences of the birthmother. Many agencies are now facilitating open adoptions, where the birthparent(s) actively participate in the selection process and perhaps meet the adoptive parents before the birth. She (or they) may indicate a preference such as religious affiliation or the presence of a sibling in the adoptive home. Many professionals feel this participation reassures the birthmother that she is making the right choice, and helps her cope with the grief of relinquishing her baby.

Once placement occurs, there is usually a supervision period of six to twelve months. To ensure that each family member is adjusting well to the adoption, the agency will contact and visit your home during this interim. If the child's adjustment is acceptable to agency, parents, and child, the adoption will be legally finalized in court. If not, agency personnel will work with the family to try to resolve the problem.

BIOLOGICAL FATHER'S LEGAL RIGHTS

Recent court decisions and statutes, such as the Uniform Paternity Act of 1975, are changing the legal rights of biological fathers in the adoption process. Both public and private adoption agencies now make a determined effort to have both biological parents sign relinquishment papers before the child is placed. If the birthparents are married, the birthfather is assumed to have equal parental rights. If they are not, the biological father may be given the option of denying paternity or waiving further notice to him of adoption planning. If he cannot be located, the agency tries to trace him through the Department of Motor Vehicles, his last three known addresses, the military, and his social security number. The adoptive parents are notified whether the birthfather has been located and if he has consented to relinquishment. Either agency personnel or involved attorneys are expected to make reasonable and diligent efforts to locate him. If he cannot be located, or if he has not filed for paternity rights, his parental rights are usually legally terminated within a year.

SEALED RECORDS

In most states, agency adoption records are sealed by statute when the adoption is legally finalized in court. This preserves the anonymity of the triad members. Some of these parties prefer the permanent secrecy of closed records, while others, frustrated in their attempts to find birthparents or adoptees, favor legislative changes to open these records to concerned parties.

Agencies that have handled thousands of adoptions over the years report an overwhelming number of requests for identifying information from all triad members. These agencies are bound by the laws of confidentiality and cannot disclose the identities of any party without the written permission of *all* triad members. An increasing number of states, however, will open sealed records when the adoptee reaches majority. Other states are considering legislation to open adoption records. Check with an adoption attorney or the department of social services for information about the status of closed records in your state.

Records regarding independent adoption are usually open to adoptive parents and adoptees. Birthparents should receive a copy of the signed consent papers that contain the names and addresses of the adopting parents.

Fost-Adopt Programs

❦ Only six weeks after our home study, we received a call about a two-month-old infant, Gary. We were interviewed by four social workers and were scared to death. We tried to psych them out. What questions would they ask? The only one I remember is "How soon can you be ready?" They passed us pictures of the baby and I passed them right back. I couldn't bear to look at them for long. He was so beautiful — big eyes, olive complexion, and dark hair. He could have been our biological son.

They explained Gary's history. His mother had abandoned him at birth, but he was not legally free yet. He would be in the fost-adopt program until the court terminated the parents' legal rights. We were one of several hundred couples screened for Gary. Several others were interviewed, but we were chosen! Shock, tears, and relief overwhelmed us. We took him home two months later.

Gary was sixteen months old before he was legally freed by the court. It was a very difficult time. Then it took another eight months before his adoption was finalized by the court.

Since that time, we've had another son placed with us through fost-adopt. Tommy had similar circumstances at birth as Gary, but his birthmother did relinquish rights to him. We did not have to go through the hearing process and are now in the six-month waiting period for finalization of his adoption.

The most important message we have for others is that there are children available through county fost-adopt programs. We felt embraced by the system, were treated with respect, and thought all legal matters were attended to properly. We never felt alone or confused.

Fost-adopt programs, which may vary in character between states, are usually administered by county social service agencies. A child who has been surrendered by, or removed from, his or her biological parents can be placed in a home as a foster child. Significant social worker contact is involved, including a screening process to qualify as fost-adopt parents. Children placed through fost-adopt may also have medical or emotional problems related to their prenatal or early childhood experiences. There may be a delay of up to two years, while the county completes its investigation and prepares reports and recommendations, before legal proceedings begin and the adoption is finalized in court. In cases where the child is not yet legally freed for adoption, there is a risk that he or she will be returned to the birthparents. Check with your state or county department of social services for information about these programs.

Special-Needs Adoption

Special-needs adoptions include older children (usually older than six years of age), newborns with HIV or in utero drug- or alcohol-related problems, kids of all ages with handicaps of a physical, emotional, or psychological nature, and sibling groups. There is usually a short wait and low initial expense for this type of adoption. There may also be state and federal funds available for health and educational needs. However, greater emotional energy and additional expense are often needed to raise special-needs children.

Older children can be especially challenging. Many have been abandoned, rejected, and perhaps physically, emotionally, or sexually abused several times in their young lives. When placing these children, most agencies look for parents who understand their history and the behavior it may elicit. Experienced parents are often sought since special-needs adoptions may be overwhelming for first-time parents. However, many individuals and couples do begin their parenting — happily and successfully — by adopting a special-needs child. AASK America (Aid to Adoption of Special Kids) is a California-based organization that facilitates special-needs adoptions and offers counseling and referral services to interested families (see Resources). They also offer a program that matches adoptive parents with a compatible special-needs child.

International Adoption

❦ After my unsuccessful surgery Steve surprised me by suggesting
adoption. We decided to adopt a Korean child and have asked for a
girl. With finally terminating our treatment, and our orientation
meeting with the agency coming up, I feel we are at the same point
for the first time in three years. I already love the tiny child I will
adopt and it seems very unimportant that she be born from our
bodies. After much pain and struggle, I now feel my infertility has
made me a unique and special person. Resolving with international
adoption has reinforced those feelings.

International adoption, in which a U.S. couple or individual adopts a child
from another country, is an increasingly popular form of adoption, accounting
for 10,000 placements in 1986. Many are drawn to the idea of parenting a child
from another culture for several reasons. It is a way to circumvent the scarcity of
infants available through agencies and the increasing competition for independent adoptions. Some also feel that their infertility struggle has deepened their
sensitivity and compassion toward all people, heightened their sense of adventure, and created an opportunity for adopting a child from another culture.

These adoptions are often handled through private agencies and involve
the U.S. Department of Immigration. A home study is required and a couple's
motivation to adopt a foreign child will be carefully evaluated before they are
accepted. As with any type of adoption, you must be cautious about selecting an
agency. Your county social services department or RESOLVE chapter may be
able to provide referrals; a partial list of international adoption agencies is also
included in the Resources section.

Some U.S. families have taken the initiative themselves of finding a child
from another country to adopt (private inter-country adoption). They arrange
for a home study by a local, licensed agency, negotiate with an agency or
orphanage abroad, meet that country's legal requirements and other red tape,
and then pick up their child in his or her native country. You can obtain more
information about this type of international adoption from Adoptive Families
of America (formerly OURS), listed in Resources.

International adoption of any sort may be quite a challenge. Those who
pursue this path must be flexible, adventurous, highly motivated, and not easily discouraged by delays, bureaucracy, or the chaos of other societies — many
of them impoverished and to varying degrees, corrupt by U.S. standards. In
addition, any American affluent enough to travel to a Third-world country is
rich by their standards, and may encounter hostility and resentment because of
this. Prospective adoptive parents may also be approached by unscrupulous
parties, and must be wary of scams or illegal practices. For these reasons, most
international adoption experts advise working with a reputable U.S. agency
that can provide support, assistance, networking, and sound advice.

Adoptive parents must also satisfy a multitude of U.S. agency, county, state, and federal requirements, as well as those of their child's country. They will be asked about their age, income, budgeting abilities, other children, marital history, health and medical insurance, race, sexual orientation, employment, and religion, among other things. They should be prepared to produce birth, marriage, and divorce certificates, employment verification, tax returns, health examinations, proof of criminal record checks by a law enforcement agency, and perhaps character recommendations and letters verifying their infertility. At least one parent should plan to travel to the country of adoption and to stay for at least four weeks. This is an invaluable way to confirm your commitment to your child and learn a bit about his or her heritage. Requirements of the Immigration and Naturalization Services, and perhaps the U.S. embassy, will also have to be satisfied. It may take a year or longer to complete the process, and costs of travel, agency fees, and other expenses may total $14,000 or more. Upon completion, an adoption decree is issued and the family can file for U.S. citizenship on behalf of their child.

Above all, prospective parents must feel in their hearts that they can love and accept a child from another culture, often of another race. There will also be a subsequent period of adjustment once you are home, the intensity depending on the age and history of the child. Many children adopted internationally have living parents and relatives and may remember them. They may have been relinquished simply because of the family's poverty and will grieve for their families and friends. Many of these children have also suffered from hunger, disease, and some type of abuse. Upon entering a new and strange society, culture shock is also common. In many ways, these are special-needs children and present similar challenges to adoptive parents.

You may or may not be able to discover the birthfamily's identities or continue contact with them. As your child grows, he will be curious about his ancestry, origins, and native culture. Parents who have adopted internationally emphasize the importance of providing information about the history and culture of the child's native country and incorporating this heritage into your family life.

As with transracial adoption, your family may confront intolerance and racism from relatives, friends, and community. It is important that you feel able to cope with prejudice and cruelty, and have support from other adoptive families. Despite its challenges, parents emphasize that international adoption is also a loving, joyful, fulfilling, and rewarding way to create a family.

Transracial Adoptions

❦ We adopted a little girl while living in India and two children of mixed black and Caucasian parentage after we returned to the United States. Our children are now fifteen, nineteen, and twenty-two.

> Our families were strongly opposed to our decisions at first and the early days were quite painful. It has taken many years for them to come around.
>
> We've lived in several different cities over the years and found racism and cruelty in each place as well as love and acceptance. When our children were small, strangers would approach us and ask if these were my kids. When I nodded, they would stare and ask, "What did you do that for?" I was furious that they were so cruel in front of my kids and wanted to protect my children. We've also had criticism from both white and black acquaintances.
>
> The early teenage years were pretty tough at times, with both racial and identity issues to confront at once! My kids were also confused about which racial group to identify with both in and out of school. I think anyone considering interracial adoption should give careful thought to their decision. The fact of adoption is a constant visible issue in an interracial family.
>
> We love our kids and wouldn't trade them. I feel we've weathered the tough times and will remain a close family in the years to come.

Although many social workers recommend placing children with racially compatible families, transracial adoption is occurring through both agency, identified agency, and independent adoption (see previous discussion and section below). Many agencies are not always able to find families of the same racial background with which to place children. Rather than exposing these kids to indefinite foster care, or multiple temporary placements, they are placing them with families of other races. In addition, many adoptive parents and birthparents are arranging transracial adoptions themselves, based on their respect and trust for each other, through identified agency or independent adoptions.

Couples and individuals considering this option must be quite honest with themselves about its challenges. That they are an adopted family is highly visible to the rest of the world; they cannot "pass" as other ethnically matched adopted families, or "slide" as members of the dominant majority, in a society that remains, sadly, racially prejudiced. Those who have adopted children of other races suggest that parents begin by acknowledging not only our culture's racism, but their own. Although they may view themselves as liberal, consciousness about racial differences is instilled in everyone in our society. Like their children, adoptive parents will be vulnerable to the cruelty and ignorance of others, manifested in bewildered or hostile looks or unpleasant comments or questions. They learn to react with directness, and sometimes humor, to insensitive remarks, and above all, to value their children's feelings and privacy. Gretchen Hathaway offered these comments about handling inappropriate questions or remarks in an OURS newsletter: "If you are asking me if she is our daughter, the answer is yes." Should the questions continue, Hathaway responds, "That information belongs to my daughter. When she is older, she may decide to share it with you."

Parents who adopt transracially, and in many cases internationally, have the additional responsibility of fostering pride in their children for their heritage and background. Parents are encouraged to seek role models of their children's race for their families, to be aware that one must constantly sort out normal childhood development from racial identity issues, and to seek support from other transracial families. (See the Bibliography and Resources for further readings and support organizations for transracial adoptive families.)

Although it is undoubtedly a challenge to adopt transracially, many families have happily done so over the years. There are certainly lifelong issues, as with any family — adoptive or otherwise. There is also love, joy, and fulfillment for both parents and kids. Seth Steinberg writes of such a family — his own:

> ❦ I am adopted. I am white. I have an older sister who is Amer-Asian, and an older brother and a younger sister who are Black. From the beginning, we all knew we were adopted. The interracial situation was something I never struggled with until the age of thirteen. It was at that time I periodically felt different. I remember conversations about hair, eye color, height, and other genetic things that I couldn't wholeheartedly participate in. There were times I felt awkward and yearned to have a "normal-looking" family. But for the most part, I was happy. As kids, we fought for our parents' attention and about the same stupid things all kids do. Still, we were close. I understood the idea of a mother and father out there who couldn't take care of me. I felt grateful to be in my family. I think we all did, including our Mom and Dad.
>
> As time went on, I began to feel lucky to have an interracial family, because I began to realize that I was ahead of my peers in learning about racial prejudice, equality, love, and acceptance. It was great to read about Martin Luther King Jr. in high school and be able to say, "He's not just talking about a good idea. He's talking about my life. We're all brothers and sisters . . . we're all God's kids. Look at my family, if we can live with each other and be a family together, so can the rest of the world."
>
> What a great feeling of pride I have. Being in a racially integrated family where unconditional love reigns supreme has given me hope that the world can become better.
>
> At the age of twenty-three, I decided a thank you was in order to the birthparents who helped me into the world. With the help of a search consultant, I found my birthmother and birthfather. What a neat process. It was healing for all of us. The thing I am most happy about is that my birthparents went on to make the most of their lives. They found new relationships, careers, and didn't get stuck in their pain. They identified the solution — to

move on as best as possible, and to live happy, joyous lives, just as I have. I wouldn't want it any other way!

Independent Adoption: A Northern California Case Study

❦ I pursued an independent adoption lead while lying in my hospital bed recovering from a surgery that left me, like my husband, clinically sterile. The lead did not work out, but it did convince me that adoption was our answer and that there was a child out there for us. Nothing was going to stop me from finding him or her.

We told all our friends and family about our decision and joined an adoption support group. We were able to verbalize, not only to the group but also to each other, all our fears and apprehensions about adoption and finally conclude that it was not birthing, but parenting that we wanted more than anything else. As couple after couple began to search privately for infants to adopt, we gained more courage to reach out and test our vulnerability again. This time we were operating with a strong support system and that made all the difference.

Every couple in our group who decided to adopt independently became parents within a year. We all worked hard, supported each other, and turned the infertility experience into an amazing and joyful miracle. We were rewarded with beautiful children and the fulfillment of our dreams of parenthood.

Over the past fifty years, the practice of independent (also called private) adoption has grown with the increasing practice of open adoption and the decreasing number of newborns available through agencies. In 1986, according to the latest figures available from the National Committee for Adoption, about 16,000 children were adopted independently, many of these infants.

In the independent adoption process, the birthparents and adoptive parents arrange the adoption themselves, usually with the assistance of an intermediary such as an attorney or facilitator. An adoption agency is not involved in the selection of the adoptive parents, although the state's department of social services performs a home study to validate the birthparent's choice.

The child is placed directly with the adoptive parents, often immediately after discharge from the hospital or shortly after. In most cases, the adoptive parents' attorney performs the necessary legal steps. The birthmother is entitled to independent counsel to represent her interests and adoptive parents are required to pay for these attorney's fees, usually up to a certain limit ($500 in California). Most experts feel it is a conflict of interest for an attorney to represent both birthparent(s) and adoptive parents.

In many cases, the parties mutually decide to meet one or more times. Some birthmothers stay with the adopting couple during part of their pregnancies, and many adoptive parents attend the baby's birth; other birthparents or adoptive parents choose not to meet. In any case, the names and addresses of each party are known to the other. Independent adoption is open adoption in that sense; the amount, frequency, and duration of contact after the child's birth varies with each family. (See discussion of "The Evolution of Open Adoption" above.)

A number of northern California families, birthmothers, and adoption professionals have generously shared their perspectives, experiences, and expertise for this chapter. The procedures mentioned refer specifically to California, and may differ in other states. In some states, independent adoption may not be legal. Before deciding on this option, obtain current, accurate legal information about your state's laws, and those of the birthparents if they reside elsewhere.

HOW TO ADOPT A CHILD INDEPENDENTLY

❦ Nobody wants to find a baby for you as much as you do, and there are birthparents who want to find good homes for their babies. Tell everyone you can think of that you want to adopt a baby.

You have something to offer too. You may think, "I'm so needy. I want to solve my problem." You will be solving your problem, true, but you'll also be solving someone else's. You're providing a good home. You're going to all this trouble to adopt a child because you think you can be a damn good parent. That's something to offer a birthmother.

Write letters to doctors, attorneys, and those who counsel pregnant women. If you send enough letters to enough people, you will find the right one.

In many states, birthparents have a legal right to place their own child for adoption. Some couples find a child to adopt by themselves, others pay a fee to an independent adoption program or facilitator to help them with the process, and some attorneys also seek birthmothers interested in placing their babies with adoptive parents. Either way many people have happily adopted infants at birth, or shortly afterward, through independent adoption.

Initially, most people feel overwhelmed and wonder how to contact pregnant women interested in private adoption. Once they have a "lead" (a referral to, or a response from, a pregnant woman possibly interested in adoption for her child), they often worry about making a good impression on the birthmother. Many infertile couples already feel inadequate and vulnerable, and fear rejection or further disappointment with independent adoption. Experts note that just as most couples don't get pregnant on the first or second try, it may take adoptive parents several leads before they find the right situation. Couples who have grieved their infertility and its losses, are committed to honesty and trust, remain flexible and determined, and accept the risks, usually adopt a baby within a year or two.

Fortunately there are many resources for both information and support. Thousands of successful independent adoptions have occurred. The experts in this field — adoptive parents, birthparents, attorneys, and facilitators — offer the following advice to interested couples.

STEP 1: **Tell everyone you know that you want to adopt a child.**

Some couples fear "going public" about their infertility and worry about the reactions of friends and family. This step, however, often yields several positive benefits:

- ☐ This openness indicates that you have grieved the loss of your fertility to the point of being comfortable about discussing it and your desire to adopt.
- ☐ It is often a relief to acknowledge your fertility problem publicly. Friends and relatives, who often felt helpless during your infertility, now have a positive way to be involved. Most will react favorably to your decision and lend assistance and moral support. Their participation also engenders enthusiasm and acceptance of your child before he or she is adopted.
- ☐ It can lead directly to a child. For example, your aunt may work with a man whose friend's niece wants to find adoptive parents for her unborn child. Many such leads come from friends of friends.

STEP 2: **Engage a reputable attorney.**

Find an attorney in your state experienced with both the legal aspects and the emotional issues of independent adoption. Some of these attorneys may help you search for a baby; all will provide expert legal advice about adoption laws and perform the required paperwork once you have reached an agreement with a birthmother.

As with any professional, you should feel philosophically compatible and comfortable working with your attorney. Clarify, in advance, his or her policy regarding availability, phone consultations, failed leads, trust account arrangements, and other charges. Some attorneys charge an hourly rate, which may range from $175 to $300 per hour. Many are now facilitating adoptions for a flat fee of $3,000 to $4,000. Sources of referral include your local Bar Association, American Academy of Adoption Attorneys, and RESOLVE (see Resources).

STEP 3: **Compose a letter.**

> ❧ Independent adoption meant composing a personal letter and mailing it to people I did not know: doctors, lawyers, hospitals, social workers, high school counselors, clergy, and women's centers. Could I handle this amount of exposure? Did I have enough energy left to compose and mail a thousand letters? Could I handle the returned mail and contacts from people upset with my method? How would I handle contact from a birthmother? How would I cope

if this didn't work? All of these thoughts scared me, but I wanted to parent and I found release for my anger in working in this direction.

With the assistance of an attorney I composed our letter; with the help of my husband, I mailed a thousand of them. I also realized I now had to direct my energy elsewhere while waiting for a positive reply.

Many couples or individuals, either themselves or with the help of a facilitator, compose a one-page letter, flyer, or "brochure" to mail nationwide to those in contact with birthmothers who may wish to place their babies with adoptive families. These include family practitioners, social workers, obstetricians, clergy, high school counselors, pregnancy or abortion counselors, and college student health services. Some couples purchase pre-printed mailing labels of these professionals from independent adoption services or direct mail organizations; others consult telephone or professional directories.

There is no perfect or magic letter. Every couple and individual is special, and their letters should reflect that uniqueness. Most people include one or more natural and relaxed pictures. Instead of looking rich, beautiful, or formally posed, it is more important to look happy and in love with each other. The text might include information about yourselves, such as occupation, age, address, interests, pets, hobbies, and so forth. Some include a short sentence or two about their infertility experience, desire to parent, and feelings about open adoption. Include phone numbers for both yourself and your attorney and any preferences for contact. Mention that collect calls are welcome and set up an answering maching with a warm, friendly message. It takes tremendous courage for a birthmother to make this call. Some birthparents may want to speak with you directly; others may prefer to speak first with your attorney.

Most important, however, is to let your personalities, creativity, and sincerity shine through. Express your feelings about having children and emphasize those qualities that would make you good parents. Remember that in most cases you are trying to reach a young woman and/or her doctor or lawyer. What will demonstrate to them that you are stable, secure, and loving potential parents? The following sample letter is offered as an example; personalize your letter to convey your own uniqueness and desire to parent.

Dear Birthmother,

We have been married for eight years and have always dreamed of being parents. We've been through five years of infertility treatments without success. After a lot of tears and soul-searching, we realize that we can forgo pregnancy. We would like to parent through adoption.

We live in a small rural community in northern California. Brian is a teacher and Janine is a freelance graphic artist. We live in a comfortable home with a big backyard, with our dogs Ginger and Mack and a chirpy parakeet named Peet. We are in our mid-thirties and love art, camping, good books, getting together with our friends and families, and outdoor sports.

Please call us collect anytime at home at (916) 555-5555, or if you would be more comfortable, please contact our attorney, Sam Smith at (415) 555-5555.

Brian and Janine Davis

STEP 4: **Find the right lead.**

After mailing your letters, you should receive some leads by phone or mail. Some may not work out. Experts advise both birthparents and adoptive parents to listen to their instincts and hearts during this process. If red flags go up — something feels doubtful or not quite right to *either* party — let this lead go. Although both adoptive and birthparents may fear that they are giving up on a "sure thing" or perhaps their only chance for adopting a baby, there will be other possibilities.

Eventually, most determined couples locate a mutually compatible birthmother. Many meet, and over one or more visits, reach agreement about adopting her baby and, usually through an attorney, payment for allowable and reasonable expenses. Some adoptive parents invite the birthmother to visit their home and perhaps stay for a few days or longer; many attend the birth. This is an opportunity to establish trust and faith in each other and lay the groundwork for future relationships. Many adoptive parents regard this as a special time to take lots of pictures, and create memories of their baby's birth and adoption that they can share with her as she grows up. Birthparents, and often their families, will treasure these memories for the rest of their lives.

While waiting for the birth, many adoptive and birthparents discuss their feelings and preferences for that day. Who will be present for the birth? Does the birthmother wish some time alone with the baby, to "room in" for a day or two, or to nurse him or her? When will the adoptive parents take the baby home? How will that be coordinated with the hospital? The parties can then confer with hospital staff about their preferences. This pre-planning eliminates a lot of confusion and chaos when the baby is born. Other necessary steps, such as settling birthfather rights and, if applicable, meeting out-of-state adoption requirements can also be taken.

During this waiting period, it is also common for everyone to feel apprehensive and worry that the other parties will change their minds. In most cases this does not happen. The adoptive couple often is present at the birth and usually takes the baby home a few days later.

STEP 5: **Pay legitimate costs of independent adoption.**

In California, the adopting couple may legally pay for reasonable living, medical, and counseling expenses for the birthmother and child. Total adoption costs will vary in each case and are itemized down to the last cent to the court. Your attorney may disburse these payments, or you can pay the birthmother directly. Most of these costs will be known in advance, although medical expenses may increase if complications occur, a Caesarean birth is necessary, or the newborn requires extra medical care. An accountant can advise you on which, if any, adoption expenses are tax-deductible.

Adoptive parents do not have to agree to any proposal or expense with which they are uncomfortable. Professionals emphasize the importance of clarifying expenses and reaching a mutual agreement. It is also critical to understand that if a birthmother changes her mind, *the prospective adoptive parent(s) do not have a contractual right to sue her for any expenses already paid unless she never intended to complete the placement, or she accepted monies from more than one prospective adoptive couple or individual.*

It is also important to differentiate between a legal, independent adoption and an illegal, or "black market," adoption, which involves large sums of money for unexplained costs. The intermediary, usually an attorney, is legally entitled only to reasonable fees for services and the birthmother only to legally determined expenses that vary according to state law.

In California in 1992, for example, independent adoptions averaged between $6,000 and $12,000, depending on the birthmothers' needs for medical, living, and counseling expenses. This sum includes $3,000 to $4,000 for attorney's fees. Allowable expenses vary between states. Some, for example, only allow payment of medical expenses; others include living, counseling, and other costs. Be sure to seek expert legal advice regarding your state's policies, and if you are in doubt about any proposed expense, check with your state's department of social services.

STEP 6: **Complete the legal process.**

In California, a woman who wishes to place her child for adoption signs an "AD 22" (Health Care Facility Report of Release of Infant to other than Natural Parent or Guardian) after her baby's birth. This form, which includes a general description of her rights, the name and address of the adopting parents, and an authorization for the adoptive parents to obtain medical care for the child, is prepared by the hospital and releases the baby directly to the adopting parents. Although this paper protects the hospital, it does not give the adoptive parents legal rights to the child. After they take the baby home, their attorney files a "petition for adoption" with the court.

The department of social services then has forty-five working days to interview all parties to the adoption. During their interview, most birthparents sign the "consent to adoption" forms in the presence of an agent of the department of social services, or, if out-of-state, before a notary public. A birthmother residing out-of-state is sometimes interviewed by the appropriate state agency in her area, or contacted by telephone or letter.

During the interview process there is also an investigation by the department of social services, which includes health reports, criminal checks, and two home visits by a social worker. The goal of these visits is to verify the birthmother's placement choice; only in extreme cases would the social worker recommend against placement.

At any time until the consent to adoption has been signed, the birthparents have the right to change their minds and, in nearly all cases, the baby will be returned to them. This is the small (about 5 percent of cases) but real risk of independent adoption. Each state's laws vary regarding the rights of the biological father in the private adoption process and custody of the child if he is opposed to the adoption.

Once the consent to adoption has been signed, it may not be withdrawn without a court hearing based on the best interests of the child and any changed circumstances. Although such hearings rarely occur, adoptive parents and birthparents probably have the same chance of being granted custody of the child. The emotional toll on all parties is considerable.

STEP 7: **Receive the final adoption decree.**

Depending on the court's calendar, the adoption is legally finalized within six months of the time the original petition is filed. The adoptive parents, child, and their attorney appear in a brief, confidential hearing before a judge. They sign both an agreement with the state to raise and treat this child as their legal offspring and a request for an amended birth certificate that is issued a few months later. A final adoption decree, issued for both independent and agency adoption, is granted.

Independent Adoption Services

Over the years, private organizations have been created to facilitate independent adoptions. They offer a range of services including the sale of mailing lists of possible contacts, legal assistance, mediation, and counseling for both parties. Many couples and individuals have adopted children with the help of such services and enthusiastically recommend them. Others have had a negative experience and spent precious time and dollars without finding a single lead.

Be careful in selecting such a service and ensure that the organization is reputable and ethical. Some are not regulated or licensed by the state; others may charge large and perhaps unrefundable fees. Check with your state's department of social services or RESOLVE for referrals (see Resources).

When Independent Adoption Falls Through

❦ After five-and-a-half years of marriage, we adopted our daughter who is now eleven years old. But before her, we brought home a baby boy through independent adoption. We lost him after ten days; his birthmother wanted him back. I felt so punished, like we had done something wrong.

When our daughter was two and a half, we found out about yet another baby. This, too, was an independent adoption. We had her seven weeks until her birthmother reclaimed her the Monday before Thanksgiving. I still hurt over losing her. I felt as if doomsday had set in. Her room remained the same for four months. I felt so alone and abandoned. I kept getting a gnawing sensation in my upper stomach and it remained there for five years.

❦ We lost one adopted child about ten days after we brought him home. It was terribly painful, and although on one level I could reason that perhaps it was meant to be that he grow up with his birthmother, it was still horrible. After only a few hours of having him in your arms, you would give your life for that baby. The love and bonding are that strong.

I do occasionally correspond with his birthparents and they have sent pictures. I think this has been even harder for my wife. It took a long time for her to heal and she rarely talks about it.

Although it is a rare occurrence (an estimated 5 percent of independent adoptions), a birthparent sometimes asks for the return of the child before the adoption is legally finalized. Although most couples successfully adopt another child afterward, this is nonetheless a terribly traumatic experience. Many parents feel great love and attachment for a baby immediately, and the loss of a child from the family after one day or a hundred is a tragic event.

Those who have endured the stresses of infertility and the adoption process are especially vulnerable to such a crisis. Although the baby did not die, there has been a profound loss. The dreams, hopes, and love showered on that baby by the adoptive parents do die. One adoptive father likens this loss to a "full-term miscarriage." It is natural that deep grief follows, often for a year or longer.

Having a lead fall through can also be devastating. Even though infertility has taught them not to hope too much, a couple finds a birthmother who is interested in placing her baby for adoption. They hope and then begin to dream of adopting this baby. A lead can fall through several hours later or a few days after the birth. In the following story, one woman shares her experience:

❦ Early last week our caseworker called us: "We think we might have a baby for you." The baby's background matched ours. As a racially mixed couple we were astonished and delighted! It was due any day. The mother felt sure that adoption was the right choice for her, and she hadn't seen the father for months. It seemed a dream we had hardly dared to dream was coming true. One moment we tried to suppress joy and excitement; the next, fear and anticipated depression.

Three days ago we learned the baby was a healthy boy (we already have a girl!) and that his mother had left the hospital without him. Both our hope and fear were stronger. This morning she changed her mind and decided to keep him.

Inside I am raging with loss; at the same time I feel numb and dulled. We had made secret arrangements. I borrowed a bassinet, saying it was for a friend. We had told only two friends so that we could have someone to talk to, and now I can't bring myself to call them to say we didn't get the baby. We made social plans for the next few weeks, privately telling each other with suppressed delight that we might have to cancel them! Now I feel miserable that we can keep those dates, that I'll have time to put in a winter garden after all.

One part of my brain has been paralyzed these last days, while the rest of me mechanically cooks, cleans, goes to meetings, and writes reports. Was I more afraid of the telephone ringing or of it not ringing?

Our little girl, adopted almost two years ago, was a miracle that did happen. We had hardly dared hope for her, and she came true. Every day we marvel at her: Isn't she wonderful? Isn't she incredible? Isn't she the dearest child ever?

These are the parts of the lecture to myself:

If things worked out the way we had hoped, we might have brought home a baby tonight, a brother for our daughter, a son for us. Instead we will spend the evening together with our precious daughter. In our lives of immense good fortune, this is really a small, fleeting sadness.

Before we had our daughter, we went through four "almosts." Now that we have her, we can't help but feel that she is the right child for us, and that we are the right parents for her. It seems so natural and perfectly fitting that she should be in our family. If we had gotten one of those other children, we wouldn't have her!

We must hope that this proves to be the right decision for this baby boy and his mother. It's tempting to feel that we would have been better parents. We must let go of this self-righteousness and wish them, from our hearts, a bright future.

There are small, but real risks associated with independent adoption. In fact, there are no completely safe paths to parenting. Pregnancy itself is a risky business, with a 15 to 20 percent chance of a miscarriage or other type of loss. "Anyone who is brave enough to get pregnant," one adoptive father maintains, "is brave enough to take the risk of independent adoption." And far outweighing the risks, emphasize thousands of delighted parents, is the joy of, at long last, creating a family of your own through adoption.

The Adoptive Family

Adoption creates a new family that will experience the same joys and challenges common to all parents and children, along with several unique, lifelong issues.

TALKING ABOUT ADOPTION

Experts advise parents to discuss adoption with their children, in an honest and straightforward manner appropriate to their age, and to continue this dialogue throughout their lives. Many families begin when their children are between two and three, with simple and positive references to adoption. They explain that children come into families by birth or adoption. Neither is better than the other; they are different and both wonderful in their own way. Your child has come into your family through the love of several people — his mom, dad, and birthparents. As children grow, they ask questions and seek answers that are important to them, ones they are usually ready to hear and absorb. Letters, messages, and pictures of, and from, birthparents, written and taken during pregnancy, birth, and infancy, bring reassurance and comfort to children as they grow.

❧ Since Anne was about three years old, we have talked about her adoption and occasionally read together the letter her birthmother wrote to her about why she gave Anne to us. It is absolutely beautiful, very sad, and leaves no question about her love for Anne.

One day, when Anne was about five, I was driving her and a friend, Jenny, to a party. I heard Jenny say to Anne, "I came out of my mommy's tummy and you didn't!"

Anne was very quiet. I asked Jenny if she knew what adoption meant.

She answered, "Yeah, Anne's real mommy didn't have time to take care of her so she gave her away."

Later I spoke with Anne about her friend's remarks. I asked her if she'd like me to read her birthmother's letter to Jenny. She liked this idea.

A few days later, I read the letter to Jenny. She was pleased we shared this with her and said she now understood more about adoption. The next day Anne told her teacher that she is a lucky girl: She has two mommies who love her.

If our family had not openly talked about Anne's adoption over the years, I'm afraid she would have been very hurt by Jenny's remarks. We might not have thought of this solution and would have missed another rich experience with each other.

Parents often take cues from their kids about when and how often to discuss adoption. Many also find the counsel of adoptive parents of older children, their pediatrician, and therapists experienced with these issues, helpful in addressing their child's feelings about adoption and his birthparents. There are also many excellent children's adoption books, some of which are included in the Bibliography. A continuing dialogue about both parents' and children's happiness, loss, fears, and hopes usually lays the foundation for a trusting and honest relationship throughout their lives.

OPEN ADOPTION ISSUES

Depending on the degree of openness and whether visitation is occurring, adoptive families and birthparents may face issues regarding the amount of contact and appropriate boundaries. In some cases, one party may desire more involvement than the other. Geographic distance may make more than an occasional visit impractical. Birthparents may find contact painful, especially if they are having difficulty in other areas of their lives, or may worry that their involvement is intrusive. Adoptive parents may feel uncomfortable, and perhaps send "mixed messages" toward birthparents. If the family has several adopted children, some of the kids' birthparents may be more accessible or involved than others. This may cause confusion or hurt feelings among the kids.

To help cope with such problems, adoption expert Lois Ruskai Melina suggests that open adoption triad members need on-going support and experienced counsel, especially in the first few years.

NO FAMILY IS PERFECT

Some adoptive parents, as well as those who become biological parents after an infertility struggle, sometimes feel that they have to overcompensate and be the perfect parent — one who knows all the answers, minimizes or denies problems, never complains, never makes mistakes, and certainly never has a bad day. This goal is, of course, impossible for any parent. Parenting is probably the toughest job in the world, and no one yet has figured out how to do it perfectly. Experts encourage adoptive families to grieve the losses they have suffered, acknowledge issues that they raise, celebrate the joy they do have, and to let go of trying to be perfect.

YOU'LL NEVER LOSE US: LOVE AND REASSURANCE

Although there are no easy answers to most painful problems, love and trust are integral to all parent-child relationships. Adoptive parents who feel entitled to the responsibilities and role of parenting their kids convey love and reassurance to them. Adoption is different than being born into a family, and does involve loss. Children need reassurance that they won't lose their adoptive parents, that their parents will be there for them this day and everyday of their lives, and that adoption is a good and honorable way to belong to a family.

MOVING INTO THE MAINSTREAM

Families created from infertility — be they just-plain or high-tech biological, adoptive, third-party assisted, or child-free — eventually join the American mainstream, a melange of family varieties itself. All have lifelong issues. (*Chapter 18* offers additional thoughts on parenting after infertility.)

An adoptive family learns to differentiate between the biological and social roots of their child. While the birthparents provide a genetic history, the adoptive family provides social ancestors and a sense of community. Creating a family album or scrapbook of pictures and mementos of your child's ancestors is a way to reinforce this bond for this and future generations. Some parents create a family tree with "genetic" roots holding the names of biological relatives and "adoptive" branches holding the names of adopted parents, siblings, and extended family.

Adoptive families may also find that some in our society do not fully "approve" or "accept" the way their family was created. They learn to find support from those who understand adoption, and perhaps most important, from within themselves. From this base, they will educate others about adoption, just as they did with infertility. This includes everyone who touches their family's life: relatives, friends, teachers, neighbors, helping professionals, babysitters, and coworkers. As with infertility, it is empowering to tell them what hurts and what helps, what is myth and what is not. Feel the pride and happiness you deserve and move ahead to new horizons, triumphs, and challenges.

Like every family, adoptive families deserve respect, encouragement, and emotional and social support for the critically important and immensely rewarding work they do: nurturing our children.

CHAPTER 18

Pregnancy and Parenting After Infertility

❧ I called the lab. They said positive. I shrieked. I called back to make sure they had the right person. "Yes," she said, "positive. You're pregnant."

I asked, "How often are there false positives?"

❧ *Poem for the Broken Cup (for David and Anne)*

The way I winced as my elbow hit it,
then even before it hit the floor
the frenzy of weeping, astonishing

the children, who stared in stunned
silence for fully five seconds before
the baby wailed in fear and David

joined in sympathy while I dried my
eyes and tried to explain to him, to
ease the terror my tears had caused:

Not the cup, I said, though the cup
was lovely, white mellowed these nine
years to cream, with its Potter

pictures of Peter Rabbit, and the
sweet frieze of green leaves on the
handle: not the cup, but it was

yours, I bought it for you four years
before you were born, just at the very
beginning, just when we were starting

to recognize that getting you was going
to take more work than simply making
love: and all those barren years

in Queens, I used to drink my morning
coffee from that cup as though that cup
were magic, as though it could change

things — And I started to cry again,
closing my eyes against his frightened
uncomprehending face: the scalding

realization that even though I have them
now, those two, the scars of those years
are still with me and always will be:

And standing in spilled milk and shards
of china, crying and not even trying to stop,
scaring my children, I cried, My cup!
The cup!

Kate Jennings

Between 50 and 60 percent of couples and single women treated for infertility will become pregnant at least once, and most will successfully birth a child. A discussion of the complex physical, emotional, and psychological processes of pregnancy and birth are beyond the scope of this book. The Bibliography contains suggestions for readings on these topics.

Instead, this chapter focuses on some of the psychological and emotional aspects of pregnancy and parenting after infertility. Although those trying so hard to conceive often reason that an eagerly sought conception will banish the pain of infertility, attaining pregnancy and parenthood after such a struggle often raises its own unique issues.

Pregnant at Last!

❦ When I called the doctor's office, a voice I didn't recognize came on the line: "Mrs. James? The test is positive. Is that good news?"
Laughing and crying, I said, "Yes, that is good news!"

❦ I wanted to pull people off the street and shout, "I'm pregnant! After three years of surgery, drugs, charts, and buckets of tears, infertile me is pregnant!"

After months or years of infertility, a positive pregnancy test often evokes a spectrum of emotions, sometimes in succession or even all at once! Like marathon runners crossing the finish line, many infertile couples feel incredibly high, euphoric, and deliriously happy when a pregnancy is confirmed. This wonderful news is often greeted with screams, laughter, tears, and a delightful hysteria that may last for hours.

When a pregnancy occurs after a poor prognosis for success, months or years of treatment, a previous miscarriage, fertility surgery, or one or more Assisted Reproductive Technology (ART) attempts, it is indeed a sweet victory. Some want to shout their joy from the rooftops, call everybody they know, and openly rejoice. Other couples favor a quiet, private celebration. Whatever your inclination, savor and enjoy this moment. You've truly earned it.

Ambivalent Feelings Are Normal. After the initial euphoria and excitement recede, ambivalent or contradictory feelings may surface. After months or years of dashed hopes and disappointments, some react to pregnancy with apprehension or anxiety, as well as happiness. They may fear a miscarriage, especially after a previous pregnancy loss. Others may feel superstitious (this kind of luck or happiness can't last), fatalistic (we've had our hopes raised so many times before, only to be repeatedly disappointed), or frightened (will mother and baby get through the pregnancy and birth without problems or complications?).

> ❦ Accepting this pregnancy has been a long drawn-out process accomplished in little steps week by week. Somewhere in the back of my head has lurked the idea that if I feel too secure in this baby, God or fate may snatch it cruelly away. I find myself reacting to all the normal anxieties threefold. Any deviation from the norm has been an opportunity to worry.

You may seesaw between positive and negative feelings: excited that you're finally pregnant, yet frightened about what lies ahead. Feelings of unreality and incredulity are also common. After months or years of futile efforts, it is hard to believe that the pregnancy is real, or that such a wanted and welcome gift won't be taken away.

Those who conceive through Assisted Reproductive Technology (ART) may be especially reluctant to believe that they are finally pregnant. Many suspend belief until a heartbeat is detected by ultrasound, unwilling to put their faith in a positive hCG test. Margarete Sandelowski, Ph.D., who has studied and written extensively about pregnancy after infertility in numerous couples, notes that these women and men must cope with an "unnatural" conception accomplished in spite of considerable obstacles, a loss of spontaneous pregnancy, the intrusion of medical professionals in an intimate process, and, in procedures such as donor insemination, intrauterine insemination, and ART, a separation of the partners in the act of conception. Many of these couples must slowly and gradually assimilate the reality of pregnancy, one step at a time.

Regardless of how conception occurs, these feelings may remain throughout the first trimester, or even the first half, of pregnancy until certain perceived hurdles are passed. These may include: the first nine to twelve weeks of gestation when miscarriage most frequently occurs; the week of pregnancy when a previous miscarriage occurred; the completion of genetic testing; or perhaps when the mother feels the baby kick and move.

> ❦ Being pregnant had been a fantasy for so long it was hard not to believe it wasn't still all in my head. My family wanted to talk baby showers, and I couldn't even talk pregnant yet. My mind seemed eternally on hold. I wasn't about to believe anything until I was past the time I had previously miscarried. Then I found myself thinking I'd wait to get excited after I had passed twelve weeks; then, after I felt the baby move. At six months I walked into a store and a clerk asked, "When is your baby due?" Surprised, my first thought was, "How in the world did she know I was expecting a baby?"

Every woman's and couple's feelings toward pregnancy are unique, as are reactions among previously infertile couples. Those who haven't followed the normal path to pregnancy may understandably react differently from women who conceive easily. There is often a mixture of poignancy, fear, worry, gratitude, and blissful joy with pregnancy after infertility. Some bask in the glow of this much-sought experience, while others feel ambivalent, anxious, or frightened during some or most of the pregnancy.

> ❦ When I was pregnant with my second baby, my doctor said sympathetically, "You've never gotten a chance to bloom, have you? You were so anxious with the first, and now you're so tired chasing your toddler. You've never bloomed."

Sandelowski notes that pregnancy feelings may be related to the degree with which the partners identified with being infertile, and observes that the work of pregnancy after infertility involves relinquishing this identity, and normalizing their pregnancy while making the transition to parenthood. Couples experienced varying degrees of difficulty in letting go of a negative identity, accepting the conception, and moving toward a normal pregnancy and parenting experience. Interestingly, an infertility history was just one of many factors that affected this process among the couples studied.

During this transition, it may be helpful to compare your reactions with other infertile women who have become pregnant. Hearing that many share similar feelings is reassuring and calming. Counseling, as a couple, with an infertility therapist may also provide insights that will help you both heal from your infertility struggle.

> ❦ Let it be known there is happiness and joy to be measured against those moments filled with anxiety and fear. There are days when I do feel the glowing picture of motherhood, days I want to shout aloud how beautiful I feel to be growing this baby at long last. And always it is worth the years it took to get here. It will not erase them; they will always be a part of me. But I can look forward and accept that this pregnancy starts a new time in my life with new battles to be won.

Changes During Pregnancy

> ❦ Of course I had years of expectations saved for this momentous occasion. I was to be the glowing Madonna, wind in my hair, maternal smile on my lips. Instead, I have been tired, pimply, gaseous, crabby, and sick.

> ❦ Except for a little indigestion, I felt wonderful during my entire pregnancy. I loved being pregnant, enjoyed watching the baby grow and move, and felt productive in every area of my life.

During the forty weeks (more or less) of pregnancy, tremendous hormonal, physical, psychological, and emotional changes rapidly occur as the baby develops and your body prepares for birth and lactation. Every woman's pregnancy is unique, and those who have birthed more than one child often remark that their pregnancies differ from each other. Some women look and feel wonderful, blessed with the proverbial Madonna glow. Others experience nausea, fatigue, indigestion, and other physical discomforts for two, three, or even six months. There is no way to predict whether this will happen to you. In addition to these considerable changes and unpredictable sensations, those previously infertile may also notice other feelings, stemming from their experience, as they progress through the three trimesters of pregnancy.

First Trimester. Ambivalent feelings are normal throughout the first trimester for all pregnant women. Those previously infertile may be especially worried about miscarriage or other complications. Constance Hoenk Shapiro, Ph.D., who has written extensively for mental health professionals in this field, notes that — depending on the duration and severity of their fertility problems — some couples have learned to expect disappointment and failure and carry this attitude into early pregnancy.

Feeling extraordinarily lucky and blessed, they also hesitate to complain about discomfort or feelings of anxiety — even if they last for months! As one woman remarked, "After all, hadn't I always envied that look of nausea on other women's faces?" Throughout gestation, infertile couples tend to highly treasure and value their pregnancies and often worry, should something go wrong, that they won't be able to conceive again.

Early pregnancy is also the time to establish a relationship with an obstetrician. Those who have worked with an infertility specialist for a number of years may feel awkward changing to a new doctor, one unfamiliar with their history and fight with infertility. If that relationship was especially close and supportive, these patients will also sorely miss contact with their specialist and his or her staff. Shapiro notes that some infertile patients may have internalized their previous relationship with their specialist — for better or worse — and bring these feelings, perhaps unconsciously, to the obstetrician's office. It is also strange, even under the best of circumstances, to enter such a pregnant world — increasingly frequent obstetrical appointments, waiting rooms filled with other pregnant women, childbirth lectures and classes, maternity clothes, baby showers, and pregnancy and parenting books — after being infertile for so long.

Second Trimester. Physical nuisances, such as fatigue and nausea, often recede in the second trimester. Fetal growth is noticeable, maternity clothes are proudly donned, any elected prenatal testing is completed, and the baby's kicks and moves can be felt. As the pregnancy becomes real, acknowledged, and absorbed, the couple also begins to realize the import of this event. For so long, the goal was to conceive. Once that is accomplished, the thought of impending *parenthood* may indeed be a sobering notion:

❧ One day it dawned on me: Not only was I pregnant, I was going to have a baby! After several years of infertility, I was more than prepared for pregnancy, but was I ready to be a mother?

The partners may now realize that parenthood will profoundly impact every facet of their lives, including their marital relationship and careers. Again, ambivalence and fear is common to any parent-to-be contemplating these changes. Those previously infertile may feel confused at these powerful feelings and stoically reluctant to complain or voice any doubts.

Genetic Testing

❧ After six long years of trying and several surgeries, I conceived my son at the age of thirty-six. I opted not to undergo chorionic villus sampling or amniocentesis. I did have the alphafetoprotein test since that only involved a blood test. I was not willing to take the risk, although I knew it was small, of miscarriage associated with CVS or amniocentesis. I made this decision early in the pregnancy, felt sure about it, and never looked back. I believed, deep within myself, that this baby was fine and that I probably wouldn't ever conceive again.

❧ I became pregnant, through IVF, when I was forty. I was also at risk for Tay Sachs disease. I wanted to know if there was any problem with the baby and had no doubts at all about having genetic testing. Although I was glad it was available, it did feel like another medical obstacle to overcome. I was nervous until the results came back, around the eighteenth week. Once I received the good news that everything was all right, I relaxed and enjoyed my pregnancy.

Our era of advanced technology offers a number of prenatal tests, such as chorionic villus sampling (CVS), amniocentesis, and alphafetoprotein blood analysis, that detect such genetic problems and birth defects as Tay Sachs disease, Sickle Cell Anemia, Down's Syndrome, neural tube defect (spina bifida), and anencephaly (an absence of part of the brain). CVS is usually performed in the first trimester and amniocentesis in the second, usually between the fourteenth and sixteenth weeks of pregnancy. Because the incidence of certain genetic problems increases with maternal age, either test is often recommended for women older than thirty-five years. Amniocentesis involves the withdrawal of amniotic fluid through a syringe, guided by ultrasound through the woman's abdomen and into the amniotic sac. CVS, usually performed transvaginally, scrapes a small sample of villi cells from the developing placenta. Both procedures carry a slight risk of miscarriage: Depending on the testing center, usually less than 1 percent for amniocentesis, and, because it is done earlier in the pregnancy and by a different technique, roughly double that for CVS. AFP testing requires a blood sample. Results are usually available in two to three weeks for amniocentesis, and within a week for CVS and AFP testing.

Barbara Katz Rothman, Ph.D., author of *The Tentative Pregnancy: Prenatal Diagnosis and the Future of Motherhood*, has noted that the availability of, and decision-making about, genetic testing has significantly affected many couples considering pregnancy in their mid-thirties and forties. Some are grateful for the technology and wish to know of any fetal problems beforehand, others feel obliged to use it although they fear the risks, and many note a delay, until the results are available, in accepting the pregnancy and their feelings for the coming baby. For these women and couples, their pregnancy experience is, in a sense, interrupted until testing is completed.

Because many couples are in their late twenties or early thirties when fertility problems are detected and treated, they are often thirty-five or older when they conceive. In deciding whether to undergo genetic testing, both partners must assess the risks and advantages and their feelings about therapeutic abortion if a problem is detected. Margarete Sandelowski, Ph.D., notes that an infertility history has a significant effect on couples' responses to these issues. All highly value their pregnancies and fear they won't conceive again easily or quickly, if ever. Many feel ambivalent about undergoing yet another medical procedure and waiting in limbo until the results come back. But like all pregnant couples, some previously infertile opt for the testing, while others decline.

Genetic testing is a confusing and frightening prospect for many couples, and especially for those who have waited years to conceive. When considering these options, your obstetrician can be an important source of information and support. Ask for pamphlets or literature about the genetic testing procedures and their advantages and risks, and discuss your questions or concerns with your physician or a genetic counselor. (Your obstetrician can refer you to prenatal testing experts.)

High-Risk Pregnancies

❦ My last trimester was quite stressful. I had frequent ultrasounds to check the baby's growth and monitor a uterine problem. I was grateful to be pregnant, of course, but I was also confused and frightened by this unexpected "problem" pregnancy.

A small percentage of pregnant women, previously infertile or not, develop medical problems that may threaten the viability or safety of mother or baby. Such a development brings sadness, disbelief, or fear. These feelings are common to *all* pregnant women.

These patients may be referred to high-risk obstetrical care. Limited activity, frequent office visits, testing, bed rest, medications, or hospitalization may be advised for part of the pregnancy. Although this is a difficult situation for any pregnant couple, Shapiro notes that for those previously infertile, familiar feelings of alienation and loneliness may be reinforced, and fears and fantasies about loss intensified.

As a result of fertility drug treatment or an ART attempt, some women may become pregnant with twins, triplets, or in rare cases, quadruplets. Ellen S. Glazer, LICSW, notes that, after years of infertility, many may initially welcome or relish the prospect of a multiple pregnancy, reasoning "the more the merrier; we'll complete our family in one pregnancy." If this does happen, however, the reality of carrying multiple fetuses can be quite stressful, both physically and emotionally. In some cases, bed rest, limited activity, medications, or Caesarean births may be necessary. These women have lost the experience of a normal, uncomplicated pregnancy. Some women also experience pregnancy loss, either naturally or through selective termination. While still pregnant with one or more fetuses, they may also grieve for the loss of others. (See chapters 13 and 14 for further discussion of pregnancy loss and selective termination.)

Securing emotional support is essential when coping with any high-risk pregnancy or pregnancy loss. Many RESOLVE chapters (see Resources) have created phone support networks for women facing these issues. Several pregnancy loss organizations, which offer information, support and referrals, are also included in the Resources section.

Third Trimester. The third trimester is usually an exciting and busy time as parents prepare for the arrival of their child. Those who were infertile may postpone, until well into this trimester, such rituals as decorating the nursery, choosing names, buying clothing and equipment, and packing the suitcase for the hospital. "I just had to wait until the beginning of the ninth month, when I felt somewhat assured that the baby would survive, before I could do any of that," one woman recalled. "I was just so afraid something would go wrong."

As the due date approaches, most couples have worked through a myriad of feelings. Anticipation and excitement build as their child's birth approaches. They are ready, as much as anyone can ever be, for parenthood.

The Couple's Relationship

❦ The hardest thing to accept has been that this would not be the pregnancy I had wished for and imagined for so many years. I could never breeze through this, like those women who got pregnant easily or accidentally, and act as if nothing dramatic was taking place. In my second month I made the dreadful mistake of running (horrors!) to meet my husband, only to find him furious with me for taking such a "chance." This pregnancy was too precious for us to take nonchalantly.

❦ During Susan's pregnancy I had two different contradictory thought systems operating. At one level I "knew" nothing would go wrong. I reasoned that because we had so much trouble getting pregnant, there just couldn't be miscarriage problems as well. I guess it was a sense that bad luck gets spread around and we neither had, nor deserved, a monopoly on it.

On an entirely different level, I was quite anxious throughout the pregnancy. During the first few months, when Susan went to the bathroom and was gone for what seemed a long time, I became quite concerned that she was miscarrying. This happened on more than a few occasions. In addition, whenever we had a test to take, like the Tay Sachs or the amniocentesis, I was quite nervous until the results came in. Paradoxically, when I was nervous, I would think: We had been extraordinarily lucky in getting pregnant on the first IVF try. Not only that, we had been fortunate in having only one fetus, and luckier still that it was the girl we hoped for. So I reasoned good luck gets spread around and we'd already had our share — now we might be due for some bad.

Achieving pregnancy after an infertility struggle can deeply affect the couple's relationship. In many cases, either or both partners may have difficulty relaxing and enjoying the pregnancy. This feat took so long to accomplish, at such a high emotional and perhaps physical price, that they worry endlessly. What if something goes wrong and they miscarry? They may never have another chance. Some men may resist acceptance or excitement about the pregnancy, determined to remain "in control" if problems arise.

Partners may also identify in different ways with the pregnancy, depending on the duration and extent of their particular fertility problems. If donors are involved, or high-tech procedures were utilized, the infertile partner may retain some feelings of grief, inadequacy, or shame. They may be affected more deeply by the circumstances of the conception than their partners.

And depending on the way the baby was conceived (ART, egg donor IVF, or donor insemination), the couple may have different feelings about sharing this information with others. Some partners may regard these as medical or technological details and are comfortable with sharing their triumph with those supportive during their struggle. Others view the circumstances of any conception as a highly personal and intimate matter. "We wouldn't go into graphic descriptions if we conceived Beth the old-fashioned way," argued one expectant father. "Why 'tell it all' with an ART pregnancy?"

The transition of pregnancy also marks an evolution in the couple's, and soon-to-be family's, intimacy and commitment to each other. The details about this conception are also a birthright that belongs to their child. Protecting his or her privacy, or the feelings of one's partner, may be more important than confiding in close relatives and friends — even those who have been supportive during infertility.

After achieving the nearly impossible dream, couples also find that real life — with its inevitable pressures and problems — goes on. After the excitement subsides, they may be surprised that pregnancy hasn't brought complete happiness or healing from infertility. They still have bad days, worries, frustrations, and arguments.

❦ For all the times I have said to myself, "If only I were pregnant," this long-sought pregnancy has yet to pay the bills, remodel our living room, or change the weather. Life still goes on. Reality could never live up to the idyllic scene I had painted for myself.

Although pregnancy after infertility undoubtedly poses challenges and stresses, it also provides an opportunity to become closer. Experts encourage couples to meet with other expectant parents and, if appropriate, consult a counselor to improve communication skills, facilitate decision-making, obtain suggestions for stress reduction and relaxation, and mend some of their infertility wounds.

The confirmation of pregnancy marks the onset of the transition to parenthood. With any pregnancy, but especially as you anticipate the arrival of your first child, a couple or single woman are truly expecting a change that will forever alter their lives — one that will bring new, exciting, challenging, and awesome roles, responsibilities, and identities. This first baby makes you a mommy and a daddy. It is a time to witness, and feel stretching, fluttering, tumbling, and kicking within your body, the development and growth — from a single fertilized cell — of a uniquely wonderful human being, unlike any other ever conceived. As much as possible, given your infertility experience and how it may understandably affect your emotions and relationship, try to savor, enjoy, and marvel at the unfolding of this miracle. For most American couples of this generation, infertile or not, it only happens once or twice in a lifetime.

Joining the Fertile World

❦ I realize that there are problems common to both infertility and pregnancy to deal with. One was the feeling of being cut off from the very network of people who have been supportive. On the other hand, I found that when we announced our pregnancy to family and friends, suddenly an abundance of people wanted to share in the good news and bask in the excitement. It was difficult to deal with everyone being so positive. Where were they when the going was tough? When I needed to talk? When I was worried and depressed? Although their enthusiasm was genuine, it was easy to resent it so late in the game.

After long-term infertility, many experience a rather disconcerting identity crisis when they become pregnant. Once the news is out, and especially after their pregnancies begin to show, the world perceives and treats them quite differently. Many people — relatives, friends, and even strangers — wanting to share and enjoy their happiness, will smile warmly at their growing bellies and shower them with approval, interest, and support.

At last they have arrived, pregnant ladies in a fertile world. Ready or not, the transitional tidal waves of pregnancy and parenthood sweeps them to new shores — obstetricians or midwives and prenatal appointments; exercise and childbirth classes; birthing suites; diapers, an endless array of equipment, breast pumps, and bottles; new mothers' support groups; automatic membership in the worldwide, ageless club of motherhood; tot parks, babysitting cooperatives, and preschools. Although they will meet new and friendly people, few will have personal experience with infertility or understand the road they have traveled.

Because of this, these new card-carrying members of the "prego club" may still identify, and feel more comfortable with, those who are infertile. Yet despite these emotional tugs, their pregnancies set them apart. Remembering their envy and awkwardness with pregnant friends or relatives, they understand why it is painful for infertile friends to share their happiness. They also fear that these treasured and sustaining bonds and friendships may dissolve.

> ❦ Every time I heard of a fellow infertile's pregnancy, I remember thinking, "Hurray, there's one for our side," and a feeling of hope would come over me. So when I learned I was pregnant, why did I sit in the back of our support group meeting, wringing my hands, heart pounding, afraid to share the good news? How could I tell all these people that I had something we all wanted so badly? I worried that this meant leaving a group of people I had learned to love and cherish for their never-ending support and encouragement. What would happen now that things had changed?

In this situation, an honest exchange of feelings is usually the best approach: a discussion often filled with tears, laughter, joy, and envy. Many of these friendships will probably weather the pregnancy and continue afterward.

For a time, many of those pregnant after infertility feel they don't fit in either world. These ambivalent feelings are normal and recede as the pregnancy advances and becomes more real. Ties with relatives and friends can be reestablished by sharing news of the pregnancy, getting together to celebrate, and asking advice about hospitals, pediatricians, and postpartum survival. Parenthood and community involvement also expand personal horizons and provide contact with others who have traveled alternate paths to parenthood: single and adoptive parents, families with disabled or challenged children, and those coping with secondary infertility. After they become parents, many continue to lend support to those still struggling with infertility through volunteer work with RESOLVE (see Resources).

Birthing and Parenting After Infertility

> ❦ I'm exhausted. I can't get anything done during the day because my son insists on being held and rocked. My dishes and laundry are piled up. I long for just fifteen minutes to call my own and a hot cup of coffee.
>
> Still, all of this is much easier to bear than three days of infertility. As I rock, I think about what makes infertility so different from other life problems.

Now that I'm a parent I have met dozens of people who empathize with me. It seems everyone knows what it's like to be up all night with a crying baby. All I need to do is reach out and there are friends and family saying, "We've been there ourselves, you'll make it through." That is the difference between now and then. Where was all that support and understanding before? I faced my infertility on my own. It was, and still is, the most isolating, lonely, frustrating experience I have ever had.

❦ Tess and Rory are precious to us, and we are grateful that we have them. But yes, parenting wears thin at times. My husband is off at work ten or more hours a day, and I constantly juggle the never-ending demands of motherhood with my own pursuits and work. I never have a moment to myself, I'm almost always tired, and I often feel overwhelmed. Quality child care is hard to find. When one of the kids is sick, I'm the one who stays home and changes my plans for that day and maybe the next. It's hard for even one parent to find a job with the flexibility needed for life with young children. In many ways, this is definitely not a "family-friendly" society.

Yet feelings linger that those who conceive easily don't understand. Every night I stand in each of my children's rooms for a few minutes, watching them sleep, and recall the terrible childless years. I came so close to never having them. I am humbled by, and deeply thankful for, the miracle of my children.

Although childbirth classes and expert advice impart valuable information and techniques, nothing quite prepares you for the monumental, unpredictable, and miraculous process of giving birth. Neither the passage of time nor a thousand retellings of your birth story can dim its memory or power. The pain and joy inherent in labor and delivery change you forever.

Just as pregnancies vary tremendously, so do birth experiences. Aside from the often intense, and sometimes prolonged pain of labor and transition, many births progress normally and without complications. In other cases, interventions such as pain medications or anesthesia, fetal monitoring, induction of labor, forceps delivery, or Caesarean births may be advised for a variety of reasons. Many women fantasize about a perfect labor and delivery, and are dismayed if their plans go awry. Those with a history of fertility problems may especially long for an uncomplicated and perfect delivery, a normal and natural conclusion to a difficult and often medically assisted conception experience. There can be feelings of letdown or depression if the fantasy birth doesn't occur. In such cases, talking about both the joys and disappointments of your birth experience with other mothers, labor and delivery nurses, and perhaps a counselor may be helpful.

POSTPARTUM

❦ The change in our lives was unbelievable. Within a week of Jamie's birth, things were in chaos. We tried to accommodate everybody who wanted to visit, while getting up every two hours around the clock to nurse and change Jamie. When we tried to take a nap, someone often knocked on the door to deliver a package or say hello. The dog would bark and wake up all of us. The sleep deprivation was awful and we started arguing and yelling at each other.

I would cry at the slightest thing. We ran out of groceries and the laundry piled up. I was lucky if I got Jamie fed and changed, and breakfast and a shower for myself by noon. My tummy sagged and my breasts leaked everytime Jamie cried. I was still in maternity clothes and they were all stained.

We thought we could do it all by ourselves — run the house, live a fairly normal life, and take care of a newborn. After ten days of this, we realized we needed help with cooking, cleaning, and errands. Relatives and friends helped for several weeks; then we hired a service for a few weeks more. It made a big difference.

It really does take three or four months to adjust and restructure your life, even longer if your baby isn't sleeping through the night by then.

There are many courses and books available for expectant parents about pregnancy and the childbirth experience. Few of these resources, however, adequately prepare you for the postpartum period, or discuss the intensity of this critical time. In many other, so-called "primitive" cultures, relatives and neighbors recognize the needs of parents and newborns, and provide constant care for weeks. Once a baby is born in our society, the enormous need for support, reassurance, and help required by all new parents is often downplayed or even ignored. This problem is compounded when new parents live far from relatives who might lend a hand, and so many neighbors — other mothers included — now work outside the home during the day. In general, women today are bearing fewer children than their mothers and many are staying at home for only a few months, or perhaps a few years, when their children are young.

As a result, many new parents often feel isolated, overwhelmed, frightened, confused, exhausted, lonely, tearful, and without support, guidance, or resources, as they learn to care for their newborn. There will be months of sleepless nights, frazzled nerves, and tremendous personal and marital adjustment.

A history of infertility does not exempt you from the intensity and chaos of early parenthood. Now it is your crying offspring, rather than the pain of being childless, that keeps you awake at night. Few first-time parents are accustomed to being on twenty-four hour call by a self-centered, crying infant — a helpless bundle who can't tell you what's wrong so you can fix it and go back to sleep. Older parents are especially tired by nighttime feedings. By the fifth or sixth week of round-the-clock duty and overall exhaustion, you may forget your own name along with the fact that you actually struggled for this opportunity!

Seasoned parents recommend advance planning before the baby is born. It can make a huge difference in the postpartum experience. The idea is to make things as easy as possible for a few months, since taking care of yourselves and a newborn is more than a full-time job. A few suggestions:

☐ Freeze dinners or quick meals for a month or two before your due date, get the nursery organized, bills paid to date, and any car or home repairs taken care of.

☐ Ideally, your mate might plan several weeks or more of vacation or parental leave after the baby's birth. If that is not possible, try to arrange for someone whom you trust and feel comfortable with to stay with you for at least three weeks. If you have a Caesarean delivery, you may need help for several weeks longer.

☐ Arrange for assistance with cleaning, shopping, errands, the delivery of nutritious, home-cooked meals, and occasional babysitting so you can rest or take a walk. If friends or family pitch in and help, you can return the favor later when they have babies. If they are unavailable, consider hiring temporary help for at least two weeks. If you can afford it, arrange for weekly cleaning help for several months.

Baby Blues. Tremendous hormonal changes occur, in only a few days, as a woman's body recovers from childbirth. In themselves, they can contribute to mood swings, irritability, and increased emotional sensitivity. Sleep deprivation, marital stress, isolation, and perhaps lowered self-esteem or identity issues intensify these feelings in many women, and often result in a syndrome known as the "baby blues." Experts estimate that up to 85 percent of American women experience some form of baby blues in the first two to six weeks after delivery. Usually these symptoms are fairly mild, subside within a few weeks, and are alleviated by frequent, nutritious meals, the love and company of supportive mates, relatives and friends, humor, some type of mild, daily exercise, and adequate rest. Adoptive parents of newborns, subject to the same emotional stresses and adjustments, may also experience a "post-adoption" letdown.

Any previously infertile parent may be reluctant to acknowledge this mild depression or complain about it, assuming they must again be stoical through a difficult time. All new parents deserve validation and the opportunity to verbalize their feelings. Parent support groups — a place where you can meet others going through the same chaos and freely socialize, laugh, complain, and cry — are heartily recommended by many new parents to ease the stress of this time. The formation of playgroups, babysitting exchanges, and lifelong friendships are often added benefits.

Postpartum Depression

❦ About a week after Margaret's birth, I abruptly descended into postpartum depression. I had never felt so miserable and trapped in my life. I was like a baby myself. I wanted to cling to John and not have to face Margaret's cries and demands. I wanted to feel like a strong, competent woman again, not like this helpless creature who could barely walk (after a Caesarean delivery) and yet had to be responsible for another helpless creature. However much help my husband provided, I couldn't shake the feeling that I was solely responsible for our daughter. After all, I had miscarried her predecessors, so her well-being must also depend on me.

It was pretty ghastly. I would sit in my rocking chair and stare at Margaret as she nursed, wondering why on earth I had overturned John's and my comfortable life together for a shrieking, red-faced creature who couldn't even respond to us, however much attention we showered on her. I finally gave up trying to look pleased with motherhood and just wept. It was worse yet when I got beyond weeping and went numb. The only thing I was sure of was that I was a rotten mother who didn't love her child.

The only analogy I could come up with was mourning the loss of someone I had loved, and yet I had ostensibly *gained* someone to love. I suppose now that the loss was the death of my old self, which had to change when I became a mother. Overall, for me, postpartum depression felt like intense grief. I started feeling better and enjoying Margaret at about five weeks. Perhaps my hormones had settled down as well. I'm still not completely over the depression, which creeps back every few weeks, but at least it no longer frightens me. I've learned how to cope.

Melanie Lawrence

Perhaps 10 to 15 percent of new mothers may experience a more severe emotional reaction, commonly termed postpartum depression (PPD). Medical experts disagree about whether PPD is physiological (perhaps an extreme hormonal imbalance or glandular dysfunction) or psychological in nature, or a combination of both. Regardless, PPD may surface from several weeks to twelve months after birth with symptoms that range in severity. Anxiety, prolonged crying, difficulty with concentration, feelings of loss of control or identity, or even thoughts of harming oneself or the baby may accompany this problem. If symptoms are severe or feelings of depression persist, *seek help immediately*. Call your obstetrician and discuss the problem. In many cases, support from other mothers or counseling with a professional knowledgable about PPD is enough. Rarely, medication or hospitalization may be appropriate.

A woman may be especially vulnerable to postpartum blues or depression after an infertility experience, considering her radically shifting hormones, long struggle to have this child, the desire to be a good, if not perfect, mother, and reticence to complain. There isn't much room for the normal feelings of ambivalence, helplessness, fear, and occasional panic that new parents often feel. Every parent, during the postpartum period, must reconcile their fantasies of parenthood with the reality of caring, day and night, for their baby — who may nurse easily or fret constantly during feedings, gurgle contentedly or cry for hours at a time, and sleep soundly for hours at a stretch or doze for only an hour or two at a time.

Parenting in the 1990s. Fortunately most kids eventually sleep through the night (until they're teenagers), colic recedes, and life again takes on a semblance of normality. Within six months of their baby's birth, most moms and dads weather the transition to parenthood, accept its attendant responsibilities, and adjust to the joys and demands of a raising a family.

All parents, regardless of their path to pregnancy, face considerable challenges as they raise children in this decade: balancing job and family responsibilities; lobbying for parental leave, flexible working hours and conditions, and other family benefits; maintaining energy and a sense of humor, often in midlife, while parenting young children and perhaps caring for aging parents; meeting the increasing expense of raising kids from infancy through young adulthood or college; finding loving, caring, dependable, and affordable child care; and deciding on public or private education, just to name a few. Many work with employers, legislators, community groups, and public or private school officials to address these critical family issues.

Those who parent after infertility encounter these challenges, as well as those associated with their experiences.

Overprotectiveness

❦ Even though I'm prone to all that every parent experiences — frustration, feeling trapped, impatience, and aggravation, I think we hold our children a little more dear and treat them with a little more care than those who haven't suffered infertility. We have tried not to spoil, although I'm the spoiling type no matter what! We try not to overprotect. I still feel somewhere in my heart that fate has another cruel trick to play on us. It's a feeling I have to suppress and that I usually forget, but it does come upon me sometimes. I don't think I'll ever be rid of it.

Many new parents feel protective of their baby, and worry about illness or accidents. Those who parent after infertility often feel especially so, and share the apprehensions natural to all parents. At the same time, they realize that because medical intervention usually bypasses fertility problems rather than cures them, they may not be able to bear another child. This may intensify their fears about leaving their baby with a sitter or child-care provider on a regular or occasional basis, returning to work after a leave of absence, or even going out for the evening.

Those who have waited a long time to parent may also strive for perfection. They not only want to do the best job possible as parents, but also to shield their child from hurt, disappointment, and pain. Although understandable, this is an impossible task. As they grow up, children have to learn to accept disappointments and failures as part of life. If parents overly focus on the child or become too protective, it will be difficult for her to learn to accept life's inevitable setbacks and bounce back.

As the baby grows, the important and necessary task of teaching limits to their cherished, yet opinionated and determined toddler may also be painfully difficult for many parents, whether previously infertile or not. For a myriad of reasons, many struggle to achieve a balanced parenting style that includes love, approval, and the setting of reasonable limits. If inappropriate or unacceptable behavior is not curbed at this time, parents may foster what Ellen S. Glazer, LICSW, author of *The Long Awaited Stork*, terms "the crown prince syndrome" — a child who perceives his treasured status and believes himself exempt from the rules and limits others must follow. If he is intended to be an only child, or if secondary infertility delays the arrival of a sibling, it may be increasingly more difficult for parents to consistently and effectively set limits.

Many find consultation with parent educators, family therapists, teachers, pediatricians, and other child-rearing experts invaluable during the early childhood years. This is also another opportunity to join with other parents struggling with the same issues.

More Children? Those previously infertile may not have the luxury of planning the two- to four-year spacing between children often recommended by experts. Family planning becomes a confusing, somewhat ironic issue. Should they try for another pregnancy fairly soon, and risk having two children closely spaced? Some have tried this approach, and found themselves with two children twelve or fifteen months apart — an experience similar to raising twins. Or should they wait a few years to try again and possibly face a struggle with secondary infertility? Should they stop with one child or adopt another? The age of the partners and their fertility factors may also influence their decision.

Issues for Alternative Families. There has been discussion in other chapters about some of the issues faced by families created through adoption (both closed and open), and such options as Assisted Reproductive Technology (ART), donor insemination, egg donor IVF, and surrogacy. All of these families face lifelong issues; among them is coping with the reactions of those who know, or will learn over the years, about their child's conception or genetic origins, and their relationship with donors or surrogate mothers. Establishing or maintaining contact, and defining or modifying boundaries with birthparents or involved donors, along with feeling fully entitled to parental roles and responsibilities, may also be issues that recur within the family over time.

As the family moves into the social mainstream, they may also discover that not everyone will necessarily approve of, or accept, their method of family-building. They may seek role models and support from similarly created families. Perhaps more than other families, they must build esteem and pride among themselves, rather than relying on validation or approval from others.

Letting Go. Despite the challenges faced by those who parent after infertility, family therapist Sheri Glucoft Wong, LCSW, notes that every family — regardless of its origins or configuration — shares more similarities with other families than differences. For all parents, this job initially involves assuming total care and responsibility for a completely dependent human being, making decisions for him, and controlling his early environment. The child's job is to internalize his parents' love, values, judgments, and controls and shape them into his own. As he grows, he will gradually assume responsibility for himself and you will slowly let go.

The task and meaning of parenting affects everyone differently, depending on their emotional make-up, childhood experience, and fertility history. Perhaps the hardest thing for many parents to do — from the time the umbilical cord is cut to the day their children leave home as young adults — is to give them both roots, to know themselves and realize their potential, and wings, to take flight, when they're ready, from the nest. This is an especially poignant task for those who struggled and fought to be parents. As their child grows, each developmental stage — smiling, sitting up, cutting and losing baby teeth, crawling, toddling those first steps on wobbly legs, going off to nursery school and then kindergarten and beyond — is wonderful, amazing, and often bittersweet. They are aware of how quickly these years will pass, how they might not have another chance to parent, and how very long they waited for this experience. The challenge lies in recognizing, enjoying, and cherishing these moments while they are here.

The Legacy of Infertility

❦ You'd think that now that our vivacious, handsome little two-year-old son is bounding about our house that those infertile feelings would never creep into our lives again. Well, believe me, they do. Amidst all our joy and happiness, a part of us still grieves about our infertility and for all those sad couples out there, especially those afraid to share their burden. Our experience of infertility helped shape who we are today.

An infertility experience underscores both the fragility of life and the miraculous chemistry and orchestration of conception, gestation, and birth. These parents may indeed treasure their children in a different way from those who conceive easily. Without medical help and a great deal of luck, they would have missed this experience, and few ever forget that. This is perhaps the reward of an infertility struggle: From the moment of your baby's birth, you have the wisdom that you have been given a precious and irreplaceable gift, a child to love, treasure, and enjoy.

Infertility is a different and unique path to parenting, be it accomplished through old-fashioned biology, high-tech procedures, adoption, or third-party assistance. All who travel this road undoubtedly acquire a variety of assets, among them inner strength, flexibility, perseverance, determination, and compassion. They have also sustained losses and wounds that require healing. The depth and severity of the wound differs with every individual, as does the time needed to heal. The certainty lies in the resiliency of the human spirit. We do heal and move forward in our own time, reestablishing our identities, boundaries, and privacy, and absorbing and reinterpreting both the gifts and the losses of infertility throughout our lives.

CHAPTER 19

Surrogate Mothers

❦ Denise, a wife and mother of two, felt great compassion for couples who could not bear children. Her own kids, Shelley and Brian, meant the world to her and she couldn't imagine missing the experience of parenthood. Both her pregnancies had been healthy with normal deliveries. As time passed, and she heard and read about infertile couples who desperately wanted children, she thought about being a surrogate mother. She wanted to give a gift of life to a couple who couldn't bear their own child and one who wanted a baby to love and cherish, rather than as a status symbol or for inheritance purposes. As she thought about it, she realized her motivation was not to make money but to give a gift. If she did this, she would want to meet the couple and stay in contact with the family.

For a year, she considered becoming a surrogate mother. Denise thought she would be able to emotionally detach herself from the pregnancy and relinquish the baby to the adopting parents. Denise also felt that surrogacy was a perfectly acceptable and ethical alternative for those unable to become pregnant or birth a child. She couldn't think of anything more wonderful than being a child this wanted and loved, even before he was conceived.

She first discussed this with her husband, Jack. Disabled the year before by a work-related accident, Jack did not want any more children. He would, however, support her decision if she chose to be a surrogate mother. She then spoke with Shelley and Brian, telling them that she loved them so much that she couldn't imagine life without them, and that she would like to have a child for a couple who couldn't have their own baby.

Denise also spoke with her minister, parents, and several close friends. Her mother had great difficulty with the idea, and said she would feel a genetic bond with any child Denise conceived and birthed. Her father said, "I wouldn't choose this for you and I don't applaud it, but I won't condemn you if you do this." Her minister felt that she was giving a gift of life and lent his emotional support. Her friends had varying reactions; some approved and others were critical or angry with her for considering surrogacy. Their disapproval did not deter her.

Denise called a contract surrogacy agency. At the interview, she was uncomfortable with a number of things, but especially with the agency's insistence of anonymity among the parties and the high fees involved. After several referrals, she found a reputable independent adoption attorney who also facilitated surrogacy arrangements. At their first meeting, they discussed her motivations for becoming a surrogate mother. He told Denise that he followed the independent adoption model with surrogacy: that as a birthmother in California, she would be entitled to reasonable living, medical, and counseling expenses disbursed in monthly payments and that, if she chose, she could legally and voluntarily terminate her parental rights. In that event, the genetic father's wife would legally adopt the baby. Denise would receive no fee as a surrogate mother, and any agreements or contracts signed would not be legally enforceable. He considered surrogacy as an "adoption planned in advance." As with adoption, she and the couple would have to trust each other. They spoke at length about the legal, psychological, and ethical issues of surrogacy. Denise also filled out a detailed questionnaire concerning her family history and health background. She told the attorney that she wanted to meet any interested couples, rather than bear a child for strangers she would never know. He too felt that all parties should meet beforehand to share their feelings and expectations.

Soon after, the attorney arranged meetings with several couples, but Denise didn't feel comfortable with either situation. Several months later, he called again and suggested she meet Suzanne and John.

A SURROGATE MOTHER IS A WOMAN who agrees to intentionally conceive and bear a child that she plans to relinquish to someone else to parent — in most cases, a couple with female-factor infertility who has been unable, after medical treatment, to become pregnant or carry a child to term. The surrogate mother usually conceives through artificial insemination with the contracting husband's sperm. He is recognized as the child's genetic father, and if she conceives with her own egg, the surrogate is both the genetic and gestational mother of the child. If she agrees to terminate her parental rights, the baby is legally adopted by the genetic father's wife. Another variation of surrogate motherhood has resulted from Assisted Reproductive Technology (ART). In some cases, a woman may agree to bear the genetic child of an infertile couple if the wife is unable to do so. This feat is accomplished by transferring the couple's in vitro-fertilized embryos to the surrogate gestational mother's uterus for pregnancy and birth (see chapter 14). This baby has two biological mothers: one genetic who hopes to raise her, and the other gestational who agrees to birth her.

The surrogate mother option may be facilitated either as an independent adoption in states where this is legal (as described in this chapter's case study) or, more commonly, by specific contractual agreements often written by surrogacy agencies, attorneys, or other intermediaries. Although exact numbers are difficult to ascertain, experts estimate that between 1,000 and 4,000 children have been born in the United States from surrogacy agreements in the past fifteen years, and that up to a thousand surrogate mother contracts may be arranged annually. Most have been contractual agreements, drawn up by third-party brokers, that include a fee for both their services and those of the surrogate mother.

Largely because of several highly publicized court cases, *Matter of Baby M* and *Johnson vs. Calvert* (discussed below), surrogate motherhood in general, and contractual surrogacy in particular, has received widespread media coverage and increasing public scrutiny over the past five years. In fact, this practice dates back to Biblical times and, like other forms of third-party reproductive involvement such as sperm and egg donation, has always generated controversy, support, ambivalence, and confusion among individuals and interested groups in our society.

This chapter discusses some of the complex ethical, legal, psychological, and emotional aspects relevant to the surrogate mother option, as well as considerations of decision-making, cost, and lifelong family issues. The Bibliography contains suggestions for additional readings.

Deciding on a Surrogacy Arrangement

❦ Suzanne and John had tried to conceive a child for five years. Suzanne's workup revealed blocked Fallopian tubes from a previous pelvic inflammation, possibly resulting from earlier use of an IUD. John's semen analyses were normal. Suzanne underwent a lengthy surgery to open her tubes. After a short convalescence, she became pregnant on the first try. The couple was ecstatic until they learned it was an ectopic pregnancy. Suzanne underwent emergency surgery that removed the pregnancy and attempted to repair her tube. She became quite depressed, but with the help of John and her therapist, she managed to get through the ordeal.

Their doctor thought they might be successful if they tried again. After a lot of thought and grief, they agreed. Again, Suzanne became pregnant immediately. Excited, but also cautious and fearful of another loss, she shared the news with only a few close friends. Several weeks later, she was diagnosed with another ectopic pregnancy that also required emergency surgery. Plunging from hope and excitement to despair and grief, Suzanne tried to cope with the loss of another baby that she and John so deeply wanted.

As she slowly and painfully recovered from this second loss, Suzanne felt she could not face, either physically or emotionally, any more infertility treatment or pregnancy loss. She also knew she wanted to become a parent. Although she felt comfortable with adoption, John was not. Having a genetic child was extremely important to him and although Suzanne really couldn't understand his feelings, she felt she had to respect them.

Suzanne and John were at an impasse until they met a couple who had become parents with the help of a surrogate mother. They were, all at once, intrigued, skeptical, curious, and frightened by the idea. After further thought and many long talks, they contacted the attorney who had facilitated that arrangement. At their meeting, they discussed the many aspects of surrogate motherhood and the attorney's application of California independent adoption procedures and laws to surrogacy arrangements. He emphasized that any contracts they might devise were not legally enforceable and any monies disbursed may not be recoverable. They would undertake the same risks as any adoptive parents. He also mentioned Denise and her interest in being a surrogate mother, and suggested the three meet to share perspectives and expectations. Excited, nervous, and frightened, the couple decided to meet Denise.

As with other third-party assisted infertility options, deciding on a surrogate motherhood arrangement is a difficult, painful, and often confusing process. While grieving for the loss of the wife's genetic line and a child of their union, the couple must also grapple with the considerable ethical, legal, moral, and psychological aspects of this resolution.

Although only a small percentage of surrogacy arrangements (an estimated 1 to 5 percent) are contested in court, disagreements and misunderstandings sometimes occur between the parties, as well as refusals to either relinquish or accept the baby. The surrogate mother option remains highly controversial and legally complex. Some states have banned or criminalized contractual surrogacy, others are considering legislation either banning or regulating it, and in many others, the legal status remains ambiguous. And, as with donor insemination, family, friends, and co-workers may not be supportive, receptive, or even tolerant of this choice. Feelings of isolation, lack of support, and vulnerability are often intensified for infertile couples considering this resolution.

Many mental health professionals, physicians, ethicists, attorneys, and clergy are also concerned that infertile couples, as well as gamete donors and birthmothers, considering third-party assisted reproductive options may be especially financially and emotionally vulnerable. Before making a decision, it is essential to weigh the advantages, risks, and ethical and psychological implications of these options for yourselves and any other adults and children affected by this choice.

Consideration and discussion of the following questions, as well as those pertinent to decision-making with infertility, egg donor IVF, donor insemination, and adoption (chapters 2, 14, 16, and 17), may help to clarify your feelings, as individuals and a couple, about the surrogate mother option:

- ☐ Have we pursued or thoroughly considered other appropriate infertility resolutions?
- ☐ Why is surrogacy a better option than adoption, egg donor IVF, or child-free living?
- ☐ Does either partner have any religious, moral, or ethical reservations about surrogate motherhood?
- ☐ Have I grieved for the loss of my fertility and a child of my genetic line? For a child of our union?
- ☐ Will I retain feelings of inadequacy, shame, or guilt because of my infertility?
- ☐ Do I feel my partner values pregnancy and a biological child over my feelings or our relationship? Do I feel obliged to consent to a surrogate arrangement from guilt or fear that he or she will leave me?
- ☐ Are both partners comfortable with another woman being inseminated with the husband's sperm and birthing his biological child?
- ☐ Will a surrogate arrangement create an imbalance in the couple's relationship because he is genetically connected to the child and she is not? Or that she, but not he, remains infertile?
- ☐ Am I concerned about loving and accepting this child, or about he or she bonding with me?
- ☐ Will we tell our child about his origins?
- ☐ Will we discuss our plans with extended family or friends? If so, how will they react to this decision and regard our child?
- ☐ Do we wish to meet the surrogate mother? To have an on-going relationship after our child's birth? What about the surrogate mother's children, our child's half-siblings? How will all the children be affected by this arrangement?
- ☐ What are my feelings about prenatal testing? What if a multiple pregnancy results, or the baby is born with an unforeseen handicap or birth defect?
- ☐ How will we pursue this option: through an independent adoption-type arrangement, or with a contractual agreement arranged by a third-party broker?
- ☐ What is the legal status of surrogacy in our state?
- ☐ Can I face the risk of a surrogate mother arrangement and handle the disappointment if it doesn't work out, or she is unable to relinquish the baby? Do we have the emotional and financial resources to cope with a custody challenge?
- ☐ What are my feelings about genetic and psychological screening for both the surrogate mother and ourselves? About undergoing a home study and other aspects of the adoption process?
- ☐ Can we afford the expense of a surrogate arrangement?

☐ Will we have enough emotional support?

☐ Am I prepared to choose a path fraught with legal, emotional, ethical, and social ambiguities or controversies?

☐ Are we prepared to accept the lifelong issues of a family created through surrogacy?

☐ Are we in agreement about pursuing surrogacy? Can we manage the stress, criticism or disapproval of others, and possible isolation of this experience as a couple, and support each other through the process?

While considering these issues, comparing the pros and cons may also be helpful. Proponents argue that surrogacy offers the advantages of: intentionally creating a child who is deeply loved and wanted by parents committed to this decision; having one parent genetically related to the child, and only one biological parent relinquishing her for adoption; working with a surrogate mother who is, ideally, committed to the decision and to maintaining good prenatal health and medical care; a valid reproductive choice for the infertile if practiced ethically, legally, and with the informed consent of all parties.

Those skeptical or critical of this option express concerns about: the emotional and financial vulnerability of the both the couple and surrogate mother; whether a birthmother can indeed predict her feelings about the baby before the birth and relinquish him for adoption; the lifelong effects of surrogacy on the families and children involved; the fate of babies not wanted by either party or those subject to custody battles; the inconsistency or lack of both medical and psychological screening of surrogate mothers and contracting couples and of state or federal regulation of surrogacy agencies or intermediaries; and, in many states, the legal and judicial ambiguity of the practice.

Being in Accord as a Couple. When considering these complex and difficult issues, partners frequently have conflicting or ambivalent emotions. It may take time, patience, frequent communication, and a period of grieving before they can sort through their feelings and reach a mutually agreeable decision. Experts agree that pursuing any resolution, and especially one as complex as surrogacy, while in conflict is not advisable. As with donor insemination, after the fact is not the time to decide this was the wrong choice. Partners must look within themselves and ask whether they can manage and cope with a surrogate mother arrangement and support each other through it. Professional counseling, from someone experienced with both infertility and surrogacy issues and *without any type of vested interest in your decision,* along with adequate emotional support, is advisable. Consideration of the following sections may also help clarify your feelings.

Ethical and Legal Issues

❦ John and Suzanne traversed miles of country roads, winding through acres of almond orchards, before they found Denise's rural home. Awkwardly and with some embarrassment, they shook her hand and greeted Jack, Shelley, and Brian. These feelings dissipated as the afternoon progressed. They were curious about each other and the pitfalls that might lie ahead, and over several hours, discussed their hopes and fears. Both John and Suzanne found Denise a wonderfully kind, sensitive, and giving woman. Warmth and trust began to grow between them. Over the next three months, they met a number of times to share their feelings and expectations. After each meeting, the two families went out to a park or restaurant to get further acquainted and relax a bit.

With each encounter, they realized that this relationship would be founded on trust, rather than contracts. John and Suzanne would have to trust Denise to refrain from intercourse during inseminations, to take good care of herself and the growing baby during her pregnancy, and to release the infant to them for adoption. Denise stated that their trust must last until she signed the relinquishment papers. Hers, on the other hand, would have to last a lifetime. She would trust them to respect her right to make decisions regarding her and the baby's well-being during pregnancy, labor, and delivery, and to provide financial support until she recovered from the birth. Most important, Denise would trust them to love and parent this child, as she would, for the rest of their lives.

Suzanne wondered how Denise could possibly give up the baby and whether she would be able to release him after birth. Denise explained her motivations and feelings about being a surrogate mother each time the couple visited. The women grew to admire and love one another as friends and sisters, although Suzanne had feelings of jealousy and fear that she sometimes expressed.

About four months after their initial meeting, the parties agreed to proceed. With the attorney's help, they drew up two agreements: a declaration of intent and a contract regarding payment of expenses. They stated their intention to enter a surrogate mother agreement and contingencies if Denise should miscarry or bear a child with a physical or mental handicap. The attorney emphasized that this agreement would not be legally enforceable. They also drew up a list of monthly expenses that included her mortgage payment, medical needs not covered by insurance, and food, utility, clothing, and counseling costs. Denise would be paid $1,250 per month, disbursed by the attorney in ten monthly installments. Suzanne and John would pay for all legal and adoption expenses.

Denise was artificially inseminated with John's sperm several weeks later and became pregnant on the first try.

For a number of years, the ethical, moral, and legal labyrinths of surrogate motherhood have sparked heated public debate. Both the Office of Technology Assessment (OTA) in its compendium, *Infertility: Medical and Social Choices,* and the Ethics Committee of the American Fertility Society in its report, "Ethical Considerations of the New Reproductive Technologies," include excellent summaries and analyses of the salient ethical issues of surrogacy.

Both reports noted objections cited by many religious groups, as well as individuals in our society, to any type of surrogacy arrangement, and their arguments that this practice: undermines the integrity of the family unit; inappropriately involves a third party in the private and intimate sphere of reproduction; carries unknown, long-term, and possibly detrimental consequences for any children affected; and that it may be emotionally, psychologically, or economically exploitive of both surrogate mothers and infertile couples. Concerns were also raised regarding the determination of appropriate medical criteria or indications for surrogacy; the possible misuse of this option for non-medical or convenience purposes; the minimal or non-existent medical and psychological screening of genetic fathers, surrogate mothers, and prospective adoptive parents; and the long-term emotional effects of relinquishment on the birthmother, the baby, and her other children.

Decisions Regarding Genetic Testing and Pregnancy, Labor and Delivery Management. Serious reservations have also been expressed about whether surrogate mothers should undertake the physical risks of pregnancy, labor, and delivery — which are substantially more significant than those associated with either sperm or egg donation — for someone else. Responsibility for decision-making about prenatal testing, pregnancy termination, and management of gestation, labor, and delivery poses a related ethical concern. Although many parties specify their expectations about these points in written contracts, it is unlikely that such provisions are legally enforceable.

The Committee on Ethics of the American College of Obstetricians and Gynecologists (ACOG) addressed these and other relevant concerns in their 1990 issue of *ACOG Committee Opinion*, "Ethical Issues in Surrogate Motherhood." In formulating their recommendations and their applicability, the committee did not differentiate between genetic or gestational surrogate mothers:

> ... the genetic link between the commissioning parent(s) and the resulting infant, while important, is less weighty than the link between surrogate mother and fetus or infant that is created through gestation and birth. Thus, in the analysis and recommendations that follow no distinction will be drawn between the usual pattern of surrogate parenting and surrogate gestational motherhood.

The committee further recommended that:

> ... the surrogate mother, who both carries the fetus and delivers the infant, 1) should be the sole source of consent for all questions regarding prenatal care and delivery and 2) should have a specified time period after the birth of the infant during which she can decide whether or not to carry out her original intention to place the infant for adoption. Thus, in all relevant respects the position of the surrogate mother should be the same as the position of any other

woman who, either prenatally or postpartum, has expressed the intention of placing an infant for adoption.

The Debate over Contractual Surrogacy. Some groups and individuals consider donor (compensation for incurred expenses only), non-enforceable surrogacy acceptable, but object to the practice of legally enforceable contractual surrogacy agreements that pay a fee to the surrogate mother, deeming them morally unacceptable, illegal in many states, and prohibited by both the United States Constitution and the Constitutions of each of the fifty states. They compare paid contractual surrogacy to commercialized baby-selling, arguing that it commodifies human life while degrading women and devaluating pregnancy. They also fear that poor women, both in the United States and Third World countries, may feel tempted or pressured to earn money in this way. (In the United States, OTA reported a 1988 annual income level of $15,000 to $30,000 for surrogate mothers, and $55,000 or more per year for contracting couples.) While many feminists share and support this view, others counter that women should be able to legally enter such contractual arrangements with informed consent and be fairly compensated for the considerable and honorable labor of pregnancy and birthing.

Regardless of their position, most agree that without compensation above expenses, most women would not become surrogate mothers. The OTA report notes that:

> ... whether prohibitions on exchanging money for termination of
> parental rights and custody are held to make surrogacy
> arrangements criminal or merely unenforceable, they would
> effectively prevent surrogacy from becoming a freely available
> alternative to adoption, since few nonrelated women will be
> surrogates on altruistic grounds. The constitutionality of such a ban
> on paid surrogacy remains to be determined by most States and by
> the Federal courts.

A national survey conducted by *Parents* magazine in October, 1987, reflects the division of opinion and ambivalence among Americans toward the complex ethical and moral issues of surrogate motherhood: 15 percent of respondents approved of the practice under any circumstances, 43 percent only in certain circumstances, 32 percent were opposed regardless of circumstances, and 9 percent were undecided. More than 50 percent supported the option for a married infertile woman, a woman with a genetic abnormality that might reasonably be passed to her child, or a woman with a health problem that would be worsened by pregnancy. Fifty-seven percent of the respondents felt that, despite her feelings before the birth, the bond established between mother and baby during pregnancy may affect a birthmother's ability to relinquish the baby. Of those polled, 39 percent favored legislation that would permit and regulate surrogacy arrangements, 22 percent favored banning the practice, and 35 percent opposed any legislation at all.

Judicial and Legal Issues. The legal debate over surrogate motherhood culminated in a landmark decision in 1988 by the New Jersey Supreme Court (*Matter of Baby M* [1988] 109 N.J. 396, 537 A.2d 1227). The famous *Baby M* decision involved the case of Mary Beth Whitehead, a surrogate mother who contracted to bear a child for an infertile couple, William and Elizabeth Stern. After the baby's birth, Whitehead felt she could not terminate her maternal rights. The Superior Court upheld the surrogacy contract and terminated Whitehead's parental rights. The New Jersey Supreme Court reversed the trial court decision in February, 1988, reinstating Whitehead as the baby's biological and legal mother. The OTA report, in its analysis of the legal considerations of surrogate motherhood, noted that the New Jersey Supreme Court found "that the surrogacy contract violated New Jersey law concerning baby-selling, adoption, and termination of parental rights."

An estimated 1 to 5 percent of surrogate mother arrangements are legally contested. Since the *Baby M* decision, other surrogacy cases have been decided, or are pending judicial review, in courts across the country. The OTA report concludes that:

> Courts and attorney general opinions have consistently stated in dictum that a surrogate mother has all the same rights to her child as does a mother who conceived with the intention of keeping her baby. In other words, in the event of a custody dispute between the genetic father and surrogate mother, both would stand on equal footing and the best interests of the child would dictate the court's decision. The courts reasoned that a surrogate motherhood contract, while not void from inception, is nevertheless voidable. This means that if all parties agree to abide by the contract terms, and the intended rearing parents are not found to be manifestly unfit, then a court will enter the necessary paternity orders and approve the various attorneys' fees agreed upon. If, on the other hand, the surrogate mother changes her mind about giving up her parental rights within the statutory time period provided by the applicable State law, then she has forfeited her rights to whatever fees the contract provided, but both the mother, child, and biological father now have the statutory rights and obligations as exist in the absence of contract.

More recently, a case involving surrogate gestational motherhood, *Johnson vs. Calvert*, has received widespread media attention. Both the genetic parents, Crispina and Mark Calvert, and the surrogate gestational mother, Anna Johnson, brought suit in 1990 to establish parental rights to the baby gestated and birthed by Johnson after the transfer of the Calverts' in vitro-fertilized embryos. A California superior court rejected Johnson's claims to parental rights on the grounds that she is not genetically related to the baby. The California Supreme Court, agreeing to hear the case on appeal, has temporarily set aside this ruling. A precedent-setting decision, the first case regarding surrogate gestational motherhood in the United States, is expected by 1993.

Although attempts to pass federal legislation banning contract surrogacy have been unsuccessful to date, there is no state in which contract surrogacy is legally enforceable. In the wake of these emotional and complex court cases, a number of states have proposed or passed legislation specifically regarding surrogacy contracts. At this time, contractual surrogacy is illegal, void, and unenforceable in Florida, Indiana, Kentucky, Louisiana, Michigan, Nebraska, Utah, North Dakota, Arizona, Washington, New Hampshire, and Virginia, and in some cases, its practice may carry fines or criminal penalties. In other states, legislation is being considered that will either ban or regulate the practice. Couples considering this option should carefully research the laws of their state regarding contractual surrogacy and independent adoption arrangements, and seek counsel from a reputable attorney *with no vested interest in this contractual relationship.*

Financial Considerations

If a couple agrees to pursue this resolution, they must decide whether to seek a donor arrangement similar to an independent adoption, or work with a contractual surrogacy agency in states where these options are legal. Expenses can vary widely between the two alternatives. In this chapter's case study, Denise was paid $12,500 in ten monthly installments for allowable adoption expenses that were itemized to the court. John and Suzanne also paid $3,000 in legal fees to the attorney, bringing the total cost to $15,500. Working with a surrogate agency or broker is considerably more expensive — often $35,000 or more. Of this sum, agencies estimate that $10,000 to $12,000 is paid to the surrogate mother, $15,000 or more is applied to expenses, and $10,000 or more to agency fees. Expenses for prenatal care and delivery may also be added to either arrangement if the surrogate mother does not have medical insurance.

The procedures, fees, ethical standards, and reputation of both attorneys and surrogate agencies vary considerably. Before consenting to any arrangement or paying any fees, research the reputation and methods of the lawyer, intermediary, or agency. In many cases, deposits or other monies paid may not be refundable. To ensure that they employ competent staff and operate within the law, check with the district attorney's office of their county and state.

Emotional and Psychological Aspects of Surrogacy

❦ For the next nine months, Suzanne and John spent many weekends visiting Denise and her family. Suzanne also attended each prenatal visit and tried to be as involved as she could with the pregnancy. Suzanne and John's affection and respect for Denise grew with every passing month. The baby was due in mid-December, and by mutual agreement, Suzanne packed a suitcase and came to stay with Denise and her family shortly after Thanksgiving. John drove up to visit each weekend. The two women grew even closer as the birth approached. The couple continued to have fears and occasional sleepless nights, wondering whether Denise would be able to relinquish the baby. Yet they also felt reassured by their on-going contact.

The baby was quite large and Denise had a painful back labor of six hours. Suzanne, John, and Shelley stayed by her side. Suzanne encouraged Denise and, with tears running down her face, continuously rubbed and pushed against Denise's back trying to ease some of the pressure. Suzanne's hands and arms ached from the effort; Denise was completely exhausted. John Carl, weighing more than ten pounds, squalling, and a tad blue, finally emerged amid tears and wild cheering. The doctor administered a little oxygen, and still screaming lustily, he quickly acquired a pink glow. John cut the cord and Suzanne, cradling the baby in her aching arms, showed him to Denise. They spent the night in Denise's hospital room and took turns holding and admiring John Carl.

Before they were discharged the next day, Denise requested a little time alone with John Carl, Shelley, and Brian. They each held the baby. Denise told him she loved him and would always be available to him, and wished him a wonderful life with his parents.

Before Suzanne and John left the hospital with the baby, the two mothers spent a few minutes together. Tearfully, Suzanne embraced and thanked Denise, saying there were no words to express her love and gratitude for the gift of John Carl. John wrote her a note: "Most children are fortunate indeed if they have one loving mother. John Carl got two."

The two families, each ecstatic and joyful over John Carl's birth, prepared to go home. They promised to get together soon. Neither could imagine discontinuing contact or ending their relationship.

The Surrogate Mother and Her Family

A surrogate mother and her family often cope with a number of emotional and psychological issues. Motivation is undoubtedly an important determinant in how this experience will affect a surrogate mother, and the degree and intensity of its lifelong effects. For some women, altruism, financial reward, attaining a life achievement, and narcissism are primary incentives. Others may be guided by more complex factors, such as subtle or overt pressure from mates or relatives, or a wish to alleviate guilt or remorse over a past pregnancy loss or abortion. Many mental health experts strongly advise women to seek counseling, *with a therapist experienced in these issues who does not have a vested emotional or financial interest in her decision,* both before consenting to a surrogacy arrangement and after relinquishment.

The experiences of pregnancy and birthing may also change a woman's feelings toward the baby and her thoughts about releasing him or her. In some cases, surrogate mothers do underestimate the emotional and psychological impact of this experience. They may feel depressed or grief-stricken for some time, especially if they do not have an opportunity to see the child again and ensure that he or she is happy and well cared for. Some wish to retain parental rights or deeply regret their decision to relinquish the baby afterward. Fighting for legal custody or visitation is often a physically, emotionally, and financially draining ordeal.

Other surrogate mothers feel fulfillment and joy in giving the gift of life to a couple unable to birth a child. In some cases, contact continues and they are recognized as a respected and treasured part of the family.

Social Criticism. Many in our society consider surrogacy immoral or adulterous in nature, and physically, emotionally, or economically exploitive of birthmothers. They also question whether a woman can relinquish a baby without lifelong damage to herself and the child. Surrogate mothers and their families often hear such criticism, and feel judged or ostracized by others. In some cases, relationships and friendships may be jeopardized or lost. This may understandably take a toll on individual esteem and the marital relationship.

Children Affected by Surrogacy. Little research has been published about the effects of this option on a surrogate mother's children — both the baby she relinquishes and those she parents. Many experts have raised concerns about how this experience affects children and whether they may fear being relinquished themselves. Young children, especially, are unable to understand the nature or complexity of surrogacy. The kids often consider themselves siblings, regardless of how their parents define the situation, and feel love and ties with each other. If an on-going relationship has not been established between the families, the children may desire contact with each other. If any of the children affected by a surrogate arrangement express or display confusion or fear, counseling is strongly recommended.

The Infertile Couple

Those pursuing a surrogacy resolution may confront, as individuals and a couple, several emotional and psychological issues. As with donor insemination (DI), sexual problems may develop during the surrogacy process. In this case, the infertile wife may feel inadequate and perhaps sexually jealous of the surrogate, who is being inseminated with her mate's sperm. Some women who are not clinically sterile may also fantasize that they could still become pregnant. The couple's sex life may also be partially controlled by the surrogate's menstrual cycle. To ensure sperm that are optimally fertile, they may have to refrain from intercourse a day or two before inseminations. This is a poignant reminder of both her infertility and their inability to bear a child as a couple. Inseminations are often emotionally and sexually difficult for an infertile couple, times when partners need even more patience and understanding. DI couples have found that showing and expressing love for each other in different ways — like long talks, walks, thoughtful gestures, romantic dinners, touching, and holding — can bring you closer together during a stressful time.

Although many wives take an active role during this time — perhaps attending prenatal visits, trying in other ways to be involved with the surrogate mother's pregnancy, and helping with the legal or adoption process — this may also be a poignant and bittersweet personal transition. The baby will be the husband's biological child, and although a wife often shares this happiness, she also grieves for the loss of her lineage. Unlike her partner, she must also cope with the doubts and stresses of an adoptive parent-to-be.

The couple must also make important decisions about who, if anyone, to tell about the surrogacy arrangement. Should they share this information with relatives and friends, or those who have supported them during their infertility struggle? If they do, others will know about the child's origins before he or she is able to understand it. They must also decide if, how, and when they will discuss this with their child, and whether they wish on-going contact with the surrogate mother and her family. If contact is not continued, search issues may arise as their child grows up. If the parties wish to maintain contact, they will need to discuss the type, degree, and frequency of communication each desires and perhaps a delineation of boundaries. (See chapters 2, 14, 16, and 18 for further discussion of these issues.)

Pursuing and coping with a surrogacy arrangement is often an intense and complex experience. Partners may have differing perspectives and feelings that can contribute to misunderstanding and friction between them. Experts emphasize that these are lifelong issues and strongly encourage counseling and on-going support during this process and, as needed, in the future.

Lifelong Issues

    ❧ Since John Carl's birth nearly five years ago, the families have remained close. They speak frequently on the phone, and since they live a two-hour drive away, visit on holidays, John Carl's birthday, and other occasions.

    The adults aren't really sure how John Carl views Denise and the idea that she is his birthmother. Shelley remarked that this whole idea took some getting used to, but she thinks her mom did something wonderful. The children regard and love each other as siblings. John Carl speaks of Shelley and Brian frequently and is always eager to see them. His half-brother and sister, in turn, love him, look forward to seeing him, John, and Suzanne, and urge Denise to arrange a get-together if too much time passes between visits. Brian and John Carl, only five years apart, tousle, tumble, and delight in each other's company as most siblings do. Suzanne and John take all the kids camping every summer.

Suzanne and John are delighted that John Carl feels such deep affection and family connection with Shelley and Brian. They look forward to the times when their families get together. They have been open and straightforward with John Carl about his origins and will continue this discussion throughout their lives. They realize that what they and Denise created together is very special, goes beyond the bounds of family and friendship, and will be with them all forever.

Denise feels a lifelong responsibility toward John Carl and will always be available to him. She remains proud of her role and feels she, Suzanne, and John did something honest and wonderful that continued the miracle of life. She realizes that many people will never understand why she became a surrogate mother in the first place, and why she didn't demand a fee in the second. She knows that some disapprove of her for doing it at all. She thinks that if these people spent a few hours with an infertile couple who desperately want a child, they might understand.

As with any type of parenting after infertility, creating a family through surrogacy carries lifelong issues and challenges. The partners must heal from the wounds of their infertility, reclaim their privacy as individuals and a couple, and perhaps reinstate boundaries that were weakened by medical investigation, the curiosity and well-intentioned inquiries of friends and relatives, and the pursual of a controversial family-building resolution.

Those involved with third-party reproductive alternatives must also define their future relationships with each other and the type of contact they wish to maintain. The feelings of all the children involved, and their relationship as half-siblings, must also be considered and evaluated. The legacy of the couple's infertility and the surrogate mother's involvement, and their effects on the children are lifelong issues and may periodically surface. Counseling for any involved party may be appropriate at various times throughout their lives.

The family will also join the mainstream of American life — new mothers' groups, babysitting co-ops, preschools, soccer and baseball teams, and scout troops. Again, the child's and family's privacy is important to respect. Not everyone will approve of, or even understand, a couple's or birthmother's involvement in a surrogacy arrangement. Experts advise being selective in whom you confide, requesting confidentiality from those you do, and seeking role models in other families created through alternative means. Above all, they suggest enjoying and cherishing the unique family that you have created, and the joy, struggle, challenge, and triumph of parenthood. Chapter 18 includes further discussion and suggestions for parenting after infertility.

CHAPTER 20

Child-Free Living

❧ My fantasies of motherhood had soft rosy edges that four or five hours of being with real-life children quickly dispelled. It made it easier to enjoy the parts of my day that were there precisely because I had no children. People with small children don't have the luxuries of time with their spouses, leisurely dinners, spur-of-the-moment shopping trips, or the quiet to curl up with a good book or even the newspaper. It was nice to remember that all the advantages were not on one side; both lifestyles have their pros and cons.

TRADITIONALLY THE TERM *childlessness* has been used to describe a lifestyle without biological or adopted children. Until recently couples without children accepted society's notion that their lives were empty, boring, unhappy, and less than fulfilled. This stereotype has been challenged, and now the term *child-free living* better describes the decision not to parent.

Many infertile couples who attach great importance to pregnancy and birthing as well as those who, for a variety of reasons, do not feel adoption is an appropriate resolution, consider child-free living. It is a concept, however, that is still being formulated and refined. In discussion groups across the country, interested couples and professionals are exploring and attempting to clarify the issues and legacy of the child-free choice — one they envision as a valid and viable resolution that can lead to a happy, positive, and enriching lifestyle.

In a sense, these couples are the most courageous of all infertility pioneers. They are challenging a deeply entrenched and perhaps worldwide cultural tradition of pronatalism that, throughout the ages, has strongly pressured couples to become either biological or adoptive parents. Until recently, they have found little emotional support for the child-free choice in either the fertile or infertile worlds.

As we approach the twenty-first century, social attitudes about child-free living are slowly changing. More couples are voluntarily choosing this lifestyle for a variety of personal, financial, and ecological reasons. Within the infertile community, the child-free choice is also receiving increasing validation and discussion. Recently the meaning, decision-making process, and complex issues of this option have been crystallized and thoughtfully analyzed in a groundbreaking and significant treatise, *Sweet Grapes: How to Stop Being Infertile and Start Living Again*. Authors Jean Carter, M.D., and Michael Carter, Ph.D., a couple who have chosen a child-free lifestyle after their own infertility experience, have graciously contributed their insights to the following discussion.

What Is Child-Free Living?

The Carters, along with other infertility experts, suggest that child-free living is a positive, life-affirming, and ultimately empowering *choice*. It is chosen for its own attributes and rewards rather than assumed by default because "we just never got pregnant" or "adoption wasn't right for us."

In making this choice, a couple transforms the way they perceive their situation. For so long a devastating and painful reality, their infertility now provides an opportunity for positive change and growth. This is, ultimately, a decision not to *want* to parent children. Instead, the couple prefers to formulate and achieve other life goals. Rather than identifying themselves as failures at having children, they collectively and individually regard themselves as successful achievers of rewarding, fulfilling, and realistically *attainable* goals.

Lynn Brokenshire, MFCC, an expert on child-free living and child-free herself, observes that the pursuit of pregnancy, though theoretically possible, can become too costly — physically, emotionally, financially, and spiritually. Everyone has the right, at any point during their infertility struggle, to redirect their energies toward a child-free resolution.

Clearly, reaching this orientation is a difficult and painful process. A couple who has invested years of extraordinary effort, thousands of hard-earned or borrowed dollars, and buckets of tears *trying* to have a child does not make the leap to *not wanting* to have a child quickly or easily. And those who have endured the stresses and devastation of infertility do not share the same perspective as couples who, at the onset of their union, agreed that parenting was not right for them. Jean Carter observes that although all of these couples are child-free, they certainly did not travel the same path to get there.

Rather, most infertile couples approach this option after years of medical procedures and emotional stress. Some have endured numerous in vitro fertilization (IVF) attempts; others have unsuccessfully tried a variety of male-factor treatments. At some point, some women experience a physical, almost visceral reaction to the thought of continued medical treatment. They recognize an accumulation, within their hearts and bodies, of fear, apprehension, memories of painful procedures, and subsequent feelings of disappointment, despair, and grief. The idea of yet another cycle of fertility drugs, donor insemination, or IVF often elicits, from deep within, responses of sobbing, shaking, and a forceful voice that says "No more!"

❦ My last in vitro fertilization attempt was really a turning point — physically and emotionally. In previous IVF cycles, I had been excited, as well as apprehensive and frightened. That excitement gave me the energy and hope to get through each procedure. But that last attempt was different and I soon realized something was very wrong. Through each step, I felt like I was fighting myself. I cried with each injection, through every ultrasound, and during the aspiration and transfer. And then I fell apart when I got the negative pregnancy test results. As I started to pull myself back together once again, I knew it was time to look for other answers and to get on with my life.

Both women and men may feel chronically sad or angry and find little joy in their daily lives. Even long-time, stable marriages can be jeopardized when partners are unable to communicate effectively or comfort each other.

This stage often prompts a reassessment of their goals and options. Many stop medical treatment, investigate adoption, and choose this path toward parenting; others are attracted to the child-free alternative. Often, the cessation of treatment and the consideration of a child-free life initiates a period of intense mourning for one or both partners.

The Mourning Process

❧ This spring I celebrated my fortieth birthday, and along with it, began to accept the probability that I will never bear a child of my own. While I resolved long ago that I would not allow this circumstance to turn my life into a tragedy should it come to pass, I am only just beginning to experience the sadness, the regret, and the self-blame that it precipitates as I move into the next era of my life. I will never see myself reflected in my child's face. I will never hold grandchildren that share my gene pool.

All women and men experience varying degrees of sadness and grief when they learn of their infertility and struggle to cope with it. This early stage of the resolution process is described in chapter 1.

When a couple or single woman approaches the child-free option, this initial mourning often resurfaces and is intensified by the import of this decision. A number of losses will be experienced, some unique to the child-free choice. The couple or woman must let go of the dreams of pregnancy, birthing, and biological children. And, because they will not adopt children, they must also release the dream of parenting and its connection to the human family. This is a significant identity change for those who truly envisioned themselves as prospective parents and worked so diligently toward that goal.

After investing a number of their "younger" years into fertility treatment, many discover that this grieving coincides with the onset of mid-life — commonly a time of personal reflection and evaluation for adults in their thirties and forties. The meaningfulness, purpose, and direction of one's life, past and present relationships, career choices, and personal achievements are often examined at this juncture.

❧ At this particular point in time, it is difficult for me to view my life as truly meaningful without children. My belief — whether I like it or not — is that being a parent defines a person as a human being more clearly than does any other role in life. I see this as true for both women and men. Consequently, no matter how I struggle, I see myself as an undefined, unfulfilled, insignificant person.

I lead a good, pleasant, busy life. I enjoy good friendships and close family ties, as well as a strong primary relationship. My career is somewhat fulfilling, but it is not a passion with me. Perhaps the fact that there are no major achievements in my life — such as the discovery of a cure for cancer — and very little in the way of religious commitment, in addition to being childless, causes me to feel that I lead a life of minimal substance. While it is not unbearably painful for me to attend baby showers or to spend time with young families, doing so heightens the sense of my own life's relative meaninglessness.

This is often a painful and, for some individuals, lengthy process. Because partners often find themselves in different stages of grief, this is a time to seek sustenance from a number of sources. Those with supportive extended families often draw closer to parents or siblings, deepening and perhaps redefining those relationships. Other infertile couples who are in this stage, religious advisers, and compassionate therapists experienced with child-free issues are other resources. In addition, some individuals utilize coping and adaptive skills developed during past crises. Others simply trust in the healing process of the body and spirit.

❧ Currently, I comfort myself with the reminder that I am someone's child and that, as such, I matter deeply. In all likelihood, whatever sense of self-esteem resulted from my parents' unconditional love will remain with me for the rest of my life. I observe the close relationship between my own parents and note how many years they have enjoyed alone together since their last child left the nest. Luckily, they have not depended upon their children to infuse their lives with meaning on a day-to-day basis in the interim.

Finally, I recognize the fact that most people endure deep grief during some period of life, yet this does not preclude the possibility of living a basically happy life.

Grief is a personal and gradual process, different for every individual. Most people find that, over time, the intensity of mourning subsides as their anger and sorrow recede. Although feelings of sadness will probably remain throughout their lives, grief is no longer a dominant or daily presence. They are able to bring closure to their infertility.

Letting go of what probably cannot be attained enables one to envision the myriad possibilities that are now available. Women, especially, report a surge of esteem as a new self-image emerges. They finally believe that, in and of themselves, they are vital, effective, and important human beings; they need not bear a child to feel complete as women.

At this stage, women and men describe a welcome and joyful return of relief, power, control, privacy, intimacy, and an enthusiasm for life. Now, the Carters maintain, they are ready to consider the child-free choice.

Making the Choice

> ❦ I had an ectopic pregnancy six years ago and haven't been able to conceive since. Both my husband and I wanted to experience pregnancy and birth. We have also both witnessed painful adoption experiences among our families. After lengthy grieving we've opted for child-free living. And I can now say, "Yes! We are happy and still very much in love!"

As with any major life choice, the child-free decision is usually not made easily or quickly. For couples, it is a process of sharing thoughts, feelings, sadness, and grief with your partner and others close to you; for single women, with a counselor or trusted friends. It is critical that the couple work together, rather than "drift" or allow the stronger-willed partner to dictate their direction. It is also important to note that partners often move through the decision-making phase at a different pace and express ambivalent feelings. In many instances, men are initially more receptive to a child-free choice than women, who often favor adoption.

During such disagreement a couple may feel angry and isolated and fear they are drifting apart. Perhaps the fight against infertility has been a central focus for years and has forged a bond between them. Although it is a relief in one sense, abandoning the struggle can also be disorienting and threatening. A couple may wonder what will hold them together after their infertility is resolved.

To avoid an impasse they must ensure that their grief is completed, work together toward compromise, and reshape future goals. During this difficult time it is important to remember that you can become close again. Joining a child-free support group or working with an experienced counselor may be helpful.

Ideally the child-free choice is mutually embraced by both partners. Reaching agreement usually involves frequent and honest discussion of their opinions and feelings, along with both intuitive and intellectual consideration of the advantages, drawbacks, and myths associated with this resolution.

If they haven't already, some couples begin with an agreement to stop medical treatment or to set a time or age limit when they will. They may research the various types of adoption and weigh their merits. This is also a time to examine feelings about the possible drawbacks of child-free living. How do you each feel about not parenting in your lifetimes? Will this choice result in a negative, long-term impact on your marriage or your relationships with extended family?

Weighing the many positive and beneficial aspects of a child-free lifestyle is also an important exercise. Instead of expending enormous amounts of energy and money rearing a child, a couple or single woman can enjoy a comfortable and active lifestyle and long-term financial security. They will have the money and freedom to travel, pursue further studies, or perhaps change or advance their careers. Despite busy lives, there will still be time for hobbies, volunteer work, and friendships. Child-free living also offers both the opportunity and the privacy to foster personal growth and nurture an intimate relationship.

The myths long associated with child-free living should also be confronted and examined. Those contemplating this lifestyle are often warned that:

- Life is empty and meaningless without children.
- A child-free life ends with isolation and abandonment in old age.
- Those who do not parent will be immersed in grief and regrets forever.

Child-free advocates counter these grim predictions with the observation that having children does not guarantee a perfect, happy life. Everyone knows couples and singles who have had extremely difficult and painful parenting experiences. Conversely, there are many role-models of child-free couples who have enjoyed both long and joyful marriages and fulfilling and productive lives. There is no reason to assume that your children will reproduce themselves, care for you in your old age, or even invite you to Thanksgiving dinner!

The Carters argue that those who drift into child-free living, rather than consciously and positively choosing this lifestyle, are more likely to experience regrets. Although some sadness and feelings of loss will probably remain, those who embrace this choice will also enjoy a life rich with love, achievement, and marital contentment. Gay Becker, Ph.D., a medical anthropologist and author of *Healing the Infertile Family*, notes that studies of older child-free couples tend to validate this theory: most feel that any regrets are more than offset by the positive aspects of their lives and relationships.

Finally, it is important to remember that *all* major life decisions are questioned, reevaluated, and at times, probably regretted to some degree. A better perspective might be, "Make the choice that you will regret the least!" One woman spoke wistfully of "not being anybody's Mommy." Although saddened by this reality, she also saw its positive side. She now had the opportunity to develop an equally fulfilling identity and interests.

REVOCABLE OR NOT?

Initially many couples drawn toward child-free living find it difficult to make a permanent decision. Should they commit to a child-free life now? Suppose a new and miraculous medical treatment is developed in five years? Or, a few years down the road, they realize that they want to parent through adoption?

At the same time, they realize that their present life is an unhappy and frustrating one. Many strike a compromise by "trying on" child-free living for a period of time and then reassessing the decision before making a permanent commitment. Dr. Marsha Young, a psychologist specializing in fertility issues, observes:

> ❦ That [child-free living] is revocable also makes this decision easiest in many ways. If new technology appears in three years, you may then decide to resume your quest. In the meantime you have three years of peace. All decisions can be made with a time line for renegotiation in a year or two or three. This is a good way to make almost all decisions including decisions to marry. Recommitment endows new vitality into any decision. Assure yourself you will review the decision and this will allow your mind to rest easy in the interim.

The Carters agree that "trying it on" for a specific period of time may benefit many couples. Yet they also note that if revocability is a primary feature of the decision, there is probably less commitment to it. Thus couples may not experience the peace and closure that a permanent choice can bring.

Pivotal life events, such as the births of siblings' children, the illness or death of one's parents, and "milestone" birthdays, may trigger reconsideration or reaffirmation of the child-free decision. In reality, many couples probably interpret this choice in a very personal way. Some stop treatment and remain child-free if pregnancy does not occur. Some "try it on" for a year or longer and then decide to adopt. Others realize, at some point, that they have made a permanent decision. They now consciously embrace this lifestyle and resume birth control, or perhaps opt for vasectomy or tubal ligation.

Many who make a conscious commitment to child-free living formally celebrate their decision. This acknowledgment can be an important rite of passage, especially if they are the only ones initially enthusiastic about their choice. Some take a special vacation, perhaps to somewhere they have always dreamed of going. Others renew their marital commitment in another personal way with a ceremony, party, or other form of announcement to their loved ones. This is an opportunity to reshape your identity, personal goals, and future as a couple and individuals.

The Social Pressures and Emotional Impact of Child-Free Living

> ❦ It was difficult for my mother to accept my decision. She raised six children and now all her friends were grandmothers. She wanted grandchildren of her own.

> ❦ Strangers will ask, "Any children?" I say, "No." There is usually a silence and then, "Oh." The nosier ones will ask why not. If you state

you have a fertility problem, they want to treat you and tell you all the cures. I've learned to educate them.

REACTIONS OF FAMILY AND FRIENDS

One woman observed that while the decision to adopt is usually supported and approved by one's family, a child-free choice is often a lonely and contested one. Your decision may evoke criticism, anger, and pressure to adopt from family and friends who have strong feelings about parenting. It often feels like you are reliving your initial infertility struggle.

Individual family circumstances can also play an important role. Sociologists have found that a couple's decisions about parenting are often influenced by their extended family's attitudes. Are they from a heritage or ethnic group that is especially child-oriented? Will there be other grandchildren to continue the genetic line? Have relatives or friends placed subtle or overt pressure on the couple to reproduce?

The Carters suggest that, because of their strong orientation to parenting, most relatives and friends need time to adjust to your child-free decision. You are indeed changing identities — from a couple trying to have a child to one who will not parent — in their eyes as well as your own. It is also important that you are clear about your choice. Those who are not at peace with their child-free life probably send mixed messages that may confuse and worry concerned friends and relatives — prompting even more questions and discussion. It may also be helpful to talk privately with those who matter most to you. If you are truly content with your decision, that happiness will be noted and ease the doubts of those who love you.

With time, most social pressures subside as others accept your decision. Over the years, many child-free couples develop an extended family network of both family and friends, creating a much needed sense of community. They seek out others they admire and enjoy, including those with and without children, single folks, and those older and younger. They discover that many people in their lives — relatives, church or club acquaintances, working colleagues, and neighbors — are eager for friendship and company.

As your peer group ages and their children grow up, there will also be less focus on pregnancy, birth, and parenting in your daily life. In fact some child-free couples later find themselves supporting friends and relatives when their children leave home. The "empty nest syndrome" can be similar to the loneliness of infertility.

OTHER INFERTILE COUPLES

The infertile soon discover that most emotional support is geared toward achieving pregnancy or adoption. In fact the child-free choice is often a taboo subject among those still undergoing treatment or waiting to adopt. Those who consider or select child-free living often feel outnumbered, overwhelmed, or even ostracized by those favoring adoption, donor insemination, high-tech medical assistance, surrogacy, or other alternatives.

> 🐦 Our first infertility support group meeting heavily emphasized adoption. I left thinking, "That's how they fix infertility. Adoption must be the only cure and solution."
> Later we drifted away from the group. Adoption just wasn't the answer for us.

Those still in the midst of an infertility struggle may feel threatened by child-free couples. They often believe these women and men have given up hope or do not approve of their continued quest for a child. Conversely, child-free couples often feel shame or guilt about stopping treatment or preferring biological parenthood over adoption. Sadly, this situation often results in a breakdown of communication and support within the infertile community. There is, however, increasing interest among infertile couples in exploring and supporting the child-free choice. In response, many RESOLVE chapters are sponsoring child-free support groups and workshops.

COPING WITH COMMENTS AND QUESTIONS

There will be relatives and friends, as well as new acquaintances and strangers, who will continue to question your choice. Perhaps because the medical aspects of their infertility experience have weakened privacy boundaries, many couples feel compelled to justify, defend, and explain their decisions time and again to anyone who asks.

They especially dread that question so casually posed at cocktail parties or other social events: "Do you have children?" Michael Carter wryly observes that this query may not necessarily indicate an interest in your personal life. Rather it is often an invitation to ask about *theirs*! A response of, "No, do you?", may launch loquacious Moms and Dads into a lengthy discourse about their parental triumphs or woes and get you off the hook.

After discussing your choice with those important to you, refrain from arguing or defending it with others. Rehashing your decision is exhausting, frustrating, and unnecessary, because most fertile people won't understand or empathize with your situation. Do not feel that you have to defend your child-free choice or argue its merits: You owe no one any apologies or explanations. Over time, child-free couples find some of their relationships endure; in other instances, they develop friendships with those, with and without children, who value and respect their choice.

Making Children a Part of Your Life

> 🐦 A very special friend put her baby in my arms and left us alone. I cuddled that infant and fell in love. That child and I have had a special relationship ever since.

❦ I was furious when my younger sister got pregnant. My mother's delight was very painful to see. But I have faced my envy and now love my role as Auntie. I dote on my nieces and nephews and then give them back!

Your child-free life-style provides many opportunities to share the joy and special company of kids. There are children everywhere and countless ways to include them in your daily activities. Nephews, nieces, cousins, and friends' children enjoy spending time with fun-loving adults. Outings to the playground, zoo, swimming pool, sports arena, circus, theater, or amusement park create wonderful memories for you and the kids and a welcome respite for their parents.

Local schools and churches welcome volunteers to work with children. Perhaps you have a special talent in music, woodworking, cooking, art, computers, or fishing to share. Many local kids' softball, football, and soccer teams need volunteer coaches and organizers. Scouting organizations, Big Brother and Big Sister programs, local YMCAs and YWCAs, tutoring services, and programs for troubled youngsters also appreciate and need volunteers.

The Legacy of Child-Free Living

Peace, contentment, and a sense of completeness are often realized gradually by child-free couples and singles. Those who consciously and purposefully embrace this choice emphasize its joyful and ultimately healing aspects. They have made an important life decision, and by gently but firmly closing one door, they have opened many more exciting ones into the future.

A FAMILY OF TWO

You are now a new and consciously chosen family of two created from the wisdom, fortitude, compassion, and understanding gained from your infertility struggle. These qualities can last a lifetime, strengthening your marriage and enabling you to master future challenges.

Like all families, yours should be cherished and celebrated! Keep scrapbooks, photo albums, and journals of your experiences, travels, triumphs, and adventures. Create holiday traditions and special birthday and anniversary rituals to celebrate your unique and loving family.

Enjoy yourselves and the advantages that come with child-free living. Travel, sleep late, indulge in spur-of-the-moment impulses and outings. Treasure each other and take advantage of opportunities to grow, spend time together, and enrich your lives in every way.

MOVING FORWARD

A child-free identity embodies both a return to a happier sense of self and a rebirth as individuals and a couple. Because you no longer wish to become parents, much of your pre-infertility essence and spirit can safely surface. You can recapture much of what you had lost during infertility.

Standing on a new and firm foundation, you can move ahead with your lives. You again regard yourselves as valued and contributing members of the human family and realize that there are many ways, in addition to parenting, to making your mark on the world in your lifetime.

Glossary

abortion — The termination of a pregnancy, initiated either spontaneously by the body or intentionally by medical intervention.

abruptio placentae — A condition in which the placenta separates from the uterus.

acrosin — An enzyme contained in the sperm head that helps the sperm penetrate the ova.

acrosome — A cap enclosed in the head of the sperm that contains enzymes that aid in fertilization.

ACTH — See adrenocorticotropic hormone.

acupressure — An ancient Eastern healing technique that applies pressure to key energy points to restore balance in the body.

acupuncture — An ancient Eastern healing art that inserts slender needles into key energy points to restore balance in the body.

acute salpingitis — Inflammation of the Fallopian tube caused by an infection.

adenoma — A small benign tumor.

adhesiolysis — Cutting of adhesions from pelvic organs or bowel.

adhesions — Scar tissue formed by the body after surgery, disease, infection, or inflammation.

adnexa — The ovaries and Fallopian tubes.

adoption — An arrangement, sanctioned by legal decree, in which an individual or couple parents and raises the biological child of others.

adoption triad — The three parties involved in any adoption: the birth-parents, the adoptive parents, and the adopted child.

adrenocorticotropic hormone (ACTH) — A hormone produced by the pituitary, which stimulates the adrenal glands to release cortisol hormone.

aerobic exercise — A consistent, uninterrupted cardiovascular workout, usually thirty to forty minutes in duration.

agglutinization — The clumping of two or more sperm together.

amenorrhea — The absence of menstrual cycles.

amenorrhea galactorrhea — The absence of menstrual cycles along with the presence of milk in the breasts.

amniocentesis — A test done during pregnancy, often in women older than thirty-five years, which examines amniotic fluid for chromosomal characteristics.

ampulla — The middle section of the Fallopian tube.

androgens — Male hormones produced by both sexes.

andrologist — A urologist who specializes in male reproductive problems.

andrology — The study of the male reproductive system.

anesthesia — The numbing of pain through drugs.

anovulation — The absence of ovulation.

anoxia — An absence or deficiency of oxygen that may affect the fetus during labor or birth.

argon beam coagulator (ABC) — Surgical tool that directs an electrical current to affected tissue through a stream of argon gas.

artificial insemination by husband (AIH) — A process in which the sperm of a husband is inseminated into his mate's uterus through intrauterine insemination (IUI).

Assisted Reproductive Technology (ART) — A variety of high-tech methods used to assist conception; includes in vitro fertilization (IVF), gamete intrafallopian transfer (GIFT), zygote intrafallopian transfer (ZIFT), and egg donor IVF.

asthenospermia — A condition in which less than half the sperm in the ejaculate are motile.

atretic process — A natural process in which most of the immature oocytes a female is born with slowly disintegrate during her childhood and reproductive years.

azoospermia — A total absence of sperm in the ejaculate.

balloon tuboplasty — A non-surgical technique that passes a catheter containing a tiny balloon or coil through a blockage in the Fallopian tube.

basal body temperature (BBT) chart — A chart used to graph daily basal (upon awakening and before any activity) body temperature during the menstrual cycle.

bicornate uterus — A congenital physical abnormality of the uterus where there is a partial duplication of the uterus.

biochemical pregnancy — Also termed "pre-clinical pregnancy," a temporary elevation of hCG hormone that only lasts for a few days; not a viable, on-going pregnancy.

birth control pills — Synthetic female hormones used as contraceptives or for treatment of some diseases, such as endometriosis.

birthparents — The biological parents of an adopted child.

bromocriptine (Parlodel) — A drug that inhibits prolactin hormone secretion.

Caesarean birth — The delivery of a baby surgically through an abdominal incision, rather than vaginally.

capacitation — A process occurring after ejaculation that alters the sperm so it can penetrate an egg.

CAT scan — An X-ray technique that produces a computerized picture of the interior of the body.

caudal anesthesia — A type of anesthetic that is injected into the air spaces around the spinal column and numbs the nerve endings leading to the legs and pelvic area.

centrifuge — A method that quickly spins an ejaculate, separating the sperm from the seminal plasma.

cerclage — A technique, sometimes utilized in cases of a threatened second-trimeter miscarriage, that secures the cervix with tiny sutures.

cervical mucus — Secretions of the cervix, which usually change character throughout the menstrual cycle and aid sperm transport, storage, and filtering.

cervix — The narrow opening (or neck) that connects the uterus to the vagina; able to dilate many times its size during labor and delivery.

child-free living — A resolution to infertility in which a couple, after a period of grieving, chooses a fulfilling and productive lifestyle without parenting.

chiropractic — An alternative healing technique that utilizes manual adjustment of the spinal column to restore balance to the body.

chlamydia — A sexually transmitted disease that can cause impaired fertility or sterility.

chocolate cysts — Ovarian cysts formed by endometriosis; also called endometriomas.

chromosome — The parts of the nucleus of a body cell that hold the parent's genetic information in twisted strands of a substance called deoxyribonucleic acid (DNA).

chronic salpingitis — Scarring or blockages of the Fallopian tube(s) caused by infection.

cilia — The microscopic, hairlike projections in the Fallopian tubes that propel the ovum toward the uterus.

climacteric — The gradual cessation of menses, usually occurring between a woman's mid-forties and early fifties, that culminates in a final menstrual period (the menopause).

clinical pregnancy — A pregnancy in which a sac of the fetus is visible on ultrasound examination.

clitoris — A female sexual organ composed of erectile tissue and highly sensitive to stimulation.

clomiphene citrate (Clomid or Serophene) — A commonly prescribed "fertility drug" that induces ovulation.

complete abortion — Expulsion of all fetal and placental tissue by the body.

Computer Assisted Semen Analysis (CASA) — Utilization of a computer to interpret a semen analysis.

conception — The fertilization of an ovum by a sperm.

contraindications — Conditions where a drug or procedure should not be used.

corpus luteum — Literally Latin for "yellow body," the formation on the ovary after the follicle has ovulated that secretes progesterone hormone.

cryopreservation — The process of freezing, preserving, and storing sperm, ova, and embryos.

cumulus oophorus — The cloudlike outer covering of the ovum.

curettage — Scraping of the uterine lining.

danazol (Danocrine) — A drug derived from male hormones used to treat endometriosis.

DES — See diethylstilbestrol.

diethylstilbestrol (DES) — A synthetic form of estrogen given to some pregnant women between 1940 and 1971 to prevent miscarriage that sometimes caused abnormalities in their offspring.

dilation and curettage (D & C) — A medical procedure, done under anesthesia, that scrapes the interior of the uterus.

donor insemination (DI) — A process in which sperm from a donor male is inseminated in a fertile woman with the hope of conception and successful pregnancy.

duct obstruction — A blockage in the epididymis or vas deferens of the male.

dysmenorrhea — Painful menses.

ectopic pregnancy — A pregnancy that implants outside the uterus, usually in the Fallopian tube, and creates a life-threatening condition.

egg donor — A woman who donates ova, usually after ovulation induction with fertility drugs, to another couple for an Assisted Reproductive Technology (ART) attempt.

egg donor in vitro fertilization — An Assisted Reproductive Technology (ART) techique that uses ova donated by another woman, fertilizes them with the sperm of the recipient's mate, and transfers the embryo(s) to the recipient's uterus for gestation and birth.

ejaculate — Semen discharged through the urethra during male climax.

electroejaculation — A procedure developed for men unable to ejaculate because of spinal injuries, which stimulates ejaculation through the use of an electrical current passed through a slender rectal probe.

electrosurgery — A microsurgery technique that uses electrical needles for cutting or adhesion removal.

embryo — A term used to describe the fertilized ovum through about the eight-cell stage of development.

embryo donation — The donation of cryopreserved embryos from one couple to another for use with in vitro fertilization, usually after the former has successfully birthed their child(ren).

embryo transfer — The transfer of embryos fertilized in the laboratory to either the uterus (IVF) or Fallopian tube(s) (ZIFT).

endocrine system — A group of glands that contribute hormones to the bloodstream.

endocrinologist — A physician who specializes in problems of the endocrine system.

endometrial biopsy — A female workup procedure in which a bit of endometrial lining is scraped or suctioned and then evaluated for maturation.

endometriomas — Ovarian cysts formed by endometriosis.

endometriosis — A condition in which the endometrial cells that normally line the uterus travel to other sites, implant, and grow during the menstrual cycle.

endometritis — Infection or inflammation of the uterine lining.

endometrium — The lining of the uterus that nurtures the fertilized embryo or is expelled during menstruation.

epididymis — The duct system that matures, develops, and transports fertile sperm.

epididymitis — Inflammation of the epididymis.

epididymovasotomy — Surgery to remedy a blockage within the epididymis.

epidural anesthesia — The injection during surgery of drugs into the air spaces of the spinal column to numb the nerve endings to the legs and pelvis.

estrogen — A female hormone, produced by the developing egg follicles during the reproductive years, that causes stimulation of the uterine lining and changes in cervical mucus.

Fallopian tubes — Also called the oviducts, a pair of tubes attached to either side of the uterus that retrieve and carry the ova from the ovary to the uterus.

fertilization — The union of egg and sperm.

fetus — The developing embryo, from the second month of gestation to birth.

fibroid tumors — Benign uterine growths composed of smooth muscle.

fimbria — The hairlike endings of the Fallopian tubes that retrieve the ovum as it is released from the ovary.

follicle-stimulating hormone (FSH) — A hormone released by the pituitary gland that triggers ovum development or sperm production; may also be used in drug form (Metrodin) for ovulation induction.

fost-adopt programs — State or county programs that place children in foster homes as a first step in the adoption process.

frozen embryo transfer (FET) — The transfer of previously frozen embryos into either the uterus or Fallopian tube(s).

fructose test — A male fertility test that checks for the presence of fructose sugar in the semen.

FSH — See follicle-stimulating hormone.

galactorrhea — The presence of milk in the breasts of a woman who is not pregnant or has not recently given birth.

gamete — An egg or sperm cell.

gamete intrafallopian transfer (GIFT) — An Assisted Reproductive Technology (ART) procedure that removes one or more eggs from the female partner, and along with her mate's sperm, places them in the Fallopian tube(s) for natural fertilization.

general anesthesia — A mixture of several drugs administered during surgery to induce and maintain unconsciousness.

genitals — External sexual organs.

GIFT — See gamete intrafallopian transfer.

gonadotropins — The hormones FSH and LH that stimulate, in women and men, the production of ova and sperm.

gonadotropin-releasing hormone (GnRH) — The hormone secreted by the hypothalamus that signals the pituitary to release FSH and LH hormones.

GnRH analogs (Lupron or Synarel) — A synthetic, more potent derivation of GnRH, sometimes used in the treatment of endometriosis and in Assisted Reproductive Technology (ART) cycles.

gonorrhea — A bacterial, sexually transmitted disease.

Graafian follicle — The dominant oocyte in the ovary that will be ovulated.

gynecology — A branch of medicine that specializes in the study and treatment of female reproduction, pregnancy, and birth.

gynecologist — A doctor of medicine who specializes in female reproduction, pregnancy, and birth (also called an ob-gyn).

habitual abortion — A medical term used to describe three or more miscarriages.

hamster egg test — See Sperm Penetration Assay (SPA).

HCG — See human chorionic gonadotropin.

hemizona assay (sperm binding test) — A test that measures the ability of the sperm to adhere to the zona pellucida of a split, non-viable human egg.

heparin lock — A device used to administer intravenous drugs.

HMG — See human menopausal gonadotropin.

HSG — See hysterosalpingogram.

home study — Part of the agency or independent adoption process, several interviews and home visits with prospective adoptive parent(s).

hormones — Secretions of the endocrine glands that trigger complex biochemical processes.

Hühner's test — See postcoital (PCT) test.

human chorionic gonadatropin (hCG) — A hormone produced by the placenta during pregnancy; also used, in conjunction with hMG or clomiphene, to trigger ovulation.

human menopausal gonadotropin (hMG) (Pergonal) — A fertility drug composed of purified FSH and LH natural hormone, derived from the urine of post-menopausal women.

hyaluronidase — An enzyme contained in the head of the sperm that aids in opening a path to the egg.

hyperprolactinism — An excessive amount of prolactin hormone in the bloodstream.

hyperstimulation syndrome — A rare side effect of ovulation induction with hMG or FSH, symptoms include ovarian enlargement, abdominal swelling, and fluid retention.

hypothalamus — The area of the brain near the pituitary gland that regulates hormonal secretions of the pituitary.

hysterectomy — A surgical procedure that removes part or all of the uterus.

hysterosalpingogram (HSG) — A work-up test that provides an X-ray picture of the uterus and tubes and checks tubal patency (openness).

hysteroscopy — Viewing the inside of the uterus through a narrow fitted telescope inserted, during anesthesia, through the cervical opening.

ICSH — See interstitial cell stimulating hormone.

identified agency adoption — An agency-facilitated adoption where birthparent(s) and adoptive parent(s) select each other.

identity-release sperm donor — A man who agrees to donate sperm for artificial insemination, with the understanding that identifying information may be released to any resulting offspring, at their written request, when they reach the age of eighteen.

idiopathic oligospermia — A low sperm count without known cause or pathology.

immobilization — A condition in which the sperm are unable to move forward; they may be immobilized or "quiver and shake" in place.

immunobead binding test — A test to check for the presence and location of sperm antibodies on the sperm.

immunoglobulins — Protein substances that form antibodies to foreign cells.

immunological infertility — Infertility caused by antibody formation to sperm that may occur in either the male or female.

implantation — The attachment of a fertilized egg to the uterine lining.

impotence — The inability to achieve or maintain an erection.

incompetent cervix — A weakened cervix that is unable to support the uterus as the fetus grows; may be the cause of second trimester miscarriages.

incomplete abortion — A miscarriage in which not all the fetal tissue is expelled from the uterus.

independent or private adoption — Adoption in which the birthparent(s) and adoptive parent(s) arrange the placement of the child themselves, usually with the assistance of a knowledgable intermediary.

infertility — The inability to conceive within one year of unprotected intercourse, or the inability to carry a pregnancy to term.

infertility counselor or therapist — A mental health professional who is knowledgable about the effects of infertility on the individual, couple, or family, and has preferably personally experienced this problem. May have a doctorate (Ph.D., Ed.D.), or be a licensed clinical social worker (LCSW) or marriage, family, and child counselor (MFCC).

infertility specialist — An obstetrician/gynecologist (ob/gyn) who has received additional experience, education, and training in the diagnosis and treatment of infertility.

inflammation — The reaction of the body's tissue to infection through swelling, pain, and/or scar formation.

infundibulum — The trumpetlike end of the Fallopian tube that nestles near the ovary.

inpatient surgery — Usually "major" surgery for which the patient is hospitalized for several days.

international adoption — An adoption of a child from another country.

interstitial cell stimulating hormone (ICSH) — The LH hormone in the male that is instrumental in stimulating sperm production.

intrauterine device (IUD) — A type of contraceptive, usually a "loop" or "shield," placed in the uterus; its use has been associated with salpingitis and infertility.

intrauterine insemination (IUI) — the insemination of specially treated (centrifuged and "washed") sperm into the uterus through a slender catheter.

in vitro fertilization (IVF) — An Assisted Reproductive Technology (ART) that extracts one or more eggs from the mother, fertilizes them with the father's sperm outside the body, and transfers the developing embryo(s) into the uterus for gestation.

in vivo fertilization — Fertilization occurring naturally within the body.

isthmus — The narrow portion of a Fallopian tube, which is attached to the uterus.

IUD — See intrauterine device.

IVF — See in vitro fertlization.

IVF Registry — An annual compilation of IVF statistics, including initiated cycles and pregnancy rates according to age and fertility factors, published by the American Fertility Society (see *Resources*).

karyotyping — A test that photographs chromosomes for genetic information.

Klinefelter's syndrome — A rare male disorder that involves an extra x chromosome.

laparoscopic linear salpingostomy — Removal of an ectopic pregnancy with laparoscopic surgery.

laparoscopy and laparoscopic surgery — A surgical procedure, often performed during the female infertility workup, in which the specialist views the reproductive organs through a telescope-like instrument, inserted through the navel during general anesthesia; many types of pelvic surgery may also be performed during laparoscopy.

laparotomy — Opening of the abdomen by incision.

laser surgery — An acronym for light amplification by stimulated emission of radiation, a type of surgery that uses a laser beam either by itself or in conjunction with other microsurgical techniques to treat pelvic disease or abnormalities.

leuprolide (Lupron) — See GnRH analogs.

Leydig cells — Cells within the testes that manufacture testosterone hormone.

LH — See luteinizing hormone.

local anesthesia — Injection of pain-numbing medicine directly into the skin or other tissues without inducing unconsciousness.

luteal (or secretory) phase — The second half of the menstrual cycle, from ovulation to menses.

luteal phase defect — A shortened luteal phase or one with inadequate progesterone production.

lutein — A yellow pigment the body manufactures from cholesterol.

luteinizing hormone (LH) — A pituitary hormone important to ovulation and progesterone production in women and testosterone production in men.

magnetic resonance imaging (MRI) — A technique that uses a magnetic field to create a visual image of the internal organs of the body.

menarche — A girl's first menstrual period, usually occurring between the ages of nine and fourteen.

menopause — The last menstrual period after years of diminishing or erratic menses (the climacteric), commonly occurring between the ages of forty-five and fifty-five.

menstrual cycle — The monthly cycle of ovulation, usually twenty-five to thirty-five days long.

menstruation — The cyclical shedding of the endometrium when pregnancy does not occur.

microadenoma — A tiny, benign pituitary tumor.

micromanipulation — Experimental techniques that create a tiny opening in the outer covering of the egg to assist sperm penetration.

Microscopic Epididymal Sperm Aspiration (MESA) — Surgical removal of the sperm from the epididymis for use in an Assisted Reproductive Technology (ART) cycle.

microsurgery — A delicate type of surgery performed through a microscope.

miscarriage — The loss of a pregnancy, most often in the first trimester.

missed abortion — A miscarriage where fetal tissue remains and symptoms have subsided.

morphology — The shape and maturity of sperm cells.

motility — The forward progression and movement of sperm.

mycoplasma — An infectious microorganism that may contribute to infertility or miscarriage problems.

myomectomy — A surgical procedure that opens the uterus to remove fibroid growths.

natural childbirth — Delivering a baby vaginally without the use of anesthesia.

natural cycle in vitro fertilization — A variation of IVF performed with natural ovulation, rather than ovulation induction with fertility drugs.

neonatal death — The death of a newborn baby within a month of birth.

neonatologist — A pediatrician who has specialized training in the care of newborn (including premature) babies.

nidation — Implantation of the fertilized ova into the uterus.

nitrous oxide — A gas used during anesthesia to maintain unconsciousness.

obstetrician/gynecologist (ob/gyn) — A physician who specializes in female reproduction, pregnancy, and birth.

occlusive radiological procedures — A male infertility treatment where a mini-balloon or coil is guided by X-ray, under anesthesia, to the spermatic vein to block blood flow to the varicocele.

oligospermia — A persistently subnormal sperm count.

oocyte — An immature ovum.

oocyte retrieval — An IVF procedure, usually performed with anesthesia, where eggs are retrieved through vaginally guided ultrasound.

open adoption — A form of adoption in which the identities of the triad members are known to each other; the degree, duration, and frequency of contact or involvement varies in each case.

orgasm — In the male, sexual climax resulting in ejaculation; in the female, sexual climax usually through clitoral stimulation.

os — Tiny opening of the cervix.

outpatient surgery — Usually "minor" surgery performed in the hospital; patient is released the same day.

ovaries — Female reproductive organs that store and release eggs during ovulation, as well as the hormones estrogen and progesterone.

oviduct — The Fallopian tube.

ovulation — The release of an egg (ovum) from the ovary.

ovulation induction — The stimulation of oocyte development and release through female hormone therapy.

ovulation predictor kit — Intended for home use, a kit that tests the LH level in the urine and "predicts" the approach of ovulation.

ovulation pump — A battery-run pump that administers gonadotropin-releasing hormone in timed pulses to induce ovulation.

ovum — A female egg; the plural of the word is "ova."

PAP smear test — Analysis of a slide of cervical cells for abnormalities.

partial zona dissection — A micromanipulation technique that mechanically creates an opening in the outer layer of the ovum to assist sperm penetration.

patration — The action of the sperm opening a pathway to the ovum for those that follow.

pelvic inflammatory disease (PID) — A catchall phrase referring to inflammation of the pelvis; most PID occurs in the Fallopian tubes.

pelviscopy — A technique utilized during laparoscopy where a half-inch incision is made through the abdominal wall to perform pelvic surgery.

penis — The male sexual organ that excretes urine and ejaculates semen.

peristalsis — Rhythmic contractions that move the sperm through the epididymis and vas deferens or move the egg through the Fallopian tube.

peritoneum — The abdominal lining.

PID — See pelvic inflammatory disease.

pipelle — A slender plastic catheter used for endometrial biopsy.

pituitary gland — An endocrine gland, located near the base of the brain, that secretes various hormones and orchestrates the complex interactions of the menstrual cycle and spermatogenesis.

placenta previa — A condition in which the placenta attaches between the fetus and the cervix.

polycystic ovarian disease — A complex hormonal problem in which the ovaries fail to ovulate and instead form numerous tiny cysts.

polyps — Small growths sometimes found in the uterus or cervix.

post-birth control pill syndrome — The body's inability to resume ovulatory cycles following use of birth control pills.

postcoital test (Sims-Hühner) — A workup test performed prior to ovulation, and several hours after intercourse, that assesses the cervical mucus and the sperms' reaction to it.

pregnancy loss — A miscarriage, ectopic pregnancy, or stillbirth.

pregnancy reduction (selective termination) — Abortion of one or more fetuses in cases of multiple pregnancy, usually resulting from an Assisted Reproductive Technology cycle or from use of ovulation induction drugs.

premature ovarian failure — A rare condition in which the ovary ceases functioning prematurely, before menopause should naturally occur.

progesterone — A female hormone produced by the ovaries in the second phase of the menstrual cycle.

prolactin — A hormone secreted by the pituitary and associated with lactation.

proliferative phase — The first half of the menstrual cycle that culminates in ovulation.

pronatalism — A value system that socially inculcates and strongly encourages pregnancy, childbirth, and parenting in adult life.

propofol — A drug often used during general anesthesia to induce immediate unconsciousness.

prostaglandins — Hormones that induce uterine contractions before menstruation or during labor.

prostate gland — A male reproductive gland that contributes seminal fluids to the sperm before ejaculation.

RESOLVE — A nationwide organization, founded in 1977 by Barbara Eck Menning, that provides referrals, support, and medical information to infertile individuals (see Resources).

resolving infertility — The complex and painful process of confronting and grieving one's infertility, and investigating and deciding on an appropriate medical, adoptive, or child-free resolution.

retrograde bleeding — The "backing up" of menstrual fluid to the tubes, ovaries, or abdomen.

retrograde ejaculation — A disorder of the male reproductive system in which semen is ejaculated into the bladder.

Rubin's test — An outdated workup procedure that tested tubal patency by blowing carbon dioxide gas into the uterus.

salpingoneostomy — Opening the closed ends of the Fallopian tube(s) with surgery.

salpingitis — An infection of the Fallopian tubes, also called pelvic inflammatory disease (PID).

scrotum — The saclike skin that covers the testicles.

secondary amenorrhea — An absence of three or more consecutive menstrual cycles after puberty.

secondary infertility — The inability to conceive or birth another child after one or more pregnancies.

secretory cells — Fluid-secreting cells within the Fallopian tubes.

secretory or luteal phase — The second half of the menstrual cycle that nourishes the fertilized egg or, if pregnancy does not occur, culminates in menstruation.

semen — The thick (viscous), cloudy ejaculate that contains sperm and seminal fluids.

semen analysis — A workup test that analyzes a sample of semen for sperm count, motility, morphology, and other characteristics.

seminal vesicles — Small glands that store sperm and contribute much of the seminal fluid.

seminiferous tubules — Tubes within the testes that produce sperm.

serum hCG test — A test used to confirm pregnancy by measuring the level of hCG hormone in the blood.

serum progesterone test — A blood test, usually taken after ovulation, that measures the level of progesterone.

sexually transmitted disease (STD) — Any of several dozen viral or bacterial diseases transmitted by genital, oral, or anal sexual contact.

sonogram — See ultrasound.

sperm — The male germ cells, carrying genetic information, that fertilize an egg.

sperm antibodies — Substances manufactured by men or women's immune systems that cause sperm damage or destruction.

sperm bank — A clinic or facility that stores and preserves frozen donor sperm for use in artificial insemination.

sperm count — A rough estimate of the number of sperm in a given "counting area."

sperm penetration assay (SPA) — Also called the hamster egg test; a male fertility test that checks the sperm's ability to penetrate a hamster ovum.

sperm washing — A technique that separates the sperm from the seminal fluid.

spermatic cord — The duct system that transports sperm from the testicle to the urethra for ejaculation.

spermatogenesis — The process of sperm production.

spermatozoon — A fertile, mature sperm.

spinal anesthesia — An anesthetic injected into the spinal fluid to produce numbness in a general area of the body, usually below the waist, used during pelvic surgery or for Caesarean birth.

Spinnbarkeit test — A test that assesses the consistency and "stretchability" of cervical mucus.

spontaneous abortion — Commonly called miscarriage, the expulsion of a fetus by the body during the first or second trimester.

STD — See sexually transmitted disease.

Stein-Leventhal syndrome — See polycystic ovarian disease.

sterility — Permanent, untreatable infertility.

stillbirth — A third-trimester fetus that has died in utero or during delivery.

subzonal injection — An experimental micromanipulation technique that injects sperm into the space surrounding the nucleus of the ovum.

superovulation — The stimulation and development of a number of eggs through fertility drug treatment; usually used for Assisted Reproductive Technology (ART) procedures.

surrogate gestational mother — A woman who gestates and births the genetic child of an infertile couple.

surrogate mother — A woman who agrees to gestate and birth a child for an infertile couple, one that is conceived with her egg and the artificially inseminated sperm of the husband.

syphilis — A sexually transmitted disease.

T-mycoplasma — A microorganism that may be associated with infertility and miscarriage.

testes — Male reproductive organs that produce sperm and male hormones.

testicular biopsy — A procedure, performed under anesthesia, that removes a sample of tissue from the testicle.

testosterone — A male hormone manufactured by the testes.

threatened abortion — Vaginal staining and bleeding during pregnancy that may or may not result in a miscarriage.

thyroid — The endocrine gland that secretes thyroxin hormone and helps maintain metabolism.

toxemia — A pregnancy complication, usually occurring in the last trimester, that may include such symptoms as high blood pressure, swelling, and protein in the urine; requires immediate medical attention.

triad — See adoption triad.

tubal embryo transfer (TET) — The transfer of embryos two days after laboratory fertilization into the Fallopian tube(s).

tubal ligation — A female sterilization procedure that severs and ties off the Fallopian tubes.

tubal patency — An open tube without signs of blockage.

ultrasound — A technique that bounces sound waves off the body to produce an image, often used to monitor ovarian activity or pregnancy.

ultrasound guided aspiration — A procedure used during an Assisted Reproductive Technology (ART) cycle to retrieve mature ova through a needle, guided by ultrasound, through the vagina to the ovaries.

unexplained infertility — A "diagnosis" given to infertile couples for whom no organic problem can be detected in either partner.

ureaplasma — A microorganism that may contribute to fertility or miscarriage problems.

urethra — The tube that carries urine and semen through the penis.

urologist — A physician who specializes in urinary tract diseases and male reproductive problems; also called an andrologist.

uterus — The female reproductive organ that nurtures the fetus from implantation until birth.

vagina — The muscular passage between the uterus and exterior vulva.

varicocele — A varicose vein of the testicle.

varicocelectomy — A surgical procedure to treat varicocele problems by tying off the affected vein(s).

vas deferens — Two long ducts that connect the epididymis to the ejaculatory duct.

vasectomy — A male sterilization procedure which severs the vas deferens.

vasectomy reversal — A surgical procedure that repairs the severed vas deferens to hopefully restore fertility.

vasography — An X-ray of the vas deferens.

vena cavae — Two large veins that carry blood to the heart.

venereal disease — A sexually transmitted disease, commonly referring to chlamydia, syphilis, or gonorrhea.

videolaserlaparoscopy — A surgical technique that utilizes laser and tiny videocameras to perform laparoscopic surgery.

viscosity — The liquidity of the semen.

visualization — A relaxation technique that employs calming, peaceful, and healing images.

zona pellucida — The outer covering of the ovum that the sperm must penetrate before fertilization can occur.

zygote — A fertilized ovum.

zygote intrafallopian transfer (ZIFT) — An Assisted Reproductive Technology (ART) technique that transfers embryos one day after laboratory fertilization to the Fallopian tube(s).

Bibliography

General Infertility Readings

Bellina, Joseph., M.D., Ph.D., and Josleen Wilson. YOU *CAN* HAVE A BABY. New York: Crown, 1985.

Berger, Gary S., M.D., Goldstein, Marc, M.D., and Mark Fuerst. THE COUPLE'S GUIDE TO FERTILITY: HOW NEW MEDICAL ADVANCES CAN HELP YOU HAVE A BABY. New York: Doubleday, 1989.

Boston Women's Health Book Collective. "Infertility and Pregnancy Loss." Chapter 21 in THE NEW OUR BODIES, OUR SELVES. New York: Simon and Schuster, 1985.

DeCherney, Alan, M.D., and Mary Lake Polan, M.D. DECISION-MAKING IN INFERTILITY. Philadelphia: B. C. Decker, 1988.

Elmer-Dewitt, Philip. "Making Babies." TIME, 9/30/91, pp. 56-63.

Franklin, Robert R., M.D. and Dorothy Kay Brockman. IN PURSUIT OF FERTILITY: A CONSULTATION WITH A SPECIALIST. New York: Henry Holt, 1990.

Garcia, C. R., M.D., Mastroianni, L., Jr., M.D., Amelar, R., M.D., and L. Dubin, M.D. CURRENT THERAPY OF INFERTILITY. Philadelphia: B. C. Decker, 1988.

Menning, Barbara Eck. INFERTILITY: A GUIDE FOR THE CHILDLESS COUPLE. Englewood Cliffs, N.J.: Prentice-Hall, 1988, rev. ed.

Mosher, William D., Ph.D. and William F. Pratt, Ph.D. "Fecundity and Infertility in the United States, 1965-88." ADVANCE DATA. No. 192, December 4, 1990. Washington, D.C.: National Center for Health Statistics, U.S. Department of Health and Human Services.

Nachtigall, Robert D., M.D., and Elizabeth Mehren. OVERCOMING INFERTILITY: A PRACTICAL STRATEGY FOR NAVIGATING THE EMOTIONAL, MEDICAL, AND FINANCIAL MINEFIELDS OF TRYING TO HAVE A BABY. New York: Doubleday, 1991.

Seibel, Machelle, M.D., ed. INFERTILITY: A COMPREHENSIVE TEXT. Norwalk, CT: Appleton and Lange, 1990.

Stangel, John H. THE NEW FERTILITY AND CONCEPTION: THE ESSENTIAL GUIDE FOR CHILDLESS COUPLES. New York: New American Library, 1988, rev. ed.

U.S. Congress, Office of Technology Assessment. INFERTILITY: MEDICAL AND SOCIAL CHOICES. Washington, D.C.: U.S. Government Printing Office, May, 1988. Ordering and information desk: (202) 783-3238.

Weckstein, Louis N., M.D. "Treating the Infertile Woman Over 40." MEDICAL ASPECTS OF HUMAN SEXUALITY. (November, 1991), pp. 22-29.

Winston, Robert M.D. WHAT WE KNOW ABOUT INFERTILITY: DIAGNOSIS AND TREATMENT ALTERNATIVES. New York: The Free Press, 1986.

The Emotional Dynamics of Infertility

Arditti, Rita (ed). INFERTILITY: WOMEN SPEAK OUT ABOUT THEIR EXPERIENCES WITH REPRODUCTIVE MEDICINE. London: Pandora Press, 1989.

Becker, Gay, Ph.D. HEALING THE INFERTILE FAMILY: STRENGTHENING YOUR RELATIONSHIP IN THE SEARCH FOR PARENTHOOD. New York: Bantam, 1990.

Berg, Barbara. NOTHING TO CRY ABOUT. New York: Seaview Books, 1983, rev. ed.

Bombardieri, Merle. "The Twenty Minute Rule: First Aid for Couples in Distress." RESOLVE National Newsletter. (December 1983), p. 5.

Burns, Cheri. STEPMOTHERHOOD. New York: Times Books, 1985.

Chiappone, Janice M., Ph.D. "Infertility as a Nonevent: Impact, Coping, and Differences Between Men and Women." Ph.D. Diss., University of Maryland, 1984.

Fleming, Jeanne, Ph.D., "Infertility as a Chronic Illness." RESOLVE National Newsletter (December 1984).

Fleming, Jeanne, Ph.D., and Kenneth A. Burry, M.D., "Coping with Infertility: How Infertile People Process Grief." Paper presented to the National Annual Convention of the American Fertility Society, Chicago, October 1985.

Glazer, Ellen Sarasohn and Susan Lewis Cooper. WITHOUT CHILD: EXPERIENCING AND RESOLVING INFERTILITY. Lexington, MA: Lexington Books, 1988.

Gold, Michael. AND HANNAH WEPT. Philadelphia: Jewish Publications Society, 1988.

Greer, Germaine. SEX AND DESTINY: THE POLITICS OF HUMAN FERTILITY. New York: Harper and Row, 1984.

Greil, A. L., Leitko, T. A., and K. L. Porter. "Infertility: His and Hers." GENDER AND SOCIETY. 2: (1988), pp. 172-199.

Johnston, Patricia Irwin. UNDERSTANDING: A GUIDE TO IMPAIRED FERTILITY FOR FAMILY AND FRIENDS. Indianapolis: Perspectives Press, 1983.

Kübler-Ross, Elisabeth. ON DEATH AND DYING. New York: Macmillan, 1969.

Kushner, Harold S. WHEN BAD THINGS HAPPEN TO GOOD PEOPLE. New York: Avon, 1981.

Liebmann-Smith, Joan. IN PURSUIT OF PREGNANCY. New York: Newmarket Press, 1987.

Mason, Mary Martin. THE MIRACLE SEEKERS: AN ANTHOLOGY OF INFERTILITY. Indianapolis: Perspectives Press, 1987.

Mitchard, Jacquelyn. MOTHER LESS CHILD. New York: W. W. Norton, 1985.

Morgan, Susanne. COPING WITH A HYSTERECTOMY. New York: Dial Press, 1983.

Nachtigall, Robert D., M.D., Becker, Gay, Ph.D., and M. Wozny. "Effects of Gender Specific Diagnosis." FERTILITY AND STERILITY. 57:1 (January, 1992), pp. 113-121.

Nsiah-Jefferson, L. and E. J. Hall. "Reproductive Technology: Perspectives and Implications for Low-Income Women and Women of Color." In Ratcliff, K. S., ed. HEALING TECHNOLOGY: FEMINIST PERSPECTIVES. Ann Arbor: University of Michigan Press, 1989.

Overall, Christine, Ph.D. ETHICS AND HUMAN REPRODUCTION: A FEMINIST ANALYSIS. Boston: Allen and Unwin, 1987.

Pepperell, R. J. THE INFERTILE COUPLE. 2nd edition. Churchill, 1987.

Pfeffer, Naomi and Anne Woollett. THE EXPERIENCE OF INFERTILITY. London: Virago, 1983.

Rubin, Theodore I. OVERCOMING INDECISIVENESS: THE EIGHT STAGES OF EFFECTIVE DECISION-MAKING. New York: Harper and Row, 1985.

Salzer, Linda P. SURVIVING INFERTILITY: A COMPASSIONATE GUIDE THROUGH THE EMOTIONAL CRISIS OF INFERTILITY. New York Harper, 1991, rev. ed.

Sandelowski, Margarete, Holditch-Davis, Diane and Betty G. Harris. "Living the Life: Explanations of Infertility." SOCIOLOGY OF HEALTH AND ILLNESS. 12:2 (June, 1990), pp. 195-215.

Sandelowski, Margarete and C. Pollock. "Women's Experiences of Infertility." IMAGE: JOURNAL OF NURSING SCHOLARSHIP. 19: (1986), pp. 70-74.

Schwan, Kassie. THE INFERTILITY MAZE: FINDING YOUR WAY TO THE RIGHT HELP AND THE RIGHT ANSWERS. Chicago: Contemporary Books, 1988.

Sha, Janet L. MOTHERS OF THYME: CUSTOMS AND RITUALS OF INFERTILITY AND MISCARRIAGE. Ann Arbor: Lida Rose Press, 1990.

Stephenson, Lynda R. GIVE US A CHILD: COPING WITH THE PERSONAL CRISIS OF INFERTILITY. New York: Harper and Row, 1987.

Stout, Martha. WITHOUT CHILD: A COMPASSIONATE LOOK AT INFERTILITY. Grand Rapids, MI: Zondervan, 1985.

Van Regenmorter, John, Van Regenmorter, Sylvia and Joe McIlhany. DEAR GOD: WHY CAN'T WE HAVE A BABY? Grand Rapids, MI: Baker Book House, 1986.

Wasserman, Marion Lee. SEARCHING FOR THE STORK: ONE COUPLE'S STRUGGLE TO START A FAMILY. New York: North American Library, 1988.

Taking Care of Yourself

Bailey, Covert. THE NEW FIT OR FAT. Boston: Houghton Mifflin, 1991.

Borysenko, Joan, Ph.D. MINDING THE BODY, MENDING THE MIND. Reading, MA: Addison-Wesley, 1987.

Bradshaw, John. HEALING THE SHAME THAT BINDS YOU. Deerfield Beach, FL: Heath Communications, 1988.

Brody, Jane. JANE BRODY'S GOOD FOOD BOOK. New York: Bantam, 1987.

Carper, Jean. THE FOOD PHARMACY. New York: Bantam, 1988.

Charlesworth, Edward A., Ph.D., and Ronald G. Nathan, Ph.D. STRESS MANAGEMENT. New York: Ballantine, 1984.

Cooper, Kenneth H., M.D. THE AEROBICS PROGRAM FOR TOTAL WELL-BEING. New York: Bantam, 1982.

_____. THE NEW AEROBICS FOR WOMEN. New York: Bantam, 1988.

Cousins, Norman. ANATOMY OF AN ILLNESS. New York: W. W. Norton, 1979.

Fonda, Jane. JANE FONDA'S NEW WORKOUT BOOK AND WEIGHT LOSS PROGRAM. New York: Simon and Schuster, 1986.

Gahagan, D. SWITCH DOWN AND QUIT. Berkeley: Ten Speed Press, 1987.

Gil, Eliana, Ph.D. OUTGROWING THE PAIN: A BOOK FOR AND ABOUT ADULTS ABUSED AS CHILDREN. San Francisco: Launch Press, 1983.

Greenwood, Sadja, M.D. MENOPAUSE, NATURALLY: PREPARING FOR THE SECOND HALF OF LIFE. Volcano, CA: Volcano Press, 1989, rev. ed.

Hasselbring, Bobbie, Greenwood, Sadja, M.D., et al. THE MEDICAL SELF-CARE BOOK OF WOMEN'S HEALTH. New York: Doubleday, 1987.

Jacobson, Michael F., Ph.D., Lefferts, Lisa Y. and Anne W. Garland. SAFE FOOD. Los Angeles: Living Planet Press, 1991.

Kushner, Harold. WHEN BAD THINGS HAPPEN TO GOOD PEOPLE. New York: Schocken Books, 1981.

Lappe, Frances Moore. DIET FOR A SMALL PLANET: TENTH ANNIVERSARY EDITION. New York: Ballantine, 1982.

Murray, Michael T., N.D., and Joseph E. Pizzorno, N.D. AN ENCYCLOPEDIA OF NATURAL MEDICINE. Rocklin, CA: Prima Publishing, 1991.

Nierenberg, Judith, R.N., and Florence Janovic. THE HOSPITAL EXPERIENCE: A GUIDE FOR PATIENTS AND THEIR FAMILIES. New York: Berkley Publishing, 1985.

Notman, Malkah T., M.D., and Carol Nadelson, M.D., eds. THE WOMAN PATIENT: MEDICAL AND PSYCHOLOGICAL INTERFACES. New York: Plenum Publishing, 1982.

Orbach, Susie. FAT IS A FEMINIST ISSUE. New York: Berkley, 1990, rev. ed.

The People's Medical Publishing House, Beijing, China. THE CHINESE WAY TO A LONG AND HEALTHY LIFE. New York: Bell Publishing, 1984.

Robbins, John. DIET FOR A NEW AMERICA. Walpole, N.H.: Stillpoint, 1987.

Robertson, Laurel, Flinders, Carol, and Brian Ruttenhal. THE NEW LAUREL'S KITCHEN: A HANDBOOK FOR VEGETARIAN COOKERY AND NUTRITION. Berkeley: Ten Speed Press, 1986.

Rosas, Debbie, Rosas, Carlos and Katherine Martin. NON-IMPACT AEROBICS. New York, Villard, 1987.

Samuels, Mike, M.D., and Nancy Samuels. SEEING WITH THE MIND'S EYE. New York: Random House, 1975.

_____. THE WELL ADULT BOOK. New York: Summit Books, 1988.

Satir, Virginia. SELF-ESTEEM. Berkeley: Celestial Arts, 1990.

Sharkey, Brian J., Ph.D. PHYSIOLOGY OF FITNESS. Champaign, IL: Human Kinetics Publishers, 1984.

Sheehy, Gail. PASSAGES. New York: Bantam Books, 1976.

Siegel, Bernie S., M.D. LOVE, MEDICINE AND MIRACLES. New York: Harper and Row, 1986.

Simonton, Carl, M.D., and Stephanie Matthews Simonton. GETTING WELL AGAIN. New York: Bantam, 1980.

Sussman, John, M.D. and B. Blake Levitt. BEFORE YOU CONCEIVE: THE COMPLETE PREPREGNANCY GUIDE. New York: Bantam, 1989.

Toguchi, Masaru and Frank Z. Warren, M.D. THE COMPLETE GUIDE TO ACUPUNCTURE AND ACUPRESSURE. New York: Gramercy, 1985.

Weil, Andrew, M.D. NATURAL HEALTH, NATURAL MEDICINE: A COMPREHENSIVE MANUAL FOR WELLNESS AND SELF-CARE. Boston: Houghton-Mifflin, 1990.

Weiss, Kay, M.P.H., ed. WOMEN'S HEALTH CARE: A GUIDE TO ALTERNATIVES. Reston, VA: Reston Publishing, 1984.

Winstein, Merryl. YOUR FERTILITY SIGNALS: USING THEM TO ACHIEVE OR AVOID PREGNANCY, NATURALLY. St. Louis: Smooth Stone Press, 1990.

Zoldbrod, Aline P., Ph.D. GETTING AROUND THE BOULDER IN THE ROAD: USING IMAGERY TO COPE WITH FERTILITY PROBLEMS. For ordering information contact the author, c/o Lexington Books, 70 Lincoln St., Boston, MA 02111.

Hormonal Problems and Their Treatment

Diamond, Michael P., M.D., DeCherney, Alan, M.D., and Bill Yee, M.D., "Ovulation Induction." INFERTILITY AND REPRODUCTIVE MEDICINE CLINICS OF NORTH AMERICA. 1:1 (October 1990).

Filicori, M., M.D., Flamigni, C., M.D., Meriggiola, P., M.D., et al. "Endocrine Response Determines the Clinical Outcome of Pulsatile GnRH Hormone Ovulation Induction in Different Ovulatory Disorders." JOURNAL OF CLINICAL ENDOCRINOLOGY AND METABOLISM. 72 (1991), p. 965.

Graedon, Joe, and Teresa Graedon. THE NEW PEOPLE'S PHARMACY: DRUG BREAKTHROUGHS OF THE 80s. New York: Bantam, 1985.

Long, James W., M.D. THE ESSENTIAL GUIDE TO PRESCRIPTION DRUGS. New York, Harper, 1992.

Rayburn, William F., M.D., Zuspun, Frederick, M.D., and Jeanne Fitzgerald. EVERY WOMAN'S PHARMACY. New York: Doubleday, 1984.

Seibel, Machelle, M.D. "Update on Polycystic Ovary Syndrome." RESOLVE NATIONAL NEWSLETTER. 16 (1991), p. 5.

Pelvic Abnormalities and Microsurgery Treatment

Arias, Fernando, M.D. "Cervical Cerclage for the Temporary Treatment of Patients with Placenta Previa." OBSTETRICS AND GYNECOLOGY. 70:4 (April, 1988), pp. 545-548.

Ballweg, Mary Lou, Miller, Charles E., M.D., Redwine, David, M.D., Keye, William, M.D., and Robert McWilliams, M.D. "Surgery through the Laparoscope: The Future Has Arrived." ENDOMETRIOSIS ASSOCIATION NEWSLETTER. 2:4 (1990), pp. 1-7.

Clapp, Diane. "DES: Its Impact on Infertilty." Reprint available from National Office of RESOLVE (see Resources).

Englemayer, Sheldon, and Robert Wagman. LORD'S JUSTICE. New York: Doubleday, 1986.

FERTILITY AND PREGNANCY GUIDE FOR DES DAUGHTERS AND SONS. DES Action, USA, 1984. For ordering information contact: DES Action USA (see Resources).

Galen, Donald I., M.D. "A Guide to Safe Outpatient Tubal Reanastomosis." MEDICAL ASPECTS OF HUMAN SEXUALITY, 1992.

Herbst, Arthur L. "Reproductive and Gynecologic Surgical Experience in DES-exposed Daughters." AMERICAN JOURNAL OF OBSTETRICS AND GYNECOLOGY 14:8 (December 1981), pp. 1019-1028.

Kaufman, D. W., et al. "Intrauterine Contraceptive Device Use and Pelvic Inflammatory Disease." AMERICAN JOURNAL OF OBSTETRICS AND GYNECOLOGY 136 (1980), pp. 159-62.

Mage, Gerard, M.D., Canis, Michel, M.D., Manhes, Hubert, M.D., et al. "Laparo-scopic Management of Adnexal Cystic Masses." JOURNAL OF GYNECO-LOGICAL SURGERY. 6:2 (1990), pp. 71-79.

Mintz, Morton. AT ANY COST. New York: Pantheon, 1986.

Nezhat, C., M.D., Crowgey, S. R., M.D., and C. P. Garrison, M.D. "Surgical Treat-ment of Endometriosis via Laser Laseroscopy." FERTILITY AND STERILITY. 45 (1986), p. 778.

Orenberg, Cynthia L., and Robert Meyers. DES: THE COMPLETE STORY. New York: St. Martin's Press, 1981. (Available only from DES Action. See *Resources*.)

Parazzini, Fabio, M.D., LaVecchia, Carlo M.D., et al. "Epidemiologic Character-istics of Women with Uterine Fibroids: A Case Control Study." OBSTET-RICS AND GYNECOLOGY. 72:6 (December 1988), pp. 853-857.

"Safer Sex: More Preached Than Practiced." NEWSWEEK. 128:24 (December 9, 1991), pp. 52-56.

"Synarel, GnRh Drug, Wins FDA Approval for Endometriosis Treatment." ENDOMETRIOSIS ASSOCIATION NEWSLETTER. 11:1 (1990), pp. 1-3.

Vancouver Women's Health Research Collective. PID: PELVIC INFLAMMA-TORY DISEASE. Vancouver: 1983.

Endometriosis

Ballweg, Mary Lou, et al. OVERCOMING ENDOMETRIOSIS: NEW HELP FROM THE ENDOMETRIOSIS ASSOCIATION. New York: Congdon and Weed, 1987.

Davis, G. D., M.D., and R. A. Brooks, M.D. "Excision of Pelvic Endometriosis with the Carbon Dioxide Laser Laparoscope." OBSTETRICS AND GYNE-COLOGY. 72 (1988), p. 316.

Fletcher, Nancy. "Members Share their Experiences with Synarel and Lupron." ENDOMETRIOSIS ASSOCIATION NEWSLETTER. 12:2 (1991).

Houston, Diana E. "Evidence for the Risk of Pelvic Endometriosis by Age, Race, and Socioeconomic Status." EPIDEMIOLOGY REVIEW. 6 (1984), p. 167.

Lamb, Karen, R.N., Ph.D., Breitkopf, Lyle J., M.D., and Karen Hamilton, M.T. "Does Total Hysterectomy Offer a Cure for Endometriosis? An Exploratory Study." ENDOMETRIOSIS ASSOCIATION NEWSLETTER. 12:3 (1991), pp. 1-4.

Lauersen, Niels H., M.D., and Constance deSwaan. THE ENDOMETRIOSIS ANSWER BOOK: NEW HOPE, NEW HELP. New York: Macmillan, 1988.

Mains, Barbara with Mary Lou Ballweg. "Research Recap: Four Studies from the Association's Research Registry Program." ENDOMETRIOSIS ASSOCIA-TION NEWSLETTER. 10:2 (1989), pp. 2-5.

Nezhat, Camran, M.D., and Farr R. Nezhat, M.D. "Safe Laser Endoscopic Excision or Vaporization of Peritoneal Endometriosis." FERTILITY AND STERILITY. 22:1 (July, 1989), pp. 149-151.

Older, Julia. ENDOMETRIOSIS. New York: Charles Scribners' Sons, 1984.

Sachs, Judith. WHAT WOMEN CAN DO ABOUT CHRONIC ENDOMETRIOSIS. New York: Dell, 1991.

Schenken, R. S., ed. ENDOMETRIOSIS: CONTEMPORARY CONCEPTS IN CLINICAL MANAGEMENT. Philadelphia: J. B. Lippincott, 1989.

Seely, Ron. "Men and Endometriosis: What Do They Feel, How Do They Cope, How Can They Help." ENDOMETRIOSIS ASSOCIATION NEWSLETTER. 8:3 (1987), pp. 3-6.

Weinstein, Kate. LIVING WITH ENDOMETRIOSIS. Reading, MA: Addison-Wesley, 1987.

Wilson, E. A., ed. ENDOMETRIOSIS. New York: Alan Liss, 1988.

Pregnancy Loss: Medical Facts and Emotional Aftermath

Berg, Barbara. NOTHING TO CRY ABOUT. New York: Harper and Row, 1981.

Borg, Susan and Judith Lasker. WHEN PREGNANCY FAILS: FAMILIES COPING WITH MISCARRIAGE, STILLBIRTH, AND INFANT DEATH. Boston: Beacon Press, 1990, rev. ed.

Covington, Sharon N., M.S.W., LCSW. SILENT BIRTH...IF YOUR BABY DIES. 1988. (For ordering information write: 9715 Medical Center Dr., Rockville, MD 20850.)

DeFrain, John. STILLBORN: THE INVISIBLE DEATH. Boston: Lexington Books, 1986.

Doelp, Alan. AUTUMN'S CHILDREN: A REAL LIFE DRAMA OF HIGH-RISK PREGNANCY. New York: Macmillan, 1985.

Friedman, Rochelle, M.D., and Bonnie Gradstein, M.P.H. SURVIVING PREGNANCY LOSS. Boston: Little, Brown, 1992, rev. ed.

Fritsch, Julie with Sherokee Ilse. THE ANGUISH OF LOSS: FOR THE LOVE OF JUSTIN. Long Lake, MN: Wintergreen Press, 1988.

Hales, Dianne and Timothy Johnson, M.D. INTENSIVE CARING: NEW HOPE FOR HIGH-RISK PREGNANCY. New York: Crown, 1990.

Ilse, Sherokee. EMPTY ARMS: COPING AFTER MISCARRIAGE, STILLBIRTH, AND INFANT DEATH. Long Lake, MN: Wintergreen Press, 1990, rev. ed.

Ilse, Sherokee and Linda Hammer Burns. MISCARRIAGE: A SHATTERED DREAM. Long Lake, MN: Wintergreen Press, 1985.

Kübler-Ross, Elisabeth. ON CHILDREN AND DYING. New York: Collier, 1983.

_____. ON DEATH AND DYING. New York: Macmillan, 1970.

Morrow, Judith Gordon and Nancy Gordon DeHamer. GOOD MOURN-ING:HELP AND UNDERSTANDING IN TIME OF PREGNANCY LOSS. Dallas: Word Publishing, 1989.

Panuthos, Claudia. ENDED BEGINNINGS: HEALING CHILDBEARING LOSSES. South Hadley, MA: Bergin & Garvey, 1984.

Pepper, Larry G., Ph.D., and Ronald J. Knapp, Ph.D. HOW TO GO ON LIVING AFTER THE DEATH OF A BABY. Atlanta: Peachtree Publishers, 1985.

Raab, Diane, R.N. GETTING PREGNANT AND STAYING PREGNANT: A GUIDE TO INFERTILITY AND HIGH-RISK PREGNANCY. Montreal: Sirdan Publishers, 1989.

Rank, Maureen. FREE TO GRIEVE. Minneapolis, MN: Bethany House Publishing, 1988.

Savage, Judith A. MOURNING UNLIVED LIVES: A PSYCHOLOGICAL STUDY OF CHILDBEARING LOSS. Wilmette, IL: Chiron Publications, 1989.

Schaefer, Dan and Christine Lyons. HOW DO WE TELL THE CHILDREN? A PARENT'S GUIDE TO HELPING CHILDREN UNDERSTAND AND COPE WHEN SOMEONE DIES. New York: Newmarket Press, 1986.

Scher, Jonathan, M.D., PREVENTING MISCARRIAGE: THE GOOD NEWS. New York: Harper and Row, 1990.

Semchyshyn, Stefan, M.D., and Carol Colman. HOW TO PREVENT MISCARRIAGE AND OTHER CRISES OF PREGNANCY. New York: Macmillan, 1989.

Shapiro, Constance Hoenk. INFERTILITY AND PREGNANCY LOSS: A GUIDE FOR HELPING PROFESSIONALS. San Francisco: Jossey-Bass, 1988.

Woods, James, M.D., and Jennifer Esposito. PREGNANCY LOSS: MEDICAL THERAPEUTICS AND PRACTICAL CONSIDERATIONS. Baltimore: Williams and Wilkins, 1987.

Male Infertility and Donor Insemination

Alexander, Nancy J., Ph.D., Sampson, John H., M.D., and Miles J. Nory, M.D. ARTIFICIAL INSEMINATION. Portland, OR: Oregon Health Sciences University, 1981.

American Fertility Society. "Revised Guidelines for the Use of Semen Donor Insemination." 56:3 (September, 1991), p. 396.

Amuzu, Betty, M.D., Laxova, Renata, M.D., and Sander S. Shapiro, M.D. "Pregnancy Outcome, Health of Children, and Family Adjustment After Donor Insemination." OBSTETRICS AND GYNECOLOGY. 75 (June 1990) p. 904.

ARTIFICIAL INSEMINATION: AN ALTERNATIVE CONCEPTION FOR THE LESBIAN AND GAY COMMUNITY. For ordering information, contact the San Francisco Women's Center, 3543 18th St., San Francisco, CA 94110.

Baran, Annette, M.S.W., and Reuben Pannor, M.S.W. LETHAL SECRETS: THE SHOCKING CONSEQUENCES AND UNSOLVED PROBLEMS OF ARTIFICIAL INSEMINATION. New York: Warner Books, 1989.

Berlind, Melvyn. SPERMATOLOGY: THE LIFE OF A SPERM. New York: Vantage, 1990.

Bronson, Richard, M.D., Cooper, George, Ph.D., and David Rosenfeld, M.D. "Sperm Antibodies: Their Role in Infertility." FERTILITY AND STERILITY 42:2 (1984), pp. 171-183.

"Forum on Donor Insemination," videocassette featuring Annette Baran, M.S.W., and Reuben Pannor, M.S.W., filmed in Kansas City in 1990. For ordering information, contact: Clinical Counseling Associates, 10550 Barkley, Suite 108, Overland Park, KS 66212.

LeDraoulec, Pascale. "Dr. Graham and his 139 Children." CALIFORNIA. 16:9 (September 1991), 46ff.

Lipschultz, Larry I., M.D., and Stuart S. Howard, M.D. INFERTILITY IN THE MALE. New York: Churchill-Livingstone, 1983.

Mahlstedt, Patricia P., Ed.D. and Kris A. Probasco, M.S.W., LSCSW. "Sperm Donors: Their Attitudes toward Providing Medical and Psychosocial Information for Recipient Couples." FERTILITY AND STERILITY. 56:4 (October, 1991), pp. 747-753.

Mascola, Laurene, M.D., and Mary E. Guinan, M.D. "Screening to Reduce Transmission of Sexually Transmitted Diseases in Semen Used for Artificial Insemination." THE NEW ENGLAND JOURNAL OF MEDICINE. 314 (1986), pp. 1354-1359.

Matot, J. P. and M. L. Gustin. "Filiation and Secrecy in Artificial Insemination by Donor." HUMAN REPRODUCTION. 5:5 (1990), pp. 632-633.

McClure, R. Dale, M.D. "The Zona Free Hamster Egg Penetration Test: Its Usefulness in Male Infertility." SEMINARS IN UROLOGY 3:2 (May, 1985), pp. 78-84.

Moghissi, Kamrah S., M.D. "Reflections on the New Guidelines for the Use of Semen Donor Insemination." FERTILITY AND STERILITY. 53 (March 1990), p. 400.

Morse, G. "Sperm Antibodies Frustrate Fertility." SCIENCE NEWS. 126 (July, 1984), p. 38.

Noble, Elizabeth. HAVING YOUR BABY BY DONOR INSEMINATION. Boston: Houghton Mifflin, 1987.

Oskowitz, Selwyn P., M.D. "Tyerburg Strict Criteria or Kruger Sperm Morphology Test." RESOLVE NATIONAL NEWSLETTER. 16:5 (December 1991), p. 4.

Probasco, Kris A., LCSW. LUCAS' BEGINNING STORY. Children's book about donor insemination, 1992.

Sharlip, Ira D., M.D. "Male Reproductive Disorders." In THE HANDBOOK OF ENDOCRINOLOGY. Palo Alto: Appleton-Lange, 1991.

Snowden, R. and G. D. Mitchell. THE ARTIFICIAL FAMILY: A CONSIDERATION OF ARTIFICIAL INSEMINATION BY DONOR. London: Counterpoint, 1983.

Spark, Richard E. THE INFERTILE MALE. New York: Plenum Medical Books, 1988.

Walzer, H., M.D. "Psychological and Legal Aspects of Artificial Insemination: An Overview." AMERICAN JOURNAL OF PSYCHOTHERAPY. 36 (1982), pp. 91-103.

Assisted Reproductive Technology (ART)

American Fertility Society. "Ethical Considerations of the New Reproductive Technologies." FERTILITY AND STERILITY. 53:6 (June, 1990).

"And Donor Makes Three." NEWSWEEK. 118:14 (9/30/91), pp. 60-61.

Andrews, Lori B. NEW CONCEPTIONS: A CONSUMER'S GUIDE TO THE NEWEST INFERTILITY TREATMENT. New York: Ballantine, 1985.

Annas, George and S. Elias. "In Vitro Fertilization and Embryo Transfer: Medicolegal Aspects of a New Technique to Create a Family." FAMILY LAW QUARTERLY. 17 (Summer, 1983), pp. 199-223.

Arditti, Rita, Klein, Renate Duelli, and Shelley Minden. TEST-TUBE WOMEN: WHAT FUTURE FOR MOTHERHOOD? Boston: Routledge and Kegan Paul, 1984.

Asch, Ricardo, M.D., Ellsworth, J.R., M.D., and Wong, P. C. "Preliminary Experience with GIFT (Gamete Intrafallopian Transfer)." FERTILITY AND STERILITY. 45 (1986), p. 366.

Callan, V. J., and J. F. Hennessey. "Emotional Aspects and Support in In Vitro Fertilization and Embryo Transfer Programs." JOURNAL OF IVF AND EMBRYO TRANSFER. 5:5 (1988), pp. 290-295.

Callan, V.J., Kloske, B., Hashima, Y. and J. F. Hennessey. "Toward Understanding Women's Decisions to Continue or Stop In Vitro Fertilization: The Role of Social, Psychological, and Background Factors." JOURNAL OF IVF AND EMBRYO TRANSFER. 5:6 (1988), pp. 363-369.

Clapp, Diane, R.N., B.S.N., and Merle Bombardieri, LCSW. "Easing Stress for IVF Patients and Staff." CONTEMPORARY OB/GYN 24:4 (October 1984), pp. 91-99.

CONSUMER PROTECTION ISSUES INVOLVING IN VITRO FERTILIZATION CLINICS. Proceeds of the hearing before the Subcommittee on Regulation, Business Opportunities and Energy, House of Representatives, 101st Congress. Washington: U.S. Government Printing Office, 1989. For ordering information: Superintendent of Documents, U.S. Government Printing Office, Washington, D.C. 20402.

Corea, Genoveffa. THE MOTHER MACHINE: REPRODUCTIVE TECHNOLOGIES FROM ARTIFICIAL INSEMINATION TO ARTIFICIAL WOMBS. New York: Harper and Row, 1985.

Fugger, E., Ph.D. "Clinical Status of Human Embryo Cyropreservation in the United States." FERTILITY AND STERILITY. 52 (December, 1989), pp. 986-990.

Jones, Howard W., Jr., M.D., Jones, Georgeanna Seegar, M.D., Hodgen, G., M.D. and Zev Rosenwaks, M.D., eds. IN VITRO FERTILIZATION. Baltimore: Williams and Wilkins, 1986.

Kennard, E. A., Colliers, R. L., Blankenstein, J. et. al. "A Program for Matched, Anonymous Oocyte Donation." FERTILITY AND STERILITY. 51:4 (1989), pp. 655-660.

Lasker, Judith N. and Susan Borg. IN SEARCH OF PARENTHOOD: COPING WITH INFERTILITY AND HIGH-TECH CONCEPTION. Boston, MA: Beacon Press, 1987.

Macklin, R. "Artificial Means of Reproduction and Our Understanding of the Family." HASTINGS CENTER REPORT. (January-February, 1991). pp. 5-11.

Medical Research International, Society for Assisted Reproductive Technologies, The American Fertility Society. "In Vitro Fertilization/Embryo Transfer in the U.S.: 1988 results from the National IVF/ET Registry." FERTILITY AND STERILITY. 53:1 (January 1990).

Meyer, C. "Cry in the Wilderness: The Ethics of Embryo Freezing." THE WITNESS. 6:9 (February, 1990), pp. 22-23.

Perloe, Mark, N.D., and Linda G. Christie. MIRACLE BABIES AND OTHER HAPPY ENDINGS. New York: Rawson Associates, 1986.

Poplawski, N., and G. Gillett. "Ethics and Embryos." JOURNAL OF MEDICAL ETHICS. 17 (1991), pp. 62-69.

Power, M., Baker, R., Abdalla, H. et al. "A Comparison of the Attitudes of Volunteer Donors and Infertile Patient Donors in an Ovum Donation Programme." HUMAN REPRODUCTION. 5:3(1990), pp. 352-355.

Pressman, S. "The Baby Brokers." CALIFORNIA LAWYER. 30:34 (July, 1991), p. 105.

Raymond, Janice G. "Women as Wombs: International Traffic in Reproduction." MS. 1:6 (May, 1991), pp. 29-33.

Robertson, J.A. "Ethical and Legal Issues in Human Egg Donation." FERTILITY AND STERILITY. 52:3 (1989), pp. 353-363.

Robinson, J. N., Forman, R. G., Clark, A. M. et al. "Attitudes of Donors and Recipients to Gamete Donation." HUMAN REPRODUCTION. 6:2 (1991), pp. 307-309.

Rothman, Barbara Katz. RECREATING MOTHERHOOD: IDEOLOGY AND TECHNOLOGY IN A PATRIARCHAL SOCIETY. New York: W. W. Norton, 1989.

Royal Commission on New Reproductive Technologies. "Update." (January, 1992).

_____. What We Heard: Issues and Questions Raised During the Public Hearings. Ottawa, Canada: Royal Commission on New Reproductive Technologies, 1992.

Sauer, M. V., M.D., Paulson, R. J., M.D., and R. A. Lobo, M.D. "A Preliminary Report on Oocyte Donation Extending Reproductive Potential to Women over Forty." NEW ENGLAND JOURNAL OF MEDICINE. 323:17 (1990), pp. 1157-1160.

Sauer, M. V., M.D., Rodi, I. A., M.D., M. Scrooc, M.D., et al. "Attitudes Regarding the Use of Siblings for Gamete Donation." FERTILITY AND STERILITY. 49:4 (April, 1988), pp. 721-722.

Sauer, M. V., M.D. and R. J. Paulson, M.D. "Oocyte Donation for Women Who Have Ovarian Failure." CONTEMPORARY OB/GYN. 34 (1989), pp. 125-135.

Seibel, M., M.D. and S. Levin. "A New Era in Reproductive Technology: The Emotional Stages of IVF." JOURNAL OF IVF AND EMBRYO TRANSFER. 4:3 (1987), pp. 135-140.

Shannon, T. "Time for Regulation: Questions about In Vitro Fertilization." CHRISTIANITY AND CRISIS. (9/10/90), pp. 268-270.

Sher, Geoffrey, M.D., Marriage, Virginia, R.N., and Jean Stoess. FROM INFERTILITY TO IN VITRO FERTILIZATION: A PERSONAL AND PRACTICAL GUIDE TO MAKING THE DECISION THAT COULD CHANGE YOUR LIFE. New York: McGraw Hill, 1988.

Singer, Peter and Deane Wells. MAKING BABIES: THE NEW SCIENCE AND ETHICS OF CONCEPTION. New York: Charles Scribner's Sons, 1987.

Stanworth, Michelle, ed. REPRODUCTIVE TECHNOLOGIES: GENDER, MOTHERHOOD, AND MEDICINE. Minneapolis: University of Minnesota Press, 1987.

Vatican. CONGREGATION FOR THE DOCTRINE OF THE FAITH: INSTRUCTION ON RESPECT FOR HUMAN LIFE IN ITS ORIGIN AND ON THE DIGNITY OF PROCREATION. Vatican City: Vatican Press, 1987.

Wisot, Arthur L., M.D., and David R. Meldrum, M.D. NEW OPTION FOR FERTILITY: A GUIDE TO IN VITRO FERTILIZATION AND OTHER ASSISTED REPRODUCTION METHODS. New York: Pharos Books, 1990.

Zaner, R. M., Boehm, F. H., and G. A. Hill. "Selective Termination in Multiple Pregnancies: Ethical Considerations." FERTILITY AND STERILITY. 54:2 (August, 1990), pp. 203-205.

Adoption

GENERAL READINGS

Adamec, Christine. THERE ARE BABIES TO ADOPT: A RESOURCE GUIDE FOR PROSPECTIVE PARENTS. Lexington, MA: Mills & Sanderson, 1987.

American Council on Adoptable Children. ADOPTION BOOKLET. A free guide on state departments of social services, adoptive parent groups, and transracial and intercountry adoptions. Write to NACAC, 1346 Connecticut Ave., N.W., Suite 229, Washington, D.C., 20036.

Brown, Dirck W., et al. DIALOGUE FOR UNDERSTANDING: A HANDBOOK FOR ADOPTIVE AND PRE-ADOPTIVE PARENTS. Palo Alto, CA: Post Adoption Center for Education and Research, 1982.

Canape. Charlene. ADOPTION: PARENTHOOD WITHOUT PREGNANCY. New York: Henry Holt, 1986.

Chase, Mary E. WAITING FOR BABY: ONE COUPLE'S JOURNEY THROUGH INFERTILITY TO ADOPTION. McGraw-Hill, 1990.

Festinger, T. NECESSARY RISK: A STUDY OF ADOPTIONS AND DISRUPTED ADOPTIVE PLACEMENTS. Washington, D.C.: Child Welfare League of America, 1986.

Gilman, Lois. THE ADOPTION RESOURCE BOOK. New York: Harper and Row, 1987, rev. ed.

Hormann, Elizabeth. AFTER THE ADOPTION. Old Tappan, NJ: Revell, 1987.

Kaplan-Roszia, Sharon and Carol Land. "Winning at Adoption." A packet of video and audio tapes and a workbook for prospective adoptive parents. For ordering information, contact: Family Network, P. O. Box 1995, Studio City, CA 91614, (800) 456-4056.

Martin, Cynthia D., Ph.D. BEATING THE ADOPTION GAME. New York: Harcourt Brace Jovanovich, 1988, rev. ed.

Melina, Lois Ruskai. ADOPTION: AN ANNOTATED BIBLIOGRAPHY AND GUIDE. New York: Garland, 1987.

_____. MAKING SENSE OF ADOPTION: A PARENT'S GUIDE. New York: Harper and Row, 1989.

Paul, Ellen. ADOPTION CHOICES. Detroit: Visible Ink Press, 1991.

Plumez, Jacqueline Hornor. SUCCESSFUL ADOPTION: A GUIDE TO FINDING A CHILD AND RAISING A FAMILY. New York: Harmony Books, 1987.

Posner, Julia L., ed. CWLA'S GUIDE TO ADOPTION AGENCIES: A NATIONAL DIRECTORY OF ADOPTION AGENCIES AND ADOPTION RESOURCES. Washington, D.C.: Child Welfare League of America, 1989. For ordering information, write to CWLA: 440 First St., NW, Suite 310, Washington D.C. 20001-2085.

Rillera, Mary Jo and Sharon Kaplan. COOPERATIVE ADOPTION: A HANDBOOK. Westminster, CA: Triadoption Publications, 1984.

Roberts, January, and Diane C. Robie. OPEN ADOPTION AND OPEN PLACE-MENT. Brooklyn Park, MN: Adoption Press, 1981.

Smith, Jerome, Ph.D., and Franklin Miroff, J.D. YOU'RE OUR CHILD: A SOCIAL/PSYCHOLOGICAL APPROACH TO ADOPTION. Washington, D.C.: University Press of America, 1981.

Sorosky, Arthur D., Baran, Annette, M.S.W., and Reuben Pannor, M.S.W. THE ADOPTION TRIANGLE: SEALED OR OPEN RECORDS: HOW THEY AFFECT ADOPTEES, BIRTH PARENTS, AND ADOPTIVE PARENTS. San Antonio: Corona Publishing Co., 1989.

CHILDREN'S BOOKS ABOUT ADOPTION

Angel, Ann. REAL FOR SURE SISTER. Indianapolis: Perspectives Press, 1988. For the eight-to eleven-year-old child whose family is about to adopt a child.

Brodzinsky, Anne. THE MULBERRY BIRD. Indianapolis: Perspectives Press, 1989. For five to ten year olds; describes a birthmother's adoption plan for her baby.

Dellinger, Annetta E. ADOPTED AND LOVED FOREVER. St. Louis, MO: Concordia Publishing, 1987. A religious perspective of adoption for young children.

Fisher, Iris L. KATIE BO: AN ADOPTION STORY. New York: Adama Books, 1987. The story of an adoption of a Korean child told by the older sibling.

Gabel, Susan. FILLING IN THE BLANKS: A GUIDED LOOK AT GROWING UP ADOPTED. Indianapolis: Perspectives Press, 1988. A workbook for helping children understand adoption.

_____. WHERE THE SUN KISSES THE SEA. Indianapolis: Perspectives Press, 1989. For six to ten year olds, the story of an international adoption of a young boy.

Girard, Linda Walvoord. ADOPTION IS FOR ALWAYS. Niles, IL: Albert Whitman & Co., 1986. The perspective of an adopted child's anger at her birthparents.

_____. WE ADOPTED YOU, BENJAMIN KOO. Niles, IL: Albert Whitman and Company, 1989. The story of a Korean child's adoption.

Gordon, S. THE BOY WHO WANTED A FAMILY. New York: Harper and Row, 1980. For ages six and older, a story about a seven-year-old foster child adopted by a single mother.

Koch, Janice. OUR BABY: A BIRTH AND ADOPTION STORY. Indianapolis: Perspectives Press, 1985. For three to seven year olds, a book about conception, birth, and the adoption process.

Krementz, Jill. HOW IT FEELS TO BE ADOPTED. New York: Alfred A. Knopf, 1982. Photos and essays in adopted children's own words.

Lifton, Betty J. I'M STILL ME. New York: Alfred A. Knopf, 1981. Fiction story about an adolescent girl's search for her birthparents; for ages fourteen and older.

Nerlove, E. WHO IS DAVID? THE STORY OF AN ADOPTED ADOLESCENT AND HIS FRIENDS. Washington, D.C.: Child Welfare League of America, 1985.

Nixon, Joan Lowery. A FAMILY APART. New York: Bantam, 1987. For eight years and older, the story of the "orphan trains," which brought children to Midwest families for adoption in the 1800s.

Nystrom, Caroline. MARIO'S BIG QUESTION. Batavia, IL: Lion Publishing Corporation, 1987. Story of a foster child and his questions about his birthparents.

Schnitter, Jane T. WILLIAM IS MY BROTHER. Indianapolis, IN: Perspectives Press, 1991. For preschool through early elementary ages; addresses issues for blended biological and adopted families.

Sobol, Harriet Langsam. WE DON'T LOOK LIKE OUR MOM AND DAD. New York: Coward-McCann, 1984. Features a family who has adopted Asian-American children.

Schaffer, Patricia. HOW BABIES AND FAMILIES ARE MADE. Berkeley: Tabor Sarah Books, 1988.

INTERNATIONAL AND TRANSRACIAL ADOPTION

Anderson, David. CHILDREN OF SPECIAL VALUE: INTERRACIAL ADOPTION IN AMERICA. New York: St. Martin's Press, 1971.

Caldwell-Hopper, Kathi. "Adopting Across Lines of Color." OURS Newsletter (July-August, 1991), pp. 23-25.

Erichsen, J., H. Erichsen and G. Galiber. HOW TO ADOPT FROM ASIA, EUROPE, AND THE SOUTH PACIFIC. Austin, TX: International Adoption Center, 1983.

Hathaway, Gretchen. "Who is She? Where Did She Come From? How to Handle Those Intrusive Questions." OURS Newsletter (July-August, 1991), p. 25.

Hopson, Darlene, Ph.D. and Derek S. Hopson, Ph.D. DIFFERENT AND WONDERFUL: RAISING BLACK CHILDREN IN A RACE-CONSCIOUS SOCIETY. New York: Prentice Hall, 1990.

International Concerns Committee for Children. REPORT ON FOREIGN ADOPTION. Boulder, CO: ICCC, 1987. Frequently updated guide about international adoption. For ordering information, write: 911 Cypress Dr., Boulder, CO 90303.

Ladner, Joyce. MIXED FAMILIES: ADOPTING ACROSS RACIAL BOUNDARIES. New York: Anchor Books, 1978.

Melina, Lois Ruskai. RAISING ADOPTED CHILDREN. New York: Harper and Row, 1986.

Powell, Azizi. "Raise Your Child with Ethnic Pride." OURS Newsletter (November-December, 1988), 26-28.

"Raising a Child of a Different Race or Ethnic Background." Audiotape. For ordering information, contact: Adopted Child, P. O. Box 9362, Moscow, ID 83843.

Register, Cheri. ARE THOSE KIDS YOURS? New York: Free Press, 1990.

Simon, Rita J., and Howard Alstein. TRANSRACIAL ADOPTION. New York: John Wiley, 1977.

Standiford, Debi. SUDDEN FAMILY. Waco, TX: Word Books, 1986.

Strasberger, L. ed. THEY BECAME PART OF US: THE EXPERIENCE OF FAMILIES ADOPTING CHILDREN EVERYWHERE. Maple Grove, MN: Mini-World Publications, 1985.

Viguers, Susan T. WITH CHILD: ONE COUPLE'S JOURNEY TO THEIR ADOPTED CHILDREN. San Diego: Harcourt Brace Jovanovich, 1986.

SINGLE PARENT/SPECIAL-NEEDS ADOPTIONS

Blank, P. NINETEEN STEPS UP THE MOUNTAIN: THE STORY OF THE DEBOLT FAMILY. Philadelphia: J. B. Lippincott, 1976.

Fahlberg, Vera, M.D. A CHILD'S JOURNEY THROUGH PLACEMENT. Indianapolis: Perspectives Press, 1991.

Hamm, W., T. Morton, and L. M. Flynn. SELF-AWARENESS, SELF- SELECTION AND SUCCESS: A PARENT PREPARATION GUIDEBOOK FOR SPECIAL NEEDS ADOPTIONS. Washington, D.C.: North American Council on Adoptable Children, 1985.

Jewett, Claudia L. ADOPTING THE OLDER CHILD. Harvard, MA: Harvard Common Press, 1978.

Marindin, Hope. THE HANDBOOK FOR SINGLE ADOPTIVE PARENTS. Chevy Chase, MD: Commitee for Single Adoptive Parents, 1987.

Morrison, Grace. TO LOVE AND LET GO. Alameda, CA: Pillar Press, 1983. (Foster care of abused children.)

ADOPTION TRIAD MEMBER ISSUES

Arms, Suzanne. ADOPTION: A HANDFUL OF HOPE. Berkeley, CA: Celestial Arts, 1990, rev ed. of TO LOVE AND LET GO.

Askin, I. Jayne, and Bob Oskam. SEARCH: A HANDBOOK FOR ADOPTEES AND BIRTHPARENTS. New York: Harper and Row, 1982.

Baran, Annette and A. D. Sorosky. "The Lingering Pain of Surrendering a Child." PSYCHOLOGY TODAY, 11:1 (1977), pp. 58-60.

Paton, Jean M. ORPHAN VOYAGE. New York: Vantage, 1978.

Brown, Dirck, et al. DIALOGUE FOR UNDERSTANDING: A HANDBOOK FOR ADOPTIVE AND PRE-ADOPTIVE PARENTS, 2 vols. Palo Alto, CA: PACER, 1981.

Campbell, Lee, ed. UNDERSTANDING THE BIRTHPARENT. Milford, MA: Concerned United Birthparents, 1978.

DuPrau, Jeanne. ADOPTION: THE FACTS, FEELINGS AND ISSUES OF A DOUBLE HERITAGE. New York: Simon and Schuster, 1981.

Dusky, Lorraine. BIRTHMARK. New York: M. Evans, 1974.

Ehrlich, Henry. A TIME TO SEARCH. New York: Paddington Press, 1978.

Fisher, Florence. THE SEARCH FOR ANNA FISHER. New York: Fawcett, 1979.

Johnston, Patricia Irwin. PERSPECTIVES ON A GRAFTED TREE. Indianapolis: Perspectives Press, 1983.

Lifton, Betty J. LOST AND FOUND: THE ADOPTION EXPERIENCE. New York: Harper and Row, 1988.

_____. TWICE BORN: MEMORIES OF AN ADOPTED DAUGHTER. New York: McGraw-Hill, 1977.

Lindsay, Jeanne W. OPEN ADOPTION: A CARING OPTION. Buena Park, CA: Morning Glory Press, 1987.

_____. PREGNANT TOO SOON: ADOPTION IS AN OPTION. Buena Park, CA: Morning Glory Press, 1980.

Lindsay, Jeanne and Catherine Monserrat. ADOPTION AWARENESS: A GUIDE FOR TEACHERS, COUNSELORS, NURSES AND CARING OTHERS. Buena Park, CA: Morning Glory Press, 1989.

Lockhart, Beth. "Adoption Adventure: A Unique Collection of Songs about Adoption." (audio tape cassette). For ordering information write: Adoptive Parents' Education Program, P.O. Box 32114, Phoenix, AZ 85064.

Musser, Sandra Kay. WHAT KIND OF LOVE IS THIS? A STORY OF ADOPTION RECONCILIATION. Oaklyn, NJ: Jan Publications, 1982.

Reilly, Jane. "Mother and Child Reunion." MIRABELLA. 29 (October, 1991), pp. 148-153.

Rillera, Mary Jo. THE ADOPTION SEARCHBOOK: TECHNIQUES FOR TRACING PEOPLE. Huntington Beach, CA: Tri-Adoption Publishers, 1981.

Silber, Kathleen and Phylis Speedlin. DEAR BIRTHMOTHER. San Antonio, TX: Corona Publishing, 1982.

Zimmerman, M. SHOULD I KEEP MY BABY? Minneapolis: Bethany House Publishers, 1983.

SURROGATE MOTHERS

Agrest, Susan. "Borrowed Bodies." SAVVY. (January, 1987), pp. 52-55.

American College of Obstetricians and Gynecologists, Committee on Ethics. "Ethical Issues in Surrogate Motherhood." ACOG COMMITTEE OPINION. 88 (November, 1990), pp. 1-5.

American Fertility Society. "Ethical Considerations of the New Reproductive Technologies." FERTILITY AND STERILITY. 53: 6 (June, 1990).

Andrews, Lori. BETWEEN STRANGERS: SURROGATE MOTHERS, EXPECTANT FATHERS, AND BRAVE NEW BABIES. New York: Harper and Row, 1989.

Arking, Linda. "Searching for a Very Special Woman." MCCALL'S. (June, 1987), 55ff.

Chesler, Phyllis, SACRED BOND. New York: Times Book Random House, 1988.

Edmiston, Susan. "Whose Child Is This?" GLAMOUR (Nov. 1991), pp. 235ff.

Field, Martha. SURROGATE MOTHERHOOD: THE LEGAL AND HUMAN ISSUES. Cambridge, MA: Harvard University Press, 1988.

Groller, Ingrid. "Parents Poll: Is Surrogate Motherhood Okay?" PARENTS. (October, 1987), p. 28.

"Infertility: Babies by Contract." NEWSWEEK (November 4, 1985), pp. 74-77.

Kane, Elizabeth. BIRTHMOTHER. San Diego: Harcourt Brace Jovanovich, 1988.

Keane, Noel P. and Dennis Breo. THE SURROGATE MOTHER. New York: Everest House, 1981.

Menning, Barbara Eck. "Surrogate Motherhood: What Are the Ethical Issues?" RESOLVE NATIONAL NEWSLETTER. (June 1981), pp. 6-7.

Overvold, Amy Zuckerman. SURROGATE PARENTING. New York: Pharos Books, 1988.

Pollit, Katha. "The Strange Case of Baby M." THE NATION. (May 23, 1987), pp. 682-88.

Powers, Rebecca and Sheila Gruber Belloli. "Most Oppose Surrogacy Ban." THE DETROIT NEWS. (Thursday, September 21, 1989), p. 16A.

Raymond, Janice S. "Women as Wombs: International Traffic in Reproduction." MS. 1:6 (May, 1991), pp. 29-33.

Rust, Mark. "Whose Baby Is It: Surrogate Motherhood After Baby M." AMERICAN BAR ASSOCIATION JOURNAL. 73 (June, 1987), pp. 52-56.

vanHoften, Ellen Lassner. "Surrogate Mothers in California: Legislative Proposals." SAN DIEGO LAW REVIEW. 18:2 (March 1981), pp. 341-385.

Whitehead, Mary Beth with Loretta Schwartz-Nobel. A MOTHER'S STORY: THE TRUTH ABOUT THE BABY M CASE. New York: St. Martin's Press, 1989.

Winslade, W. J. "Surrogate Mothers: Private Right or Public Wrong?" JOURNAL OF MEDICAL ETHICS. 7 (1981), pp. 143-144.

Pregnancy and Childbirth

Arms, Suzanne. IMMACULATE DECEPTION. South Hadley, MA: Bergin and Garvey, 1985.

Ashford, Janet L., ed. THE WHOLE BIRTH CATALOG: A SOURCEBOOK FOR CHOICES IN CHILDBIRTH. Trumansburg, NY: Crossings Press, 1983.

Baldwin, Rahima. SPECIAL DELIVERY. Berkeley: Celestial Arts, 1986.

Ballweg, Mary Lou. "Pregnancy, Labor, and Postpartum Experience of Women with Endometriosis." ENDOMETRIOSIS ASSOCIATION NEWSLETTER. 8:3 (1987).

Blatt, Robin. PRENATAL TESTS. New York: Vintage, 1988.

Comport, Maggie. TOWARDS HAPPY MOTHERHOOD: UNDERSTANDING POSTNATAL DEPRESSION. Great Britain: Corgi, 1987.

Cox, Kathryn, M.D., and Judith D. Schwartz. THE WELL-INFORMED PATIENT'S GUIDE TO CAESAREAN BIRTH. New York: Dell, 1990.

Dick-Read, Grantly. CHILDBIRTH WITHOUT FEAR. New York: Harper and Row, 1987, rev. ed.

Eisenberg, Arlene, Eisenberg, Markoff and Sandy Eisenberg Hathaway, R.N. WHAT TO EXPECT WHEN YOU'RE EXPECTING. New York: Workman Publishers, 1988.

Fay, Francesca C., and Kathy Smith. CHILDBEARING AFTER 35: THE RISKS AND REWARDS. New York: Balsam Press, 1985.

Goldberg, Larry H., M.D., and Joann Leahy, M.D. THE DOCTOR'S GUIDE TO MEDICATION DURING PREGNANCY AND LACTATION. New York: Quill, 1984.

Hotchner, Tracy. PREGNANCY AND CHILDBIRTH. New York: Avon, 1990, rev. ed.

Johnston, Susan H., M.S.W. and Deborah A. Kraut, M.Ed. PREGNANCY BED-REST: A GUIDE FOR THE PREGNANT WOMAN AND HER FAMILY. New York: Henry Holt, 1990.

Karmel, Marjorie. PAINLESS CHILDBIRTH: THANK YOU, DR. LAMAZE. New York: Dolphin, 1965.

Katz, Michael, M.D., Gill, Pamela, R.N., and Judith Turiel, Ed.D., eds. PREVENTING PRE-TERM BIRTH: A PARENTS' GUIDE. San Francisco: Heath Publishing, 1988.

King, Janet Spencer. TAKING THE BLUES OUT OF POSTPARTUM. New York: Villard, 1987.

La Leche International. THE WOMANLY ART OF BREASTFEEDING. New York: New American Library, 1987.

Lamaze, Ferdinand. PAINLESS CHILDBIRTH: THE LAMAZE METHOD. Chicago: Contemporary Books, rev. ed. 1987.

Nilsson, Lennart. A CHILD IS BORN: THE COMPLETELY NEW EDITION. New York: Delacorte Press, 1990.

Noble, Elizabeth. HAVING TWINS. Boston: Houghton Mifflin, 1991, rev. ed.

Renfrew, Mary, Fisher, Chloe, and Suzanne Arms. BESTFEEDING: GETTING BREASTFEEDING RIGHT FOR YOU. Berkeley, CA: Celestial Arts, 1991.

Rich, Laurie A. WHEN PREGNANCY ISN'T PERFECT: A LAYPERSON'S GUIDE TO COMPLICATIONS IN PREGNANCY. New York: Penguin, 1991.

Rosen, Mortimer, M.D., and Lillian Thomas. THE CESAREAN MYTH. New York: Viking, 1989.

Rothman, Barbara Katz. THE TENTATIVE PREGNANCY: PRENATAL DIAGNO-SIS AND THE FUTURE OF MOTHERHOOD. New York: Viking Press, 1986.

Samuels, Mike, M.D., and Nancy Samuels. THE WELL PREGNANCY BOOK. New York: Summit, 1986.

Sandelowski, Margarete, Ph.D., Harris, Betty G., Ph.D., and Beth P. Black. "Relin-quishing Infertility: The Work of Pregnancy for Infertile Couples." QUALI-TATIVE HEALTH RESEARCH, forthcoming, 1992.

Sandelowski, Margarete, Ph.D., Harris, Betty, G., Ph.D., and Diane Holditch-Davis, Ph.D. "Amniocentesis in the Context of Infertility." HEALTH CARE FOR WOMEN INTERNATIONAL. 12 (1991), pp. 167-178.

_____. "Pregnant Moments: The Process of Conception in Infertile Couples." RESEARCH IN NURSING AND HEALTH. 13 (1990), pp. 273-282.

Schevill, Susie and Joanne Cuthbertson. HELPING YOUR CHILD SLEEP THROUGH THE NIGHT. New York: Doubleday, 1986.

Shapiro, Constance Hoenk, Ph.D. "Is Pregnancy After Infertility A Dubious Joy?" SOCIAL CASEWORK: THE JOURNAL OF CONTEMPORARY SOCIAL WORK. (May, 1986), pp. 306-313.

Parenting After Infertility

Anderson, Kathryn. NURSING YOUR ADOPTED BABY. Franklin Park, IL: La Leche International, 1983.

Boston Women's Health Book Collective. OURSELVES AND OUR CHILDREN. New York: Random House, 1978.

Brazelton, T. Berry, M.D. INFANTS AND MOTHERS: DIFFERENCES IN DEVEL-OPMENT. New York: Delacorte Press, 1974.

Clegg, Averil and Anne Woolet. TWINS: FROM CONCEPTION TO FIVE YEARS. New York: Ballantine, 1988.

Curto, J. HOW TO BECOME A SINGLE PARENT: A GUIDE FOR SINGLE PEOPLE CONSIDERING ADOPTION OR NATURAL PARENTHOOD ALONE. Engle-wood Cliffs, N.J.: Prentice Hall, 1983.

Dix, Carol. THE NEW MOTHER SYNDROME: COPING WITH POSTPARTUM STRESS AND DEPRESSION. Garden City, NY: Doubleday, 1985.

Glazer, Ellen Sarasohn. THE LONG AWAITED STORK. Lexington, MA: Lexington Books, 1990.

Halaby, Mona and Helen Neville, R.N. NO FAULT PARENTING. Tucson, AZ: Body Press, 1986.

Hallenbeck, Carol A. OUR CHILD: PREPARATION FOR PARENTING IN ADOPTION. Wayne, IN: Our Child Press, 1988, rev. ed.

Hanscombe, G. and J. Forster. ROCKING THE CRADLE—LESBIAN MOTHERS: A CHALLENGE IN FAMILY LIVING. Boston: Alyson Publications, 1982.

Hormann, Elizabeth. AFTER THE ADOPTION. Old Tappan, NJ: Fleming Revell Co., 1987.

Hotchner, Tracy. CHILDBIRTH AND MARRIAGE. New York, NY: Avon, 1988.

Ilg, Frances L., M.D. and Louise Bates Ames, Ph.D. CHILD BEHAVIOR: FROM BIRTH TO TEN. New York: Harper & Row, 1955.

Jessel, Camilla. FROM BIRTH TO THREE: AN ILLUSTRATED JOURNEY THROUGH YOUR CHILD'S EARLY PHYSICAL AND EMOTIONAL DEVELOPMENT. New York: Delta, 1990.

Jewett, Claudia. HELPING CHILDREN COPE WITH SEPARATION AND LOSS. Boston: Harvard Press, 1982.

Kelly, Marguerite. THE MOTHER'S ALMANAC II: YOUR CHILD FROM SIX TO TWELVE. New York: Doubleday, 1989.

Kelly, Marguerite and Elia Parsons. THE MOTHER'S ALMANAC. New York: Doubleday, 1989, rev. ed.

Lawrence, Melanie. "Pregnancy and Parenthood after Infertility." PARENTS' PRESS. (February, 1990).

Lindsay, Jeanne Warren. DO I HAVE A DADDY? Buena Park, CA:Morning Glory Press, 1982.

Lockhart, Beth. GUIDELINES FOR ORGANIZING AND TEACHING ADOPTIVE PARENT CLASSES. (1980) For ordering information, write: Adoptive Parents' Education Program, P. O. Box 32114, Phoenix, AZ.

Merritt, Sharyne and Linda Steiner. AND BABY MAKES TWO: MOTHERHOOD WITHOUT MARRIAGE. New York: Franklin Watts, 1984.

Renfrew, Mary, Fisher, Chloe, and Suzanne Arms. BESTFEEDING: GETTING BREASTFEEDING RIGHT FOR YOU. Berkeley: Celestial Arts, 1990.

Schaffer, Judith and Christina Lindstrom. HOW TO RAISE AN ADOPTED CHILD: A GUIDE TO HELP YOUR CHILD FLOURISH FROM INFANCY THROUGH ADOLESCENCE. New York: Crown, 1989.

Smith, Dorothy and Laurie Sherwen. MOTHERS AND THEIR ADOPTED CHILDREN: THE BONDING PROCESS. New York: The Tiresias Press, 1988.

Spock, Benjamin, M.D., with Michael B. Rothenberg, M.D. BABY AND CHILD CARE. New York: Dutton, 1985.

White, Burton L. THE FIRST THREE YEARS OF LIFE. New York: Prentice Hall, 1990.

Child-Free Living

Bombardieri, Merle. THE BABY DECISION: HOW TO MAKE THE MOST IMPOR-TANT CHOICE OF YOUR LIFE. New York: Rawson, Wade Publishers, 1981.

_____. CHILD-FREE DECISION MAKING. Reprint available from RESOLVE's National Office.

Burgwyn, Diana. MARRIAGE WITHOUT CHILDREN. New York: Harper and Row, 1982.

Carter, Jean W., M.D. and Michael Carter, Ph.D. SWEET GRAPES: HOW TO STOP BEING INFERTILE AND START LIVING AGAIN. Indianapolis: Per-spectives Press, 1989.

Covington, Sharon, LCSW. "Child-free: The 'Closet Choice.'" RESOLVE, Wash-ington, D.C. Metropolitan Chapter Newsletter, May,1985.

Dowrick, Stephanie and Sibyl Grundberg, eds. WHY CHILDREN? New York: Harcourt Brace Jovanovich, 1980.

Elvenstar, Diane C. CHILDREN: TO HAVE OR HAVE NOT? San Francisco: Har-bor Publishing, 1982.

Faux, Marian. CHILDLESS BY CHOICE: CHOOSING CHILDLESSNESS IN THE EIGHTIES. Garden City, NY: Anchor Press, 1984.

Feldman, Silvia. MAKING UP YOUR MIND ABOUT MOTHERHOOD. New York: Bantam, 1985.

Love, Vicky. CHILDLESS IS NOT LESS. Minneapolis: Bethany House, 1984.

Matthews, Ralph and Anne Martin Matthews. "Infertility and Involuntary Chidlessness: The Transition to Nonparenthood." JOURNAL OF MAR-RIAGE AND THE FAMILY. 48 (August 1986), pp. 641-649.

Peck, Ellen. THE BABY TRAP. New York: Bernard Geis Associates, 1971.

Peck, Ellen and Judy Senderowitz. PRONATALISM: THE MYTH OF MOM AND APPLE PIE. New York: Thomas Crowell, 1974.

Poole, William E. "Fathering Without Children." SAN FRANCISCO EXAMINER IMAGE MAGAZINE (November 3, 1985).

Silverman, Anna, and Arnold Silverman. THE CASE AGAINST HAVING CHIL-DREN. New York: David McKay, 1971.

Sullivan, Judy. MAMA DOESN'T LIVE HERE ANYMORE. New York: Arthur Field Books, 1974.

Whelan, Elizabeth. A BABY? MAYBE. New York: Bobbs-Merrill, 1975.

Resources

Medical Information, Referrals, and Emotional Support

AMERICAN ASSOCIATION OF GYNECOLOGIC LAPAROSCOPISTS
11239 S. Lakewood Blvd.
Downey, CA 90241

AMERICAN ASSOCIATION OF TISSUE BANKS
1350 Beverly Rd., Suite 220A
McLean, VA 22101
(703) 827-9582

AMERICAN COLLEGE OF OBSTETRICIANS AND GYNECOLOGISTS (ACOG)
409—12th St., SW
Washington, D.C. 20024
(202) 638-5577

AMERICAN FERTILITY SOCIETY
2140—11th Ave. S., Suite 200
Birmingham, AL 35205
(205) 933-8494

Publications, referrals, and literature regarding infertility and Assisted Reproductive Technology, including IVF Registry and clinic-specific data. Write or call for ordering information.

AMERICAN SOCIETY OF ANDROLOGY
309 West Clark St.
Champaigne, IL 61820
(217) 356-3182
FAX (217) 398-4119

AMERICAN UROLOGICAL ASSOCIATION
1120 N. Charles St.
Baltimore, MD 21201
(301) 727-1100

COMPASSIONATE FRIENDS, INC
900 Jorie Blvd.
P. O. Box 3696
Oak Brook, IL 60522-3696
(312) 990-0010

A nationwide organization for parents who have lost a child of any age.

DALKON SHIELD CLAIMANTS' TRUST
P. O. Box 444
Richmond, VA 23202
(804) 783-8600

Contact for information regarding the claims process for women sustaining injury and/or infertility from use of the Dalkon Shield.

DES ACTION, CANADA
P. O. Box 233
Montreal, Quebec H3X 3T4
(514) 482-3204

DES ACTION, USA
National Office
1615 Broadway, Suite 510
Oakland, CA 94612
(510) 465-4011

DES Action organizations provide information, support, newsletters and education about DES.

THE ENDOMETRIOSIS ASSOCIATION
International Headquarters Office
8585 N. 76th Place
Milwaukee, WI 53223
(414) 355-2200 or (800) 992-3636 (USA), (800) 426-2363 (Canada)

An excellent and extensive resource for women with endometriosis, offering literature, newsletters, video and audio tapes, national support group network, conferences, referrals, and crisis line. The "800" line operates twenty-four hours a day, and callers can leave their name and address for a free information packet.

FERRE INSTITUTE, Inc.
258 Genesee St., Suite 302
Utica, NY 13502
(315) 724-4348

A non-profit organization, established through Title X family grants in 1975, devoted to the promotion of quality infertility services through professional and public education and encouragement of research. Publishes brochures, newsletters, and maintains library of infertility literature.

GYNECOLOGIC LASER SOCIETY
6900 Grove Rd.
Thorofare, NJ 08086
(609) 848-1000 or (800) 257-8290

INFERTILITY AWARENESS ASSOCIATION OF CANADA (IAAC)
1785 Alta Vista Dr., Suite 104
Ottawa, Ontario K1G3Y6
(613) 738-8968
FAX (613) 738-0159

A national charitable organization offering assistance, support, referrals, and education to Canadians with infertility concerns.

THE PLANETREE HEALTH RESOURCE CENTER
2040 Webster St.
San Francisco, CA 94115
(415) 923-3680

Consumer health library open to the public free of charge. Also offers a bookstore and medical information research service.

PLANNED PARENTHOOD FEDERATION OF AMERICA
810 Seventh Ave.
New York, NY 10019
(212) 777-2002

PREGNANCY AND INFANCY LOSS CENTER
1421 E. Wayzata Blvd.
Wayzata, MN 55391
(612) 473-9372

National non-profit organization that provides referrals, support, and literature for those suffering pregnancy loss or infant loss.

RESOLVE, INC.
1310 Broadway
Somerville, MA 02144
(617) 623-0744

Medical information, quarterly newsletter, referrals, emotional support, educational materials, and related books and articles. More than forty local chapters across the United States.

ROYAL COMMISSION ON NEW REPRODUCTIVE TECHNOLOGIES
Box 1566, Station B
Ottawa, Ontario
K1P 5R5
(613) 954-9999 or (800) 668-7060

Literature and information regarding research and policy recommendations for application of the new reproductive technologies in Canada.

SERONO SYMPOSIA, USA
100 Longwater Circle
Norwell, MA 02061
(617) 982-9000 or (800) 283-8088; Access line: (800) 326-3151

Cosponsors day-long symposia throughout the country about the many facets of infertility. Access line assists with assessing insurance coverage for fertility drug treatment.

SHARE
St. Joseph's Health Center
300 First Capitol Dr.
St. Charles, MO 63301
(314) 947-5000

Support for and information about pregnancy loss.

SHATTERED DREAMS
c/o Born to Love
21 Potsdam Rd., Unit 61
Downsviews, Ontario M3N 1N3
(416) 663-7143

Newsletter filled with media and medical articles, poems, book lists, and letters regarding pregnancy loss.

THE SPERM BANK OF CALIFORNIA
3007 Telegraph Ave., Suite 2
Oakland, CA 94609
(510) 444-2014

Information regarding donor screening, recipient education, and anonymous and identity-release donor programs.

Adoption

GENERAL RESOURCES

ADOPTED CHILD
P. O. Box 9362
Moscow, ID 83843
(208) 883-1794

Monthly newsletter to assist parents with daily realities of adoption.

ADOPTEE LIBERTY MOVEMENT (ALMA) and
ALMA International Reunion Registry Bank
P. O. Box 154
Washington Bridge Station
New York, NY 10033

A group actively working for openness in adoption; also provides assistance
with searches.

ADOPTION TRIAD NETWORK
120 Thibodeaux Dr.
Lafayette, LA 70503
(318) 984-3682

ADOPTEES IN SEARCH
P. O. Box 41016
Bethesda, MD 20014

AMERICAN ACADEMY OF ADOPTION ATTORNEYS
P. O. Box 33053
Washington, D.C. 20033-0053
(202) 331-1955

Provides referrals to attorneys specializing in adoption.

CHAIN OF LIFE
P. O. Box 8081
Berkeley, CA 94707

A feminist adoption reform and child welfare newsletter.

CHILD WELFARE LEAGUE OF AMERICA
440 First St. NW, Suite 310
Washington, D.C. 20001-2085
(202) 638-2952

COMMITTEE FOR SINGLE ADOPTIVE PARENTS
P. O. Box 15084
Chevy Chase, MD 20825

CONCERNED UNITED BIRTHPARENTS (CUB), Inc.
2000 Walker St.
Des Moines, IA 50317
(515) 263-9558

INDEPENDENT SEARCH CONSULTANTS
P. O. Box 10192
Costa Mesa, CA 92627

INTERNATIONAL CONCERNS COMMITTEE FOR CHILDREN (ICCC)
911 Cypress Dr.
Boulder, CO 80303
(303) 494-8333

INTERNATIONAL SOUNDEX REUNION REGISTRY
P. O. Box 2312
Carson City, NV 89702

NATIONAL ADOPTION INFORMATION CLEARINGHOUSE
1400 Eye St. NW, Suite 1275
Washington, D.C. 20005
(202) 842-1919
FAX (202) 408-0950

Referrals, directory of adoption agencies, speakers' bureau, and database for adoption-related books and articles.

NATIONAL COMMITTEE FOR ADOPTION, INC. (NCFA)
1933—17th St., NW
Washington, D.C. 20009-6207
(202) 328-1200; hotline (202) 463-7563

Promotes adoption as a positive family-building option. Hotline provides information and referrals.

NATIONAL ORGANIZATION FOR BIRTHFATHERS (NOBAR)
P. O. Box 1993
Baltimore, MD 21203

NORTH AMERICAN ADOPTION CONGRESS
1053 Filbert St.
San Francisco, CA 94133-2507

ORPHAN VOYAGE
2141 Rd. 2300
Cedaredge, CO 81413
(303) 856-3937

Founded and administered by Jean Paton; offers orientation to adoption as life-long experience.

POST ADOPTION CENTER FOR EDUCATION AND RESEARCH (PACER)
P. O. Box 3090
Orinda, CA 94563
(510) 935-6622

Information, referrals, and support for all adoption triad members.

RIGHTS OF ADOPTEES' PARENTS, INC.
P. O. Box 30326
Cleveland, OH 44130
(216) 572-1599

SINGLE MOTHERS BY CHOICE
P. O. Box 1642
Grace Square Station
New York, NY 10028
(212) 988-0993

TRI-ADOPTION LIBRARY
P. O. Box 638
Westminster, CA 92684

INTERNATIONAL ADOPTION

ADOPTIVE FAMILIES OF AMERICA, INC. (formerly OURS, Inc.)
3333 Highway 100 North
Minneapolis, MN 55422
(612) 535-4829
Primarily international and special-needs adoption support, information, and
educational materials; twenty-four hour phone line.

AMERICANS FOR INTERNATIONAL AID AND ADOPTION
947 Dowling Rd.
Bloomfield Hills, MI 48013

FAMILIES ADOPTING CHILDREN EVERYWHERE (FACE)
P. O. Box 28058
Baltimore, MD 21239

FRIENDS FOR ALL CHILDREN
445 S. 68th St.
Boulder, CO 80303

FRIENDS OF CHILDREN OF VIETNAM (FCVN)
600 Gilpin St.
Denver, CO 90218

HOLT INTERNATIONAL CHILDREN'S SERVICES
P. O. Box 2880
Eugene, OR 97402
(503) 687-2202

INTERNATIONAL CONCERNS COMMITTEE FOR CHILDREN (ICCC)
911 Cypress Dr.
Boulder, CO 80303
(303) 494-8333

LATIN AMERICAN PARENTS ASSOCIATION (LAPA)
P. O. Box 339
Brooklyn, NY 11234
(718) 236-8689

DAVID LIVINGSTONE MISSIONARY FOUNDATION ADOPTION PROGRAM
P. O. Box 232
Tulsa, OK 74101

LOS NINOS INTERNATIONAL AID AND ADOPTION REFERRAL
919 W. 28th St.
Minneapolis, MN 55408

LOVE THE CHILDREN
221 West Broad St.
Quakertown, PA 18951

MISSIONARIES OF CHARITY
2562—36th St., NW
Washington, D.C. 20009

INTERRACIAL ADOPTION

FAMILIES ADOPTING INTER-RACIALLY (FAIR)
989 Woodland
Menlo Park, CA 94025

PACT — AN ADOPTION ALLIANCE
3315 Sacramento St., Suite 239
San Francisco, CA 94118
(510) 530-7225
Specifically facilitating adoptions of infants of color.

SPECIAL-NEEDS ADOPTIONS

AID TO ADOPTION OF SPECIAL KIDS (AASK AMERICA)
657 Mission, Suite 601
San Francisco, CA 94105
(415) 543-2275

FAMILY BUILDERS BY ADOPTION
1230—2nd Ave.
Oakland, CA 94606
(510) 272-0204

THE NATIONAL ADOPTION CENTER
1218 Chestnut St., Suite 204
Philadelphia, PA 19107
(215) 925-0200

NORTH AMERICAN COUNCIL ON ADOPTABLE CHILDREN (NACAC)
1821 University, Suite N498
St. Paul, MN 55104
(612) 644-3036

Clearinghouse offering conferences, newsletters, and general information about children waiting for homes in the United States and special-needs adoptions.

SURROGACY

NATIONAL COALITION AGAINST SURROGACY
1130—17th St., NW, Suite 630
Washington, D. C. 20036
(202) 466-2823

THE ORGANIZATION OF PARENTS THROUGH SURROGACY (OPTS)
National Headquarters
750 N. Fairview St.
Burbank, CA 91505
(818) 848-3761

Index